世界中医学专业
核心课程教材

World Textbook Series
for Chinese Medicine
Core Curriculum

总主编 Chief Editor

张 伯 礼
Zhang Bo-li

世界中医药学会联合会教育指导委员会
The Educational Instruction Committee
of the WFCMS

（供中医学、针灸学和推拿学专业用）

（For Majors of Chinese Medicine, Acupuncture & Moxibustion and *Tuina*）

推 拿 学

Theory and Practice of *Tuina*

主 编　王之虹　王金贵
Chief Editors　Wang Zhi-hong　Wang Jin-gui

副主编　刘明军　顾一煌　李征宇　于天源　吴　山　王守东（美国）
Associate Chief Editors　Liu Ming-jun　Gu Yi-huang　Li Zheng-yu　Yu Tian-yuan　Wu Shan
Wang Shou-dong (USA)

主 译　段颖哲（美国）　林楠（美国）　克里斯·杜威（美国）
Translated by　Azure Duan (USA)　Lin Nan (USA)　Chris Dewey (USA)

U0346113

中国中医药出版社　中国·北京
China Press of Traditional Chinese Medicine
Beijing PRC

中国中医药出版社
China Press of Traditional Chinese Medicine

Website:www.cptcm.com

Book Title: Theory and Practice of *Tuina*

[*World Textbook Series for Chinese Medicine Core Curriculum (Shì Jiè Zhōng Yī Xué Zhuān Yè Hé Xīn Kè Chéng Jiào Cái,* 世界中医学专业核心课程教材)]

Contact address: Building No. 8, Zone 2, Compound 31, No. 13 Kechuang Street, Economic-Technological Development Area, Beijing 100176, P. R. China

ISBN 978-7-5132-5730-5

First Edition 2019
ISBN 978-7-5132-5730-5

Printed in P. R. China

World Textbook Series for Chinese Medicine Core Curriculum
(Shì Jiè Zhōng Yī Xué Zhuān Yè Hé Xīn Kè Chéng Jiào Cái,
世界中医学专业核心课程教材）

Compilation Committee of

World Textbook Series for Chinese Medicine Core Curriculum

(Shì Jiè Zhōng Yī Xué Zhuān Yè Hé Xīn Kè Chéng Jiào Cái,
世界中医学专业核心课程教材)

Translation Committee of

World Textbook Series for Chinese Medicine Core Curriculum

(Shì Jiè Zhōng Yī Xué Zhuān Yè Hé Xīn Kè Chéng Jiào Cái,
世界中医学专业核心课程教材)

Advisors:
Xie Zhu-fan   Nigel Wiseman (Britain)   Fang Ting-yu   Zhu Zhong-bao   Huang Yue-zhong   Huang Jia-ling   Li Zhao-guo   Eric Brand (USA)   Shelley Ochs (USA)   Wang Kui   Maya Sutton (USA)   Tom Spencer (USA)

Chief Translators (in alphabetical order by pinyin of last name):
Alicia Grant (Britain)   Angela Wei-hong Yang (Australia)   Azure Duan (USA)   Brian Glashow (USA)   Chen Ji   Chen Ye-meng (USA)   Chen Yun-hui   Chris Dewey (USA)   Eric Brand (USA)   Fan Yan-ni   Gong Chang-zhen (USA)   Guo Ping (Hong Kong, China)   Han Chou-ping   He Ye-bo   He Yu-xin (USA)   Huang Li-xin (USA)   Ioannis Solos (Greece)   James Bare (USA)   Jason Ji-shun Hao (USA)   Jessica Li Feng (New Zealand)   John Paul Liang (USA)   Kathleen Dowd (Ireland)   Kristin Weston (USA)   Laura Castillo (USA)   Leil Nielsen (USA)   Lesley Hamilton (USA)   Li Ai-zhong (Canada)   Li Can-dong   Li Ling-ling   Li Zhao-guo   Lin Nan (USA)   Liu Jiang-hua (USA)   Liu Ming   Lu Yu-bin (USA)   Maya Sutton (USA)   Robert Yu-sheng Tan (Canada)   Shan Bao-zhi   Shelley Ochs (USA)   Sun Hui   Tang Shu-lan (Britain)   Thomas Hodge (USA)   Tian Hai-he (USA)   Tom Spencer (USA)   Tong Xin (USA)   Wang Xue-min   Zaslawski Christopher (Australia)   Zhao Ji-fu (USA)   Zhao Zhong-zhen (Hong Kong, China)   Zhu Xiao-shu (Australia)   Zhu Yan-zhong (USA)

Office of Translation Committee
Director: Shan Bao-zhi
Deputy Directors: Jiang Feng   Li Ling-ling

Publisher: Fan Ji-ping

General Coordinators of Publishing Project: Fan Ji-ping   Li Xiu-ming   Li Zhan-yong   Shan Bao-zhi   Rui Li-xin

General Editor-in-Charge: Shan Bao-zhi

Editors-in-Charge (Chinese Version) (in alphabetical order by pinyin of last name):
Geng Xue-yan   Han Yan   Hao Sheng-li   Hua Zhong-jian   Huang Wei   Li Yan-ling   Li Zhan-yong   Liu Zhe   Ma Jie   Ma Xiao-feng   Nong Yan   Qian Yue   Shan Bao-zhi   Tian Shao-xia   Wang Li-guang   Wang Lin   Wang Shu-zhen   Wang Wei   Wu Ning-qian   Xiao Pei-xin   Xu Shan   Zhang Chen   Zhang Yan   Zhang Yong-tai   Zhang Yue   Zhou Yan-jie

Editors-in-Charge (English Version): Shan Bao-zhi   Shelley Ochs (USA)   Chris Dewey (USA)   Chen Yun-hui   He Ye-bo   Maya Sutton (USA)   Tom Spencer (USA)   Jason Ji-shun Hao (USA)   He Yu-xin (USA)   Geng Xue-yan

Cover Design: Zhao Xiao-dong and Beijing Lucky Computer Color Platemaking P. R. China

Layout Design: Beijing Lucky Computer Color Platemaking P. R. China

Preface

In ancient times, Chinese medicine played a major role in the cultural exchanges that took place among the diverse civilizations along the Silk Road. Today, this sharing and learning has "gone global". It is increasingly recognized and accepted among medical authorities worldwide that Chinese medicine offers an array of benefits that include preventing and treating a wide range of illnesses from common ailments to critical life-threatening diseases. Chinese medicine has enormous potential for advancing human well-being as it is adopted around the world. However, the overseas development of the education of Chinese medicine is not balanced and instruction in its principles is uneven. Given these circumstances, it is imperative to compile a series of Chinese medicine textbooks for learners, both at home and abroad, that align with the *World Standard of Chinese Medicine Undergraduate (Pre-CMD) Education* [*Shì Jiè Zhōng Yī Xué Běn Kē (CMD Qián) Jiào Yù Biāo Zhǔn*, 世界中医学本科（CMD 前）教育标准] as formulated by the Educational Instruction Committee of the World Federation of Chinese Medicine Societies (EIC-WFCMS).

On the first anniversary of the dissemination of *The Law of the People's Republic of China on Chinese Medicine* (*Zhōng Huá Rén Mín Gòng Hé Guó Zhōng Yī Yào Fǎ*, 中华人民共和国中医药法), the *World Textbook Series for Chinese Medicine Core Curriculum* (*Shì Jiè Zhōng Yī Xué Zhuān Yè Hé Xīn Kè Chéng Jiào Cái*, 世界中医学专业核心课程教材) are going to be published. The work of compiling these textbooks began in 2008 and was funded (twice) by the International Cooperation Division of State Administration of Traditional Chinese medicine. Professor Zhang Bo-li has served as Editor-in-Chief while the EIC-WFCMS has been utilized as the compilation's platform. A large number of domestic and overseas experts were convened to carefully select model textbooks from around the world. These texts were studied and compared chapter by chapter in order to learn from their respective strong points and deficiencies. The compiling outline was then formulated and the Chinese versions of the manuscripts were reviewed and modified several times. Supported by the Specialty Committee of Translation of the World Federation of Chinese Medicine Societies, experts, both from home and abroad, were selected to translate the textbooks and proofread the English manuscripts. These experts are proficient in Chinese Medicine translation, skillful in language application, and familiar with Chinese Medicine education abroad. As an ancient Chinese saying goes, "It takes a decade to grind a sword." This saying means that steady and meticulous work yields a fine product and these textbooks illustrate this kind of careful attention to detail. The textbooks, which aim to cultivate excellence among Chinese Medicine practitioners and facilitate their clinical practice, focus on the prevention and treatment of diseases that respond well to Chinese Medicine treatment and frequently occur around the world. Based on classical knowledge and practice, the textbooks are conducive to the comprehensive, systematic and accurate dissemination of Chinese Medicine to other nations.

Just as a ship was essential for a journey to Japan in ancient times, so a textbook is indispensable to a learner. The publication of this series of books will contribute to the cultivation of Chinese Medicine professionals internationally and help spread the many benefits of Chinese Medicine to the world. In its own way, the creation of these comprehensive textbooks will play a role in the "Belt and Road" initiative which seeks to revive the civilization-connecting Silk Road of ancient times. Chinese Medicine can serve as a powerful force contributing to the health and well-being of people all over the world. This project will play a significant and positive role in the history of international education of Chinese medicine.

Wang Xiao-pin
Director-General of International Cooperation
Division of State Administration of
Traditional Chinese Medicine
Bejing, P.R. China
July 2018

Foreword

The Educational Instruction Committee of the World Federation of Chinese Medicine Societies is dedicated to leading and promoting the healthy development of the international education of Chinese medicine and the standard education of Chinese medicine specialists all over the world. As early as the time when it was founded, the Educational Instruction Committee, under the leadership of the World Federation of Chinese Medicine Societies (WFCMS), organized a series of international expert meetings to analyze the future development of Chinese medicine education worldwide. The experts put forward some suggestions and solutions concerning the global development of the education of Chinese medicine, and drafted the *World Standard of Chinese Medicine Undergraduate (Pre-CMD) Education* [*Shì Jiè Zhōng Yī Xué Běn Kē (CMD Qián) Jiào Yù Biāo Zhǔn*, 世界中医学本科（CMD 前）教育标准]. At the 4th council meeting of the 2nd session of WFCMS held in May 2009, the *World Standard of Chinese Medicine Undergraduate (Pre-CMD) Education* [*Shì Jiè Zhōng Yī Xué Běn Kē (CMD Qián) Jiào Yù Biāo Zhǔn*, 世界中医学本科（CMD 前）教育标准] was issued after serious discussion and consideration.

The international education of Chinese medicine is growing rapidly and vigorously. The cultivation of professionals of Chinese medicine relies heavily on having relevant curriculum of Chinese medicine. However, due to the unbalanced development of the education of Chinese medicine in different countries, the professional curriculum varies significantly among educational institutions. Besides, the core contents are sometimes incongruent. Hence, it is imperative to determine the core curriculum for Chinese medicine.

To realize the professional education of Chinese medicine through the practice of Chinese medicine at educational institutions in different countries (regions), the Educational Instruction Committee of the WFCMS formulated the *World Core Curriculum for Chinese Medicine* (*Shì Jiè Zhōng Yī Xué Zhuān Yè Hé Xīn Kè Chéng*, 世界中医学专业核心课程) (hereinafter referred to as WCCCM) and *the Outline of World Core Curriculum for Chinese Medicin e* (*Shì Jiè Zhōng Yī Xué Zhuān Yè Hé Xīn Kè Chéng Jiào Xué Dà Gāng*, 世界中医学专业核心课程教学大纲). The characteristics of the education of Chinese medicine and professional requirements, as well as the actual conditions of the education of Chinese medicine in different countries (regions), were taken into consideration. The Educational Instruction Committee of the WFCMS decided to initiate the compilation and translation of the *World Textbook Series for Chinese Medicine Core Curriculum* (*Shì Jiè Zhōng Yī Xué Zhuān Yè Hé Xīn Kè Chéng Jiào Cái*, 世界中医学专业核心课程教材).

This series of 13 textbooks is comprised of *Fundamental Theories of Chinese Medicine* (*Zhōng Yī Jī Chǔ Lǐ Lùn*, 中医基础理论), *Diagnostics in Chinese Medicine* (*Zhōng Yī Zhěn Duàn Xué*, 中医诊断学), *Chinese Materia Medica* (*Zhōng Yào Xué*, 中药学), *Formulas of Chinese Medicine* (*Fāng Jì Xué*, 方剂学), *Chinese Internal Medicine* (*Zhōng Yī Nèi Kē Xué*, 中医内科学), *Gynecology in Chinese Medicine* (*Zhōng Yī Fù Kē Xué*, 中医妇科学), *Pediatrics in Chinese Medicine* (*Zhōng Yī Ér Kē Xué*, 中医儿科学), *Theory and Practice of Acupuncture & Moxibustion* (*Zhēn Jiǔ Xué*, 针灸学), *Theory and Practice of*

Tuina (*Tuī Ná Xué*, 推拿学) , *Selected Readings from the Yellow Emperor's Inner Classic* (*Huáng Dì Nèi Jīng Xuǎn Dú*, 黄帝内经选读), *Selected Readings from the On Cold Damage* (*Shāng Hán Lùn Xuǎn Dú*, 伤寒论选读), *Selected Readings from the Essentials from the Golden Cabinet* (*Jīn Guì Yào Lüè Xuǎn Dú*, 金匮要略选读), and *Warm Diseases: Theory and Practice* (*Wēn Bìng Xué*, 温病学).

- **The foundation for the compilation and translation of the textbooks**

The Compilation and Translation Guiding Committee of the *World Textbook Series for Chinese Medicine Core Curriculum* (*Shì Jiè Zhōng Yī Xué Zhuān Yè Hé Xīn Kè Chéng Jiào Cái*, 世界中医学专业核心课程教材) was established in 2012. It examined the "Compilation and Translation Principles and Requirements of the *World Textbook Series for Chinese Medicine Core Curriculum* (*Shì Jiè Zhōng Yī Xué Zhuān Yè Hé Xīn Kè Chéng Jiào Cái*, 世界中医学专业核心课程教材)". Many constructive suggestions and proposals concerning the "Compilation and Translation Principles and Requirements" were put forth by the experts at the meeting. In view of the proposals put forth by the experts, funded and worked on by teachers at Tianjin University of Traditional Chinese Medicine, the Secretariat of the Educational Instruction Committee of the WFCMS carried out a "Comparative Study of Chinese and Foreign Textbooks for WCCCM" from 2012 to 2013, which compared and analyzed the well recognized textbooks for Chinese medicine education in different countries.

On the basis of a complete summary of the features and advantages of the textbooks in different countries, the curriculum research teams drafted the "Contents and Sample Manuscripts of the Curricula" and sent them to different countries for examination. There were 94 pieces of advice received, covering many aspects such as the content, translation, style and layout of the textbooks. The Secretariat convened relevant specialists to examine and analyze the findings of the above-mentioned study as well as the feedback of the Chinese and overseas experts on the "Sample Manuscripts of the *World Textbook Series for Chinese Medicine Core Curriculum* (*Shì Jiè Zhōng Yī Xué Zhuān Yè Hé Xīn Kè Chéng Jiào Cái*, 世界中医学专业核心课程教材)". Afterwards, the "Compilation and Translation Principles and Requirements of the *World Textbook Series for Chinese Medicine Core Curriculum* (*Shì Jiè Zhōng Yī Xué Zhuān Yè Hé Xīn Kè Chéng Jiào Cái*, 世界中医学专业核心课程教材)" were conscientiously revised. The above-mentioned work has laid a solid foundation for the compilation and translation of the textbook Series.

- **The orientation of the textbooks**

The current reality of medical education in different countries shows that undergraduate education still plays a major role in the professional education of varied disciplines. Besides, the *World Textbook Series for Chinese Medicine Core Curriculum* (*Shì Jiè Zhōng Yī Xué Zhuān Yè Hé Xīn Kè Chéng Jiào Cái*, 世界中医学专业核心课程教材) should comply with the published educational standards of Chinese medicine, and the reality of the education of Chinese medicine and clinical needs in different countries should be considered. "The *World Textbook Series for Chinese Medicine Core Curriculum* (*Shì Jiè Zhōng Yī Xué Zhuān Yè Hé Xīn Kè Chéng Jiào Cái*, 世界中医学专业核心课程教材)" (hereinafter referred to as "textbooks") are suitable for undergraduate education of Chinese medicine all over the world as well as being reference books for postgraduate education and self-education of Chinese medicine practitioners. Regarding the scope of knowledge, the textbooks are supposed to meet the clinical requirements of a future Chinese medicine practitioner, and certain depth and breadth should be provided to ensure the extension of knowledge.

- **The compiling and translating principles of the textbooks**

This series of 13 textbooks follows the principles of medical ethics, scientific value, systematic integrity, general applications, advancement of Chinese medicine, safety, and medical standards.

Medical ethics: Chinese medicine always attaches great importance to medical ethics such as the absolute sincerity of a great physician, the virtue of benevolence, the ethical education of the students, and a devotion to people's health. They are the kernel of the cultivation of medical ethics and the key to becoming a qualified Chinese medical practitioner.

Scientific value: The textbooks should correctly reflect the intrinsic law of the system of Chinese medicine, and the concept, theory, definition and reasoning of Chinese medicine, accord with the connotation of traditional literatures, be concise, accurate and standard in expression, and try to avoid using Western biomedical terms. Chinese medicine is rooted in the development of Chinese medicine theory. Only by respecting the traditional connotation of Chinese medicine can we retain the essence of Chinese medicine and maintain the stability and continuity of the textbooks. During intercultural communication of the concept, theory, definition and reasoning of Chinese medicine, emphasis should be placed on the scientific expression of the relevant knowledge.

Systematic integrity: The textbooks should systematically contain the theories of Chinese medicine, completely present the core knowledge system of Chinese medicine , and highlight the basic theories, knowledge and skills. The course resources should be clear in arrangement, strict in logic and moderate in progression. Besides, the sections should be logically connected without duplicating or overlapping content.

General applications: Practicality is of great value in the textbooks, so it is essential to elaborate on the clinical treatment of diseases commonly or frequently occurring in different countries. Regarding the study of traditional classics, emphasis should be laid on the clinical guidance of the textbooks and cultivate the clinical thinking ability of the students.

Advancement of Chinese medicine: The textbooks should reflect the development of Chinese medicine and introduce any tested, published and acknowledged new theories, new technologies and new achievements in scientific teaching and research. For instance, some research updates on the prevention and treatment of avian influenza or atypical pneumonia can be included in the courses of warm diseases, and the research progress in acupuncture point specificity can be included in the courses of Acupuncture and Moxibustion. Advanced research reflects the vitality of a subject.

Safety: The textbooks should attach great importance to the safety and clinical requirements of treatment methods or techniques, and be specific about the indications and contraindications. For instance, the indications and safe handling of some acupuncture points should be introduced in the courses of Acupuncture and Moxibustion; the correct processing, differentiation, dosage and decoction of medicinals, as well as substitutes for banned medicinals from endangered animals should be introduced in the courses of Chinese Materia Medica; and the requirements and prohibitions of *Tuina* manipulations should be introduced in the courses of Theory and Practice of *Tuina*. In other words, the textbooks should be at the service of clinical practice, attach importance to safety, be accurate in expression, and comply with the legal requirements in different countries (regions).

Medical standards: The textbooks should use standard terms and be easy to understand without losing the flavor of Chinese medicine. The translation should conform to the principles of "fidelity, fluency and elegance", adopt the existing international standard terminology, and be accurate in expression while containing the original flavor of Chinese medicine. Besides, intellectual property rights should be protected.

Universality: The textbooks should serve the teaching of Chinese medicine, with classic content, appropriate length of chapters or sections, and moderate extension of knowledge. They should also conform to the teaching reality in different countries. In terms of layout, stylistic rules and expression, the international compiling stylistic rules should be adopted. It is advisable to make brief summaries and avoid lengthy descriptions. Sidelights to a major story are used to make the layout colorful and varied and, more importantly, to provide additional knowledge without compromising the major body of knowledge. For example, some basic knowledge of Western medicine can be added to the clinical courses, and Western chiropractic therapy can be added to the courses of Theory and Practice of *Tuina*. Moreover, figures and tables can be used for visual expression of abstract ideas.

- **The compiling and translating process of the textbooks**

In 2015, we received a total of 313 recommendation- and self-recommendation forms (89 forms from overseas). All of the recommenders, who are experts at the educational institutions of Chinese medicine in different countries, conform to the selection criteria of compilers and translators of the textbooks. Finally, 28 experts were chosen as chief editors and 64 experts as associate chief editors. A total of 290 experts were involved in the compilation and translation of the textbooks. They are from 15 countries or regions, i.e., China, the United States, Britain, France, Australia, Canada, Singapore, New Zealand, Malaysia, Holland, Greece, Japan, Spain and China's Hong Kong and China's Taiwan. Among the 59 overseas experts, 26 of them served as chief editors or associate chief editors. Participating agencies include 74 colleges and universities of Chinese medicine or research institutes. Among them, 34 agencies are from China, and 40 are from overseas.

In 2015, the chief editors were convened to discuss the compilation of the *World Textbook Series for Chinese Medicine Core Curriculum* (*Shì Jiè Zhōng Yī Xué Zhuān Yè Hé Xīn Kè Chéng Jiào Cái,* 世界中医学专业核心课程教材). At the meeting, the general compilation and translation requirements of the textbooks were determined, the writing tasks, division of work and compiling schedule were discussed in depth, and the teaching program, compiling outline and overlapping content were clarified. In addition, the solutions to possible relevant problems during the process of compilation and translation were also discussed. After 20 months of industrious work, the *World Textbook Series for Chinese Medicine Core Curriculum* (*Shì Jiè Zhōng Yī Xué Zhuān Yè Hé Xīn Kè Chéng Jiào Cái,* 世界中医学专业核心课程教材) (Chinese version) were finalized in October 2016. The textbooks are the crystallization of the wisdom of world-renowned education specialists of Chinese medicine, and are characterized by medical ethics, scientific value, systematic integrity, general applications, safety, medical standards, and authority.

The chief translators were recruited for the English translation of the textbooks and the Translation Seminar of the *World Textbook Series for Chinese Medicine Core Curriculum* (*Shì Jiè Zhōng Yī Xué Zhuān Yè Hé Xīn Kè Chéng Jiào Cái,* 世界中医学专业核心课程教材) held in October 2016.

The selection of the chief translators was based on strict criteria. The academic status and influence, authority, and geographical representation of the applicants were fully considered. After recommendation and self-recommendation, 50 chief translators (40 with doctoral degrees, 8 with master's degrees and 2 with a bachelor's degree) were approved by the Educational Instruction Committee of the WFCMS, Specialty Committee of Translation of the WFCMS and China Press of Traditional Chinese Medicine. They came from 9 countries/regions. Among the 38 overseas chief translators, 26 were from America. Most of the Chinese chief translators have overseas teaching experience. They have long been involved in the education and translation of Chinese medicine, with rich experience.

The publication of this series of textbooks is of great significance. It seized the golden opportunity of revitalizing and developing Chinese medicine at this occurrence of good timing, geographical convenience and good human relations. It helps Chinese medicine to go globally, promotes the reconstruction and sharing of Chinese medicine, and contributes to realizing the lofty goal of "basic medical services for all" advocated by WHO. Besides, the publication of the textbooks is conducive to the promotion and popularization of the international standards of Chinese medicine, and meets the growing worldwide demand for Chinese medicine when global reform of medical and health systems focuses on "prevention and healthcare". Therefore, this series of textbooks will inevitably be beneficial to the cultivation of Chinese medicine professionals all over the world, and to recognizing , popularizing and applying Chinese medicine worldwide.

The textbooks are going to be published, and here I want to express my heartfelt gratitude to the experts and scholars from home and abroad for their industrious and conscientious work, which guarantees the successful publication of the textbooks. Thanks to the State Administration of Traditional Chinese Medicine, World Federation of Chinese Medicine Societies, China Press of Traditional Chinese Medicine, and Tianjin University of Traditional Chinese Medicine

for their great support and selfless help. Thanks to all the friends who are engaged in the same pursuit and have contributed to this project. In particular, I would like to extend my special thanks to Professor Shan Bao-zhi for her great effort and brilliant contribution to the textbooks.

Zhang Bo-li,
the Editor-in-chief for
World Textbook Series for Chinese Medicine Core Curriculum (Shì Jiè Zhōng Yī Xué Zhuān Yè Hé Xīn Kè Chéng Jiào Cái, 世界中医学专业核心课程教材)
Summer, 2018

Note for Compilation

Theory and Practice of Tuina (*Tuī Ná Xué*, 推拿学）, an important component of Chinese medicine, is a crucial subject to the research of its theories and methodologies. The curriculum of *tuina*, therefore, is seen as a core curriculum and thus mandate for students majoring in Chinese medicine. Both the theory and practice are emphasized, and didactic studies and demonstration are addressed while the subject is taught. Through such training, students need to master the fundamental knowledge, theories, methodologies, and skills of diagnosis and treatment, building a foundation for treating illnesses using *tuina* in the future.

As one of the *World Textbook Series for Chinese Medicine Core Curriculum* (*Shì Jiè Zhōng Yī Xué Zhuān Yè Hé Xīn Kè Chéng Jiào Cái*, 世界中医学专业核心课程教材）, *Theory and Practice of Tuina* is compiled based on the following documents issued by the World Federation of Chinese Medicine Societies: *The World Standard of Chinese Medicine Undergraduate (Pre-CMD) Education* [*Shì Jiè Zhōng Yī Xué Běn Kē (CMD Qián) Jiào Yù Biāo Zhǔn*, 世界中医学本科（CMD 前）教育标准], the Standard of *The World Core Curriculum for Chinese Medicine* （*Shì Jiè Zhōng Yī Xué Zhuān Yè Hé Xīn Kè Chéng*, 世界中医学专业核心课程）, and *the Outline of World Core Curriculum for Chinese Medicine* （*Shì Jiè Zhōng Yī Xué Zhuān Yè Hé Xīn Kè Chéng Jiào Xué Dà Gāng*, 世界中医学专业核心课程教学大纲）. At the same time, we have learned from previous successful experience of compiling universal-use textbooks, and absorbed suggestions from education experts worldwide and in China that teach *Theory and Practice of Tuina* in colleges and universities with international viewpoint. As a result,

the textbook is aiming for students studying *Theory and Practice of Tuina* in Chinese medicine colleges and Chinese medicine clinicians worldwide, or those who come to China to study Chinese medicine, and Chinese medicine students in English programs in China.

The textbook has 14 chapters. Part One is Overview of *Tuina*, in which Chapter One, Historical Evolution of *Tuina*, introduces the concept, origin, historical development, global application and popularization, and learning methods of *tuina*. Chapter Two and Three discuss Chinese medicine and biomedical mechanisms, and the treatment principles and methods of *tuina*. Chapter Four to Six elaborate common examination methods, preparation work, cautions and forbidden situations for *tuina*. Part Two focuses on maneuvers and practice methods of *tuina* for adults. Amongst it, Chapter Seven to Eight mainly illustrate adult *tuina* maneuvers and ways to practice them by grouping the maneuvers into subcategories of swinging, frictional, vibrating, squeezing and pressing, tapping, and passive joint movements. Chapter Nine mainly explains how to apply *tuina* to treat common adult illnesses, such as locomotor, internal, and gynecological problems. Part Three, including Chapter 10 to 12, concentrates on pediatric *tuina*, its maneuvers, acupoints and treatment of common pediatric problems using specific techniques. The appendix illustrates breathing exercises and preventative methods for *tuina* therapists. Furthermore, the textbook is designed to include supplementary sections such as notes to help learners grasp the content and requirements of each chapter and deepen the understanding of it. The goals for composing the textbook are achieving a high academic level and making it closely relevant to clinical practices.

The original Chinese script of the textbook is a collective work and wisdom of *tuina* experts from a number of universities in China and abroad. Chapter One to Chapter Six are works of Wang Zhi-hong, Wang Jin-gui, Li Hua-nan, Wu Yun-chuan and Liu Shu-quan respectively while Chapter Seven and Eight are written by Wu Shan, Zhang Jun, Li Hua-dong and Liu Tie-ying. The authors of Chapter Nine are Yu Tian-yuan, Li Zheng-yu, Zhou Yun-feng, Wang Xin-jun, Wang Chun-lin, Sun Wei-liang and Chapter 10 to 12 are compiled by Liu Ming-jun, Wang Shou-dong, Lei Long-ming, Zhang Xin. The authors of Chapter 13 and 14 are Gu Yi-huang, Lu Li-jiang and Lin Nan. Last but not least, Wang Zhi-hong, Wang Jin-gui and Zhang Xin are in charge of unifying and finalizing the draft of the textbook.

There might be imperfections in the textbook due to limitations of the editors. We hope that teachers, students and other readers can provide us with feedback and improvement suggestions, so that the textbook can meet the need for overseas learners by satisfying their study and cognitive pattern.

Compilation Board of *Theory and Practice of Tuina*
August, 2016

Contents

Part Three

Appendix

Breathing Exercise for *Tuina* Physician and Preventative Methods *207*

Indexes

Part **One**

Overview of *Tuina*

Chapter One

Historical Evolution of *Tuina*

Section 1 The Origin and Development of *Tuina*

Tuina is the name of the Chinese medical massage. As an important component of Chinese medicine, *tuina* is within the scope of the external treatment modality. As a medical therapy, *tuina* is employed for the purpose of preventing and treating certain diseases, is operated according to the Chinese medicine theory. *Tuina* is performed on the human body or on acupuncture points using a variety of specific physical movements.

As the oldest medical therapy of humankind, *tuina* originated from the daily life and work of primitive people. During prehistoric times, they would inevitably fall, get injured, or sometimes even break their bones while hunting, farming, clearing land, constructing, sewing, and traveling over land and water. After the occurrence of injury, they would press and rub the area out of instinct to ease the pain. Over a long period of time, some instinctive actions for pain relief became part of life experience, and these actions were codified in the earliest forms of *tuina*.

The pre-*Qin* period was the embryonic formation stage of *tuina*, evidenced by the archaeological discovery of *Ma Wang Dui* Tombs of *Han* Dynasty in Changsha and oracle bones of the *Yin* Ruins of *Shang* Dynasty. *Tuina* constitutes the largest proportion in *Formulas for Fifty-two Diseases* (*Wǔ Shí Èr Bìng Fāng*, 五十二病方), the most important medical work unearthed in Tomb Number Three of *Ma Wang Dui* Tombs in Changsha, Hunan Province, China. The book records a large number of diseases treatable with *tuina*, such as inguinal hernia, vitiligo, warts, insect bites, skin itching, frostbite, and traumatic bleeding. *The Illustration of Guided Qi Gong* (*Dǎo Yǐn Tú*, 导引图), unearthed during the same period, is the earliest work in *Qi Gong* and guided exercises. The manuscript depicts 44 postures of guided *Qi Gong*, which include back-pounding, chest-rubbing and pressing in addition to a few dozen breathing techniques and body movements. Furthermore, an oracle shell discovered in *Yin* Ruins also has records of *tuina*. Some Chinese characters inscribed on the oracle bone were found to be related to *tuina* therapy. An example is the character " 拊 ", indicating one's hand rubbing another's body or undressed abdominal area. Later on, the same character was written as " 付 " in *Lì* Clerical Script (隶书), but the meaning remained unchanged. Therefore, the evidence suggests that *tuina* was one of the major methods in treating disease in the *Shang* Dynasty.

The *Qin* and *Han* Dynasties set an important historical watershed in the development of *tuina*, because two classic medical works were written during the period. One, *The Yellow Emperor's Inner Classic* (*Huáng Dì Nèi Jīng*, 黄帝内经), is the earliest existing work that systematically and comprehensively elaborates the theory of Chinese medicine. The other was China's first *tuina* monograph titled *Ten Tuina Volume of The Yellow Emperor and Qi Bo*, which was unfortunately lost. Nevertheless, the completion of the two books marked the formation of the therapeutic system of *tuina*.

The Yellow Emperor's Inner Classic applied *tuina* to palpation as a diagnostic method to improve the accuracy of the disease diagnosis. The book also presents a systematic summary of *tuina* treatment effects, such as moving qi to invigorate blood, dissipating cold to relieve pain, unblocking the meridians and collaterals, and dispelling heat to calm the spirit. At the same time, it pointed out that *tuina* maneuvers could be either supplementing or draining, therefore, it was appropriate to differentiate between them. In addition, *tuina* was commonly used in coordination with acupuncture, Chinese herbal medicine, and other treatment modalities. Moreover, there was a greater number of maneuvers recorded in *The Yellow Emperor's Inner Classic*, compared to those recorded in the *Formulas for Fifty-two Diseases*. It described pressing, rubbing, palpating, palm-pressing, tracing, plucking, grasping, pushing, intense-pressing, bending, stretching, rotation, and other methods. Among these maneuvers, pressing (*Àn*) and rubbing (*Mó*) were most frequently used, leading later generations to often refer to *tuina* as *Àn Mó*.

Since then, the scope of *tuina* has broadened. For the first time, Zhang Zhong-jing, a famous doctor from the Eastern Han Dynasty, listed a form of *tuina* using a cream named *gāo mó* (ointment rubbing, 膏摩), as one of the preventive health care methods in his book *Essentials from the Golden Cabinet* (*Jīn Guì Yào Lüè*, 金匮要略), and introduced the *Mó Sǎn Fāng* (Rubbing Powder Formula, 摩散方) to treat head-wind. In *Chapter Twenty-Three: Miscellaneous Formulas* (*Zá Liáo Fāng Dì Èr Shí Sān*, 杂疗方第二十三) of *Essentials from the Golden Cabinet*, are described detailed *tuina* methods for treating people who had attempted to commit suicide by hanging themselves, making it the earliest scientific record of the world's medical history of treating such condition. In the end of the Eastern *Han* Dynasty, Hua Tuo, another famous doctor, advocated the Five-Animal Exercises (*Wǔ Qín Xì*, 五禽戏) for future generations, which provided a set of effective guided-exercises (*dǎo yǐn*, 导引) for maintaining good health.

In the *Jin*, *Sui*, and *Tang* dynasties, *tuina* was recognized by the government and a department of *Àn Mó* was established. In the *Sui* Dynasty, the Imperial Medical Bureau created a doctor's title for *tuina* specialists. During the *Tang* Dynasty, the Imperial Medical Bureau was expanded with the establishment of the *Tuina* Department and three levels of *tuina* specialists: doctor, therapist, and technician. During this period, self-performed *tuina*, health cultivation, and *dǎo yǐn* gained wider attention, as is reflected in books such as *Emergency Formulas to Keep in One's Sleeve* (*Zhǒu Hòu Bèi Jí Fāng*, 肘后备急方) by Ge Hong, *Important Formulas Worth A Thousand Gold Pieces* (*Qiān Jīn Yào Fāng*, 千金要方) by Sun Si-miao, and *Treatise on the Origins and Manifestations of Various Diseases* (*Zhū Bìng Yuán Hòu Lùn*, 诸病源候论). In addition, the combination method of using Chinese herbal medicine and *tuina* were further developed. In *Life-Saving Formulas to Keep in One's Sleeve* (*Zhǒu Hòu Jiù Cù Fāng*, 肘后救卒方), Ge Hong summarized the formulas for *gāo mó* (ointment rubbing) that had been developed prior to the Han Dynasty. An example of *gāo mó* is the popular *Chén Yuán Gāo* ointment which originated from the *Life-Saving Formulas to Keep in One's Sleeve - Volume Eight* (卷八) - *The Seventy-Second of Important Emergency Formulas in Forms of Bolus, Powder and Paste That Treat A Hundred Diseases*. During the same period, a large number of *gāo mó* formulas in a variety of forms were collected in two books, *Arcane Essentials from the Imperial Library* (*Wài Tái Mì Yào*, 外台秘要) and *Important Formulas Worth A Thousand Gold Pieces*.

After recognition by the Imperial medical Bureau, the treatment scope of *tuina* continued to expand. For example, in *Six Classics of Tang* (*Táng Liù Diǎn*, 唐六典), it states that *tuina* can treat eight types of diseases, namely wind, cold, heat, dampness, hunger, fullness, tiredness, and lack of exercise. In *Arcane Essentials from the Imperial Library*, it says that "[after] the first day [from when one is affected] with cold damage, and suffers from headache and stiffness of the back, [it is] best to use *Mó* (i.e, *tuina*) method." Furthermore, the knowledge exchange in medicine between China and other countries was fairly active, and so it was at this time *tuina* was widely spread to Korea, Japan, India, Arabia, and Europe.

In the *Song, Jin,* and *Yuan* dynasties, *tuina* experienced a temporary trough. During the *Song* Dynasty, the Imperial Medical Bureau eliminated the *tuina* department, which had existed for nearly 400 years, therefore *tuina* lost support at the national level. On the other hand, the direction shifted, putting more emphasis on the research and analysis of different maneuvers. The *Comprehensive Recording of Divine Assistance* (*Shèng Jì Zŏng Lù,* 圣济总录), an extensive medical book written in the *Song* Dynasty, whose first chapter elaborates, summarizes, and categorizes *tuina* maneuvers, was the earliest and most complete monograph specifically for *tuina*. The book explained the meaning of *Àn* (pressing) *Mó* (rubbing) and the difference between the two maneuvers. It stated that "[one] can [use] *Àn* or *Mó* [separately], [though] sometimes [one can] use [the two] combined, together naming it *Àn Mó*. [Sometimes one can just use] *Àn* but not *Mó*, [other times] *Mó* but not *Àn*; *Àn* only needs hands, [but] *Mó* may [need the appliance of] medicinals; *Àn* or *Mó* is applied accordingly to [the present situation]. In general, the method of *Àn Mó* is often used to open up or suppress. Open up the obstruction to disperse, suppress the tough to calm". Second, the book differentiated Àn Mó from *dăo yĭn* by explaining that "when people in general discuss *Àn Mó*, [they] do not analyze [the disease] and treat it, but combine with *dăo yĭn* to solve it, clearly indicating [that] they do not think". In addition, the book took *The Yellow Emperor's Inner Classic* as its foundation, further elucidated the application scope of *tuina* therapy, and explained that under which circumstances "pressing stops pain, pressing has no benefit, pressing causes more pain, pressing induces comfortness". The distinctions concerning the relationship of pressing to pain provided significant guidance for the clinical application of *tuina*.

In the *Ming* and *Qing* Dynasties, the development of *tuina* faced dramatic ups and downs. In early *Ming* Dynasty, the Imperial Medical Bureau adopted the system of the *Tang* Dynasty, incorporated *tuina* as one of the thirteen medical departments, creating certain conditions for its further advancement. In the fifth year of Long Qing Emperor's reign, however, the thirteen departments were reorganized to eleven, with the elimination of *tuina* and *zhu you* (a way of curing disease by prayng, *zhù yóu,* 祝由) department.

Although the development of *tuina* encountered hardship, it managed to survive. it was during this period that the phrase *tuina* appeared for the first time, and the unique system of pediatric *tuina* was formed. The phrase *tuina* was first seen in *Elaboration of Pediatrics* (*Yòu Kē Fā Huī,* 幼科发挥) completed in 1549 in the *Ming* Dynasty by Wan Quan, a famous pediatrician. The book said that "a child suffered twitching, I told [the family] that I could not treat it. The family invited a *tuina* therapist to treat [the child]. [Then] the child tried to cover the painful area, was able to stare at others and move his mouth. The whole family was happy". From then on, the phrase *tuina* became popular in published books. The evolution of the term reflected the change and development of specific maneuvers used in *tuina*, causing the therapy to more closely approximate the characteristics of the subject matter, which was a huge leap in the history of *tuina*.

During the same period, a series of monographs was published on the topic of pediatric *tuina*, such as *Divine Techniques for Infant Care* (*Bǎo Yīng Shén Shù,* 保婴神术) by the Chen Family of the Si Ming area, *The Encyclopedia of Pediatric Tuina with Formulas, Pulse-Taking, and Infant Revival Secrets* (*Xiǎo Ér Tuī Ná Fāng Mài Huó Yīng Mì Zhǐ Quán Shū,* 小儿推拿方脉活婴秘旨全书) by Imperial Doctor Gong Yun-ling, *Secret Tips of Pediatric Tuina* (*Xiǎo Ér Tuī Ná Mì Jué,* 小儿推拿秘诀) by Zhou Yu-fan, *The Principles of Pediatric Tuina* (*Xiǎo Ér Tuī Ná Guǎng Yì,* 小儿推拿广意) by Xiong Ying-xiong, *The Secret Book in Pediatric Tuina* (*Yòu Kē Tuī Ná Mì Shū,* 幼科推拿秘书) by Luo Ru-long, and *Three-Character-Verse Classic for Pediatric Tuina* (*Tuī Ná Sān Zì Jīng,* 推拿三字经) by Xu Qian-guang. One book in particular entitled *The Iron Mirror of Pediatric Department* (*Yòu Kē Tiě Jìng,* 幼科铁镜), written by Xia Yu-zhu, was innovative, uniquely composed, and rather different from other books with the use of "verses of *tuina* as alternative of medicinal remedies". Another book, *Amendment to Key An Mo Techniques* (*Lí Zhèng Àn Mó Yào Shù*, 厘正按摩要术) by Zhang Zhen-jun, was a collection of pediatric *tuina* methods gathered from a variety of practitioners with a unique editorial style, so that it became one of the greatest monographs in pediatric *tuina*, and was reprinted numerous times prior to the fourteenth year of Guangxi Emperor's reign in the *Qing* Dynasty. The production of these books marked the formation of a unique treatment system for pediatric *tuina*.

In regards to *tuina* for adults, although it was not included in the officially-recognized medical system, it thrived over the years among ordinary people, and many different schools of it appeared, such as orthopedic *tuina*, acupoint *tuina*, single-finger-*zen tuina*, ophthalmic *tuina*, *tuina* for external diseases, qi gong *tuina*, and health maintenance *tuina*. Therefore, during the *Ming* and *Qing* Dynasties *tuina* become more comprehensive in terms of development, description, and innovation.

After the Imperial Dynasties ended and the Republic of China was created, there was a critical turning point in the process of school formation for *tuina* development. Due to the westernization advocated by the national government, advocates for the abolition of Chinese medicine emerged, which negatively impacted Chinese medicine. As a Chinese medicine component, *tuina* faced discrimination and exclusion, so that it could only exist at grassroots level. On the other hand, such an environment provided a great deal of room for the formation of distinctive *tuina* schools. Some of the schools included Three-Character-Classic Pediatric *Tuina*, Western Hunan Pediatric *Tuina*, Single-Finger-*Zen Tuina*, Meridian-Collateral *zang-fu* Organs *Tuina*, Acupoints *Tuina*, Abdominal Diagnosis *Tuina*, Internal *Qi Gong Tuina*, and Rolling Maneuver *Tuina*. The number of academic schools dealing with different approaches to *tuina* made the history of *tuina* development in China fairly special. Furthermore, due to the impact of Western medicine, *tuina* absorbed and integrated knowledge of anatomy and physiology from Western medicine, as can be seen from the two books published at the time, namely, *Practical Guide of An Mo Techniques* (*Àn Mó Shù Shí Yòng Zhǐ Nán*, 按摩术实用指南), and *An Mo Techniques of the Huas* (*Huà Shì Àn Mó Shù*, 华氏按摩术).

After the founding of the People's Republic of China, *tuina* medical science entered a new developmental period with the emergence of interest in all aspects of *tuina* including clinical, scientific research, teaching, publishing, and professional team building. The first *tuina* specialty college was opened, and the first Chinese medical *tuina* clinics were established in Shanghai. In addition to the traditional apprentice system, classroom education in colleges with various department made it possible to train a large number of *tuina* professionals, and also accelerated the development of academic research. Secondly, *tuina* therapy was widely used in clinical settings, and a series of professional education materials and monographs in this field were published. Thirdly, summaries of *tuina* practice and clinical experience were becoming increasingly science-based. Diagnosis used in *tuina* was no longer confined to the four diagnostic methods of Chinese medicine, but began to draw upon modern technologies, such as X-ray, ultrasound, EMG, CT, and MRI, which were accepted readily by the majority of *tuina* physicians. In recent years, *tuina* researchers have used modern science and technology, in combination with modern medical knowledge to investigate a broad range topics that focus on the mechanism of *tuina*, such as the reason why *tuina* could ease pain, reduce swelling, remove blood stasis, and lower blood pressure. Pinching the skin along the spine [i.e. pinching *jǐ* (spine, 脊)], a subset of pediatric *tuina*, was researched for its function in improving the absorption efficiency of the small intestine. Finally, many new *tuina* techniques were documented or invented, such as auricular *tuina*, foot *tuina*, sports *tuina*, and *tuina* anesthesia. In short, this was the unprecedented golden and prosperous age in the history of *tuina*, from clinical, researching, publishing, and educational aspects.

Note:

> Chinese culture has a very long and fascinating history, of which the development of *tuina* can be seen as an important branch. It is recommended to take a glance at the historic chronicles of China, which would make it easier for the readers to understand the development process of tuina.

Section 2   The Development and Application of *Tuina* Worldwide

I. The Development of Manual Therapy Worldwide

As an ancient non-drug therapy, *tuina* has been used for several thousand years. Since the Sui and Tang dynasties, *tuina* therapy was widely disseminated to Japan, Korea, India, Arab, and European countries, and had a far-reaching impact. Throughout the history of the development of manual therapies worldwide, although the processes and theoretical bases were different, it is possible to see the similarities between *tuina* and Swedish massage, Thai massage, Japanese acupressure and bonesetting or orthopedic procedures. Moreover, it is possible to see similarities found all over China among various schools of *tuina*.

Note:

> Manual therapy is very precious in world civilization. Historic records of massage and *tuina* can be found anywhere in all countries globally.

Swedish massage is a health maintenance manual therapy based on principles of anat-omy, physiology and clinical medicine. Although it is a product of modern medicine, its diagnosis process has similarities to that of the four diagnostic methods in Chinese medicine, with steps such as observation, inquiry, palpation, physical examination, ruling out contraindications, and making a diagnostic conclusion. The manual procedures may include Swedish massage, soft tissue techniques, tender points maneuvers, trigger points manipulations, stretching, traction, and passive movements, similar to that of the process of diagnosis and treatment in orthopedic *tuina* diagnosis.

Thai massage is an important part of traditional Thai medicine. Originating in the western part of ancient India, it is based on Indian herbal medicine and yoga. The therapy consists of two forms, one called Nuad Ra Jasamnak, a manual therapy that only uses hands, thumbs, and fingertips to press the area being treated. Another one is called Nuad Chaloeisak, with its main purpose being to relax and maintain health, using hands, elbows, knees, and heels to press, torque, drag, stretch, and to perform other manual operations. Among those, pressing and torquing are quite similar to that of *tuina*, as well as its theoretical basis, operating procedures, and the use of the meridian theory.

Japanese acupressure or Shiatsu, is a type of massage therapy based on, and evolved from, ancient acupuncture and *Àn Mó* therapy of China. The term "Shiatsu" is derived from two words meaning finger and pressure in Japanese. Clinically, besides the application of acupoints theory in Chinese medicine, it also combines modern anatomy, with acupressure areas located along pathways of some arteries. Japanese massage physician Shuyonjuu Tsutomusawa said: "[Japanese] massage was introduced from China in ancient times as *dao yin* and *an qiao* (pressing and stepping), also known as *an mo*, rubbing and pressing therapy. People were fond of it and improved it". The text is clear enough to see the historical connection between Shiatsu and *tuina*.

Bone-setting or orthopedic manipulation was created by Andrew Taylor Still, an

American physician in the late 18th century. The therapy is a complex system including adjusting motor and visceral systems that combined a variety of manual therapeutic techniques, such as reduction of fracture and dislocation, visceral adjustment, fascia relaxation, and general relaxation of nervous, skeletal and muscular systems. The philosophic theories and principles include integrity of the body, the self-healing ability and the self-regulating function of the body. The scope of orthopedic manipulations has several aspects that overlap with viscera *Àn Mó* and orthopedic manipulations of the discipline of *tuina*.

II. Application and Popularization of *Tuina* Worldwide

Sharing knowledge with other countries is an important part of the modern development of Chinese medicine. As the Chinese Economical Reformation and Opening gains momentum, international exchanges continue to increase, therefore *tuina* has entered another thriving period, possibly the most important since the Sui and Tang dynasties.

Since the Chinese Economical Reformation and Opening, the international exchange of *tuina* knowledge has become increasingly frequent. On one hand, *tuina* scholars leave the China for academic exchanges, teaching technical skills, and expanding the international market of *tuina*. On the other hand, foreign scholars come to visit and learn Chinese medicinal *tuina*. International medical experts are increasingly interested in Chinese medicine, and some countries that have previously excluded Chinese medicine have been, or are, admitting Chinese medicine therapy through proper procedures, some of which have been included in the scope of medical insurance systems. As a direct result of the increase in interest, the unique charm and appeal of *tuina* is attracting more and more *tuina* medical professionals and clients seeking treatment. In the 21st century, *tuina* will undoubtedly be recognized as one of the most promising therapies across the globe.

At present, more than 120 countries and regions have established institutions of Chinese medicine. More than one-third of the world's population uses Chinese medicine, including acupuncture, *tuina*, and qigong to treat a number of diseases. The efficacy of Chinese medicine has become trusted, affirmed, and supported in varying degrees by governments and people in general. According to an incomplete statistic, there are about 3,000 clinics practicing Chinese medicine in the United Kingdom and Canada each. Australia has more than 4,000 such clinics. In Europe, for every 15,000 people, there is one clinic of Chinese medicine, in countries like France, Germany, Spain, Italy and the Netherlands; *tuina* is one of the most commonly used treatments in these clinics. Among the 47 countries where Chinese medicine is widely disseminated, the British government has classified acupuncture and *tuina* into the category of physiotherapy, and *tuina* is further classified as a "compensation therapy," and is not covered by free medical care, requiring patients to pay from their own pocket. Germany, on the other hand, allows *tuina* therapy to be partially covered by insurance. The Swiss federal government has enacted legislation on Chinese medicine, and since 1999, the cost of treatment for Chinese medicine such as *tuina*, acupuncture, and moxibustion can be paid by medical insurance. Other countries such as the United States and Australia are also regulating the use of Chinese medicine in accordance with their respective legislation or other regulatory forms.

Although Chinese medicine, including *tuina*, shines abroad in recent years, there are still many difficulties and obstacles in the application and development of *tuina* in foreign countries due to differences in cultural background and theoretic system. In many countries, *tuina* has not yet achieved legislative status, and has gained little attention from academic fields. Concurrently, the competence of *tuina* practitioners varies due to the lack of effective and accessible industry standards and supervision mechanisms during the international development of Chinese medicine. It is therefore critical that global standards be established for regulating *tui-*

na through associations and their members worldwide. In June of 2012, the Changchun University of Traditional Chinese Medicine led an effort to establish the Professional Committee for Traditional Chinese Medical Manual Therapy under the World Federation of Chinese Medicine Society, with participants from more than 30 countries and regions in the world, recognizing that *tuina* academic exchanges have already expanded into a global setting. The authors believe that with the credibility, legislative status, insurance coverage, and other issues of Chinese medicine continuing to improve in foreign countries, *tuina* will be more widely used and further developed, to better serve the healthcare needs of people around the world.

Section 3   Ways to Study *Tuina*

As a medical discipline with a very strong practical nature, *tuina* falls within the scope of the fundamental Chinese medicine theory, because the use of manual *tuina* techniques or certain tools on specific areas or acupuncture points of the body surface are used to prevent and treat diseases. It is important to focus on both theoretical accumulation and daily practice of manual techniques, as both aspects are indispensable to becoming a competent practitioner. At the same time, the accumulation of theory is subtle, and years of practice are necessary to exercise skill. As with many professionals relying on manual work, every practitioner needs to undergo a rigorous training process, similar to that of typists, who need to be familiar with the keyboard and trained to type faster and faster, and piano students, who need more and more rigorous fingering and strengthened training in musicality daily. As a basis for *tuina* physicians, technique is a tool for them to implement therapeutic thought. The competence of the manual skills is directly proportional to the level of effectiveness of *tuina* treatment. With that in mind, what are the best practices for *tuina* maneuvers?

There are three stages in learning and practicing *tuina* maneuvers.

First, students need to learn and be trained with the basic techniques of *tuina*. Knowledge of the basic techniques, although tedious, is the initial and most critical apsect in learning *tuina*. At this stage, bad operational habits formed in learning a certain maneuver is often really difficult to correct in the future; therefore, be sure to accurately mimic instructions shown in the literature and by teachers. It will not be a good idea to casually alter or exaggerate a maneuver; rather, it will be beneficial for students to carefully understand the essentials and purpose of each action to improve accuracy while learning and performing *tuina* maneuvers. Learners need to practice with great concentration, and avoid being impetuous. In the early stage of learning it is critically important to mimic the movements of each *tuina* maneuver repeatedly, and carefully understand its essentials. Thus, in this stage, students need to "initially synchronize with the teacher."

Second, continuous and repetitive practice is the way to master *tuina* techniques. Since *tuina* requires doctors to apply physical power on certain body areas on a patient, there needs to be a certain level of strength and length of time to obtain a better effect. Therefore, after mastering the basic technique, students must practice to increase their hand power, to enhance their proficiency, strength, and durability. During this process, they must pay attention to the natural coordination of both hands, so they can operate at the same time. Another aspect of training is learning to be flexible, coherent, uniform, and durable in the applicatin of the maneuver, so as to avoid being stiff or using excessive force that may result in self-injury. Moreover, students should try to find opportunities to reinforce training in their daily lives. After a long period of practice, the student can eventually achieve the level where operation is as smooth as water. A good method of self-training is to practice on a beanbag.

Third, students need to study and train in the clinical application of each maneuver. At this stage of learning it is necessary to master a variety of techniques on the basis of the practical application, while the knowledge of each technique and its applications is refined and deepened. Through the application in this process, students can practice on each other to find what areas exist for improvement, so that they can adjust the application of the maneuvers to make themselves more flexible during actual application. After students meet the requirements of the first and second stage, they can start applying what they have learned on the human body. There is a big difference between practicing on a beanbag versus practicing with the human body due to the elasticity of muscles and the ability of a real person to vocalize how the treatment feels to them. Therefore, practitioners should always pay attention to the reaction and changes of force under their hands to gradually improve the sensitivity of the hands and make proper adjustment of applied power accordingly. In addition, it is more meaningful to carry out operations on humans, and gather feedback from the person being operated on. Through this stage of training, students can improve their sensitivity, setting a good foundation for mastering the ability and adjusting the level of strength as necessary. At this stage, students will often form a number of their own unique styles in applying the maneuvers, which is perfectly fine, as the idiom says, "eventually deriving from the teacher".

Whether it is for health prevention or for treatment purposes, whether the receiving parties are patients or people with marginal health status, *tuina*, like any other medical interventions, involves risks during its implementation. Some may experience side effects, others may even encounter life-threatening events, causing both the doctor and the patient to suffer losses. As a result, it should be top priority to reduce the risk while protecting the interests of both parties. Only in normative and safe conditions does *tuina* ensure clinical efficacy, with the safety and effectiveness of maneuvers uniformed. Therefore, it is important to have safety in mind by emphasizing the standardization of *tuina* maneuvers, their indications, and contraindications in the learning process of *tuina*.

Practicality is always emphasized when studying *tuina* discipline. Therefore, it is necessary to pay attention to the accumulation of basic knowledge of Chinese medicine and Western medicine, as well as diligently practicing during the learning process. "Practice makes perfect". By relating to relevant course content, theoretical knowledge, in-depth understanding of the mechanism of treatment, a student often needs to summarize the knowledge to finally master the rules of this discipline. While it is important to learn from past experience, students should not limit themselves to the past, there is always more to learn and new information to acquire. All of this lays a solid foundation for the clinical practice of *tuina*.

Note:

Tuina is not only a technique, but also a scientific system. Before a student studies *tuina* maneuvers, it is extremely important to get familiar with the fundamental and theoretical knowledge of Chinese medicine in order to guide the study of *tuina* maneuvers.

Chapter Two

The Principles Behind the Effects of *Tuina*

Section 1   The Principles of the Effects of *Tuina* in Chinese Medicine

Tuina is a discipline in the scope of external treatment methods in Chinese medicine, with which a doctor treats a patient using manual techniques depending on the patient's condition. *Tuina* adjusts the body's physiological and pathological conditions through various *tuina* maneuvers on the physical body, to achieve the prevention or treatment of various diseases. The treatment principles can be summarized as: regulating yin and yang, supplementing the deficienct and draining the excess, invigorating blood and dissolving stasis, dredging meridians and unblocking collaterals, and adjusting tendons and restoring bones.

> **Note:**
>
> Please review reference books, for instance, *The Yellow Emperor's Inner Classic.* Keep in mind that the principles explaining the mechanism of *tuina* are based on the theories such as Yin and Yang, Deficiency and Excess, and Tendons and Bones, and the theories need to be comprehended with consideration of the clinical aspects of *tuina*.

I. Regulating Yin and Yang

In Chinese medicine, it is believed that during occurrence and development of disease, there will be a variety of pathological changes. Yin and yang disorders are the root causes of disease and are reflected in all diseases and stages of disease. *Tuina* can adjust the deficiency or excess of yin or yang based on the properties of disease patterns, balancing of the body's yin and yang, restoring its normal physiological function and achieving the purpose of curing the disease. The function of regulating yin and yang is mainly achieved through the meridians, qi and blood. Since *tuina* maneuvers have direct effects on body areas being worked on, *tuina* techniques can unblock the meridians and collaterals, move qi and blood, moisten bones and tendons, which further impacts organs and other parts of the body through the qi, blood, meridians, and collaterals.

II. Supplementing the Deficient and Draining the Excess

Although there is no direct supplementing or draining material entering the body with *tuina* manipulations, *tuina* relies on stimulating the diseased portion of the body with hands to work on specific areas on the surface of the body. It promotes the body's normal function to reach a supplimenting effect, or inhibits the hyperactive function to achieve a draining effect. Through hand maneuvers, *tuina* changes qi, blood, body fluids, organs, meridians, and collaterals correspondingly to achieve the purpose of supplementing the deficient and draining the excess. Take the example of a sore and distended feeling of a maneuver, if a patient's feeling is strong, it is considered a heavy and draining method; otherwise, a moderate feeling is seen as a light and supplementing method. In *tuina* treatment, the frequency and direction of the manual manipulations play an important role. Generally speaking, a maneuver following the direction of a meridian is supplementing, while the ones against the direction of a meridian is draining. Therefore, when it comes to applying *tuina* to achieve the purpose of supplementing or draining effect, it is important to take all three aspects into consideration: select the appropriate treatment areas according to the condition of the illness, use either light or heavy force while working on a patient based on their constitution and disease condition, and choose appropriate maneuvers for different treatment sites.

Note:

The power of the maneuver is measured by the amount of stimulation the patient feels, rather than the pressure the practitioner applies. The same amount of strength applied on different parts of the body may cause different level of stimulation. The same amount of power can cause different amount of stimulation using different maneuvers. Therefore, we cannot simply think that the use of greater power is an intense maneuver, and a lighter application of power is a light maneuver. The gentleness or heaviness of a certain maneuver is only one aspect in determining whether a technique is supplementing or draining, especially when other aspects such as the frequency and direction are also taken into account.

III. Invigorating Blood and Dissolving Stasis

Blood stasis is a pathological result caused by coagulation of blood due to unregulated blood circulation, which becomes a pathogenic factor resulting in other illnesses. *Tuina* can adjust the contraction and relaxation of muscles, passing the effect to the blood vessel walls, causing the muscles to relax and contract rhythmically thereby promoting blood circulation around damaged tissues. Improved blood flow further increases perfusion to tissues, and improves blood rheology. Thus, by promoting the movement of qi and blood, *tuina* invigorates blood to dissolve stasis by providing direct stimulation at certain meridian acupoints or other parts on the body surface.

VI. Dredging the Meridians and Unblocking the Collaterals

The meridian and collateral system is collectively the general term of the networked conduits in the body that transfer qi and blood, connect organs interiorly and joints and limbs exteriorly, and linking throughout by running up and down the body. The system unifies all the organs, tissues and structures into a stable, coordinated and organic whole. *Tuina* operates on meridian acupoints of the body surface, causes local meridians to respond, and stimulates and adjusts meridian qi. At the same time, it affects the functional activity of organs, tissues, and limbs through the meridians and collaterals to regulate the physiological and pathological conditions of the body. As a result, a *tuina* treatment serves the purpose of dredging vessels, harmonizing all five organ systems, and restoring the normal physiological function of the human body.

V. Adjusting Tendons and Restoring Bones

In the *Golden Mirror of the Medical Tradition* (*Yī Zōng Jīn Jiàn*, 医宗金鉴), it states that "[a doctor] uses the hand to touch it, [and he would] know the condition". The *Golden Mirror of the Medical Tradition* also contains statements about tendons being distorted, broken, reversed, twisted, dislocated and other pathological changes. The book suggests that disorder and dislocation in different tissues found through palpation should be corrected and adjusted in a timely manner, returning tendons to their normal locations, so that qi and blood could run smoothly, and pain would be relieved. For soft tissue dislocation, *tuina* can create these results with external manual force. Taking tendon slippage as an example: a patient in this situation would have serious difficulty in joint movement. By using the plucking and push-torquing maneuvers, such slippage can be corrected. For those suffering intra-articular cartilage injury with joint interlocking and facing difficulties of physical movement, *tuina* can also relieve such joint disorder using appropriate techniques. For joint dislocation, *tuina* can be used for passive joint movement to have the joint returned to its normal anatomical location. An example is sacroiliac joint subluxation, where the patient will experience pain due to obstruction and stretching of local soft tissue. In this case, pain can be reduced and even disappear through passive movement such as oblique torquing, flexion, and stretching of the hip to restore the dislocated joint back to its normal location. By adjusting tendons and restoring bones, *tuina*, with its various manual techniques, corrects anatomical abnormalities caused by injuries, so that meridians and collaterals can be unblocked, joints can be adjusted, and various tissues can be restored to their normal places. Thus, *tuina* is beneficial for relieving soft tissue spasm and recovering joint function.

> *Note:*
>
> "Tendons slipped out of the slots, bones displaced" is what Chinese medicine summarized about most joints and tendon injuries, which makes an important guiding principle. Thus, the treatment of *tuina* should make "tendons return to their slots, and bones restore to their places". Often, the two need to be treated concurrently.

Section 2   The Mechanisms of *Tuina* from the View of Biomedicine

Through manipulation on the body surface or specific parts of the body, *tuina* on one hand has a direct treatment effect on a local area, and on the other hand has a certain impact on various systems via different venues such as nerves and body fluids.

I. Impact to the Motor System

Recent studies have shown that *tuina* has a unique effect for motor system damage that is mainly due to soft tissue injury. *Tuina* can directly or indirectly promote the contracting and stretching of muscle fibers to improve nutrition and metabolism for muscles, and speed up absorption or discharge of harmful metabolites such as lactic acid within muscle tissue. *Tuina* can also promote the dilution and decomposition of inflammatory mediators, so that inflammation caused by local damage is diminished and it is therefore easier for edemas and hematomas to be absorbed. At the same time, *tuina* techniques can increase the temperature and pain threshold of local tissues, while muscle spasms can be relieved with the use of muscle tractive maneuvers such as stretching, flexion, extension, and plucking.

II. Impact to the Nervous System

It has been shown that *tuina* can, to some extent, regulate the central nervous system. By observing EEG, tactile stimulation can be used to reflect the excitatory and inhibitory processes of the central nervous system through a reflex pathway. *Tuina* can also impact the release of endogenous opioid peptides to achieve an analgesic effect, eliminate anxiety, reduce pain, regulate mood, and release pleasure-enhancing endorphins. In recent years, research also found that *tuina* plays a unique and advantageous role in the repair and regeneration of nerve injury.

III. Impact to the Circulatory System

Tuina can cause protein decomposition, resulting in the production of histamine and histamine-like substances within cells, which play a role in expanding the capillaries. *Tuina* can promote the reconstruction of the vascular network for the diseased tissue, consume and remove lipids on the blood vessels wall, slow down the hardening of blood vessels and restore their elasticity. *Tuina* can accelerate flow and enhance the circulation of blood, strengthen the function of the heart, and effectively regulate heart rate and blood pressure.

IV. Impact to the Digestive System

Tuina can have both direct and indirect effects on the digestive system. First, through manual stimulation, *tuina* directly causes morphological and motor function changes to the gastrointestinal tract, and further alters the rate of gastrointestinal peristalsis, thereby speeding or delaying the movement and excretion process of gastrointestinal contents. Second, the manual stimulations of *tuina*, through the reflex effect of nerve conduction, indirectly enhances gastrointestinal peristalsis and digestive secretion, promotes the process of food digestion and absorption, and strengthens the digestive system function.

V. Impact to the Endocrine and Immune Systems

Tuina has a certain regulatory effect on the endocrine system. For example, when the body is stimulated by gentle and rhythmic *tuina* maneuvers, the parasympathetic function increases, promoting vasodilatation, gastrointestinal peristalsis, sphincter relaxation, and glandular secretion. *Tuina* also promotes sugar utilization and metabolism, so it decreases blood sugar levels. Excitement of the parasympathetic nerve also directly promotes insulin secretion. In combination, the two effects of *tuina* reduce blood sugar. Additionally, *tuina* stimulation can increase the total number of white blood cells in blood and can enhance phagocytosis. At the same time, *tuina* regulates immunoglobulin IgG, IgM, IgA and complement C3 in the serum bidirectionally, improves the potency of serum complement, and increases the number of T lymphocytes and their subgroups. *Tuina* therefore enhances the immune function of body fluids and cells.

VI. Other Impacts

Tuina can also regulate tension of the bladder and function of the sphincter to treat urinary retention and enuresis. It can improve the function of the traction receptors of the bladder wall and the excitability of the sympathetic innervation of the sphincter, and reduce the excitability of the parasympathetic innervation of the detrusor, to increase the bladder voiding threshold. In addition, since *tuina* is applied on skin, *tuina* is able to eliminate local aged epithelial cells, and improve skin respiration. It promotes decomposition of some types of skin protein, resulting in the production of histamines that activate skin capillaries and nerves, thereby improving skin nutrition and metabolism, so that the skin obtains color, luster, and elasticity. Since *tuina* improves skin elasticity, there is a reduction in wrinkles, therefore, *tuina* can be used for beauty purposes.

Chapter **Three**

Treatment Principles and Methods of *Tuina*

The treatment principles of *tuina* were developed using a holistic view and pattern differentiation of Chinese medicine that provides universal instructions in applying *tuina* to treat diseases in a clinical setting. The treatment methods of *tuina*, were also developed under the guiding principles in treating specific diseases, such as the method of sweat-promotion, emesis, or purgation. Or, it can be a method aimed to treat a specific disease pattern, such as the method of qi benefiting with blood invigorating, or qi rectifying for pain relief.

Section 1   Treatment Principles of *Tuina*

In general, the treatment principles of *tuina* consists of five aspects: preventive treatment, treating a disease from its root cause, supplementing the deficient and draining the excess, regulating yin and yang, and treating the disease according to the three factors.

I. Preventive Treatment

The term preventive treatment, referred to as *treating a future disease* (zhì wèi bìng, 治未病) in *The Yellow Emperor's Inner Classic*, involves taking some measures to prevent a disease from happening, or when the disease has occurred, take appropriate method to halt its further development and to alter its pathologic evolution. There are three treatment principles from the *tuina* perspective: prevention prior to the occurrence of the disease, preventing a disease from further change, exercising after healing of the disease. Disease

prevention refers to using specific methods and taking certain measures to prevent a disease from happening. *Dao yin* exercise, health maintenance *tuina*, and subjective adjustment of body positions are commonly-used prevention methods in the scope of *tuina*. Disease change prevention refers to preventing a disease from developing further after its occurrence, and striving to achieve both an early diagnosis and timely treatment. Exercising after healing from a disease refers to using functional exercises to enhance a treatment effect when the disease is partially relieved or considered clinically cured; or, when a chronic disease is in its remission phase, and the treatment is not yet completed. Healing exercise is also an important means of treatment to prevent a disease from recurring. Patients can be treated with *tuina*, and concurrently perform *dao yin* exercise on their own to maintain and consolidate treatment effect in an effort to prevent the recurrence of the disease.

> *Note:*
>
> *Dao yin*, as an ancient disease prevention and treatment method, is an active physical exercise coordinated with breathing and regulating mental activities. Five Birds Play and Tendon Alternation Classic are *dao yin* exercise in traditional Chinese medicine. The latter is also required prior to the study of *tuina* discipline.

II. Treating the Root Cause of the Disease

Treating the root cause of any disease refers to the principle of tackling the nature and principal challenge of a disease, which is one of the fundamental principles in pattern differentiation while applying *tuina* within the scope of Chinese medicine. The clinical use of this principle is to apply targeted treatment in accordance with the specific cause of the disease besides relieving clinical symptoms of the disease. For example, frozen shoulder is characterized by pain and dysfunction of the shoulder. It is generally believed that the occurrence of the disease is due to deficient qi and blood, externally contracted wind, cold, and dampness, and traumatic strain. Therefore, the treatment method should include supplementing qi to generate blood, dispelling wind-cold, dissolving dampness, and dredging the meridians and collaterals to relieve the shoulder pain and dysfunction. In addition, the principles of "treating the branch when it is urgent," and "treating the root when it is eased" should be obeyed while applying *tuina* clinically in order to treat the root cause of a disease. In general, the principle of "treating the branch while urgent" is more suitable for acute illnesses. For instance, when a joint dislocation causes severe pain, it is not a good time to perform reduction. Therefore, the first measure to take is to relieve pain with *tuina* maneuvers, thus "treating the branch". When the pain is reduced, reduction maneuvers are used to fix the dislocated joints, thus "treating the root" when the urgent condition has been eliminated.

III. Supplementing the Deficient and Draining the Excess

The occurrence of a disease involves the process of the healthy qi (a.k.a. right qi) combatting pathogenic qi. *Tuina* uses a series of maneuvers to support the healthy qi, dispel the pathogenic qi, and alter the ratio of the two. Thus, the healthy qi gradually increases while the pathogenic qi weakens. When the ratio is altered in favor of the healthy qi, the condition will be transformed to the direction of benefiting health and eliminating the disease. Therefore, supplementing the deficient and draining the excess is one of the fundamental guiding principles in the clinical practice of *tuina*.

IV. Regulating Yin and Yang

Regulating yin and yang is another basic principle in the clinical practice of *tuina*. There are several common types of yin and yang imbalance: yin deficiency, yang deficiency, yin and yang deficiency, yin deficiency with hyperactive yang, and yang deficiency with hyperactive yin. Therefore, a practitioner should regulate yin and yang according to specific circumstances by applying appropriate methods accordingly, such as nourishing yin, benefiting yang, supplementing both yin and yang, nourishing yin to conquer yang, and warming yang to control yin. By way of example, when there is excessive yang, yin is weak; and vice versa. As the result, the body will exhibit either hypofunction or hyperfunction respectively. It is appropriate to use low frequency and light pressure *tuina* maneuvers that excites the body while treating hypofunctional problems to supplement the deficiency. On the contrary, it is suitable to apply suppressive *tuina* maneuvers with high frequency and heavy pressure to drain the excess.

V. Treating the Disease According to the Three Factors

Treating diseases should be based on the three etiologic factors: time, place, and person, more specifically, the treatment plan should be made in accordance with the season, the region, and a person's specific condition including body constitution and age. From the clinical standpoint of *tuina*, the individual patient's circumstances are particularly important, because *tuina* applies external force on the body surface, causing direct effects. Therefore, it is reasonable that a practitioner take into account differences of each person since the differences are mainly reflected in the age, gender, occupation, physical fitness, past history, family history and other aspects. For example, moderate stimuli for young adults may be beyond the tolerance level for elderly people and children.

> ### Note:
>
> The principle of treating a disease based on three factors of time, place and person is an important principles of *tuina*. For example, the amount of stimulation from *tuina* is different between summer and winter, and associated with the tolerance level of patients. At the same time, when treatment time becomes longer, the patient's tolerance level will change, which is another aspect of treating the disease based on the condition of each individual.

Section 2   Treatment Methods of *Tuina*

By using manual treatment methods, *tuina* works on specific areas of the patient's body to treat certain diseases. It is an important external medical treatment of Chinese medicine. According to the nature and quantity of the maneuver, combining them with treatment area, *tuina* therapy can be categorized into eight basic types: warming, unblocking, supplementing, draining (purging), sweat-promoting, harmonizing, dispersing, and clearing.

I. The Warming Method

The warming method is applicable to patients showing the deficiency-cold pattern. It often uses maneuvers such as swinging, rubbing, squeezing, and pressing with a relatively slow, gentle and rhythmic execution. On the area or acupoint receiving the treatment, the continuous application of certain maneuvers should last longer, causing the patient to experience stimulation with a deep and thorough warm feeling. Such method has effects of warming the meridians, unblocking the collaterals, and replenishing yang qi.

II. The Unblocking Method

The unblocking method is used to unblock the body's conduits. Chinese medicine believes that "blockage causes pain", and "the unblocking method relieves pain". Thus, the manifestation of meridian blockage is often pain, so the unblocking method should be applied. Common unblocking *tuina* methods include squeezing and frictional maneuvers, with the force alternating between strong and soft during the manual application. While applying pushing, grasping, and foulage on the four limbs, it can unblock and regulate meridians and collaterals. In addition, grasping *jiān jǐng* (GB 21, 肩井) area can unblock stagnant qi and moving qi and blood.

III. The Supplementing Method

Supplementing, which is also known as nourishing and tonifying, is to supplement deficient qi, blood, body fluids, and weakened organ functions. Clinically, methods of swinging and frictional types of maneuvers are mainly employed. At the same time, techniques need to be applied out lightly and gently, rather than excessively strong stimulation. The technique is mainly used in qi and blood deficiency, spleen and stomach weakness, lack of kidney yin, yin-deficient night sweats, or nocturnal emission.

IV. The Purging Method

Purging is a laxative method used for excess patterns of the lower-*jiao*. The corresponding manipulations include swinging, rubbing, wiping, squeezing, and pressing that should be applied with comparatively intense power. The frequency of the manipulation should start slow and gradually increase. Although the stimulation of the purging method is relatively strong, it achieves the purpose of purging the pathogenic excess by regulating the functions of the internal viscera; therefore, generally there is no side effects.

V. The Sweat-promoting Method

The purpose of the sweat-promoting method is to induce sweat and disperse pathogens, so that pathogenic factors are removed from the exterior level. The main maneuvers used clinically are of squeezing, pressing, and swinging types. *Tuina* has a strong effect of sweat-promoting and exterior-releasing, with manipulation on the patient's skin and muscles to open up the pores and interspace of the skin. A further result is that the pathogenic qi will be released from the exterior level, and the healthy qi will return to a peaceful status.

VI. The Harmonizing Method

The harmonizing method has the effect of regulating qi, blood, and *zang-fu* organs. Some manipulations used are vibrating, rubbing, pushing, and wiping. The harmonizing method is designed to treat patterns such as liver and stomach qi stagnation, irregular menstruation, disharmony of the spleen and stomach, distending pain all over the body caused by qi and blood disharmony, and meridian stagnation.

VII. The Dispersing Method

Dispersing means to scatter. In general, main *tuina* maneuvers for dispersing are swinging and frictional methods, with gentle, agile, and soft execution. The dispersing method unblocks the conduits, and allows for qi and blood to run smoothly, which disperses masses in organs, stasis of qi and blood, and the stagnant accumulation of phlegm and food. For instance, the dispersing method can be used to treat fullness, distention, and suppression of the chest and abdomen, which are the result of excessive eating, or the transporting and transforming inability of the spleen.

VIII. The Clearing Method

The clearing method is used to clear heat. Clinically, squeezing and frictional maneuvers are used, with soft but firm force. To clear and drain excessive heat at the qi level, perform the pushing maneuver gently along the *du mai* from *dà zhuī* (DU 14, 大椎) to the coccyx. For patient with deficient heat, the physician needs to wipe the lower back area to foster yin and clearing the deficient fire. For those with excessive heat in the blood level, apply the pushing maneuver with a good level of power from *dà zhuī* (DU 14) to the caudal vertebrae to clear heat and cool down the blood. For people with excessive exterior heat, use light pushing method along the bladder meridian on the back, from bottom to top, and the same method is used with the opposite direction from top to bottom for patients with deficient exterior heat, both to clear the heat and release the exterior.

Note:

A student should not make one-to-one link between a particular maneuver with a specific *tuina* method introduced in this section. To the contrary, we should understand the three factors generating the effect associated with a specific manipulation: the nature and amount of the manipulation, the specificity of a certain body area or acupoint receiving the stimulation, and the functional status of the body. Only after identifying the functional status of the patient's body, is a *tuina* physician able to achieve different treatment effects using different treatment methods according to the nature and amount of force, and the specific treatment area.

Chapter **Four**

Common Diagnostic Methods Used in *Tuina*

Clinically, *tuina* can be widely used to treat diseases including orthopedic, internal, external, gynecological, and pediatric conditions. However, correct diagnosis is an important prerequisite for the application of *tuina*. Therefore, the clinical examination must follow the holistic viewpoint of Chinese medicine diagnosis and treatment combined with the basic knowledge of modern medicine. At the same time, there should be the use of the six diagnostic methods: observation, listening/smelling, inquiry, pulse-taking, passive movement, and measuring, which is a comprehensive examination to distinguish the primary and secondary problems in determining the condition. What must be emphasized is that the clinical physical examination is only a diagnostic method, so it must be combined with the patient's medical history, imaging examinations (ultrasound, X-ray, CT, MRI, etc.), laboratory tests, and other necessary information acquired with a comprehensive analysis. Only with a comprehensive understanding of the patient's general condition and specific signs and symptoms, can a physician obtain a correct and comprehensive diagnosis to lay a good foundation for an effective *tuina* treatment.

Section 1   Examination of the Head and Neck

I. Examination of the Head and Face

(I) Observation

The observation of the head and face is mainly to observe the vitality, complexion, and local morphological changes.

1. Observe the Vitality and Complexion Vitality (*shen*-spirit, 神) is the general term for human vital activities, and is also a high level summary of external performance of the mental, consciousness, thinking, and functional activities of qi, blood, and viscera. As pointed out in *The Plain Questions - The Discussion of Transforming Essence and Altering Qi*, "[those] who got *shen* [would] thrive, [and those] who lost *shen* [would] die". By observing vitality, a physician can determine the rise and fall of the healthy qi in the transformation process of a disease. The complexion of the face is therefore the outer expression of qi and blood of internal organs.

In general, a disease is either not very serious or superficial, or the functions of *zang-fu* organs are not feeble when a patient has clear consciousness and quick response, both eyes are flexible and bright with sufficient vital signs, and can distinguish objects well. The patient should also have a vivid facial complexion and normal facial luster. Even if the illness is somewhat serious, the patient should have a positive prognosis.

On the other hand, the disease can be serious and the prognosis of the patient is not good when he is apathetic, unresponsive, or has a gloomy expression, sluggish pupils, and a dull facial complexion lacking of luster. The prognosis of a patient is poor when they have symptoms such as unconsciousness, coma, delirium, pale complexion, dull eyes, fuzzy gaze, dilated or constricted pupils, cold limbs, sticky sweat, feeble constitution, and extremely withered appearance. Those who suddenly show improved vitality deserve extra attention after being sick for a long time, or having a severe illness, with an extremely low level of essential qi. This phenomenon is the so-called "fake *shen*", with common analogy "the last radiance of the setting sun".

Clinically, if a patient has a pale and puffy face, it is usually the indication of yang deficiency seen in patients who have lost a large amount of blood or suffer from asthma. Pale face lacking of luster with an emaciated figure generally indicates blood deficiency. In acute situations, if a patient's face suddenly turns paler, mostly it indicates sudden loss and escape of yang qi, which is often seen in shock caused by a variety of reasons. If the face, eyes, and body has a yellow tint, it is known as the *huang* pattern. The pattern showing bright yellow is called yang *huang* pattern, mostly pertaining to damp-heat. When it shows a dull yellow, it is named yin *huang* pattern, generally caused by cold-damp. If the facial complexion looks bluish with lips presenting a grayish color, it mostly indicates qi stagnation. When a child suffers febrile convulsions or seizures, the facial complexion appears to be bluish and dull in most cases. Headache of wind-cold pattern and abdominal pain of cold-sluggish pattern with severe pain shows a dull, pale or bluish facial complexion. Zygomatic flush on both malar bones seen in the afternoon indicates mostly deficient heat pattern owing to yin deficiency and yang hyperactivity. If dark circles are seen around the eyes, most commonly it indicates water retention caused by kidney-yang deficiency, or leukorrhea pertaining to the downward pouring of cold- damp pattern.

2. Observation from Morphologic Standpoint Whether the shape of the body is strong or weak is a uniform reflection of the functional level of internal organs. Generally speaking, interior strength determines exterior strength, and interior weakness results in exterior weakness. Bulging frontal cheekbones on both sides, flat and square-shaped vertex, and sparse hair are commonly seen in children with rickets. In patients with peripheral facial paralysis, symptoms include inability to close one eye, disappearance of ipsilateral forehead wrinkles, the mouth becoming deviated to the contralateral side

when trying to show the teeth, and the disappearance of ipsilateral nasolabial groove. Conversely, if a patient has central facial paralysis, the mouth deviates to the ipsilateral side with the lower part of the face paralyzed. In ankylosis of the temporomandibular joint (TMJ), if it is unilateral, the chin seems skewed to the affected side, causing asymmetry of the face with ipsilateral puffiness and contralateral flatness. In a patient with congenital bilateral ankylosis of TMJ, the entire mandibular has dysplasia with a shrunken, showing bird face deformity. If the condition happens in an adult, the deformity will not be significant, however, movements such as opening the mouth are difficult.

For patients suffering trauma, the physician should check if the nasal bridge is crooked or depressed, whether there is hematoma and ecchymosis of the nasal area, or whether the respiratory tract is blocked. If there is a nasal bone fracture, there will be obvious local tenderness, and a depressed nasal bridge can be felt. Eyes should also be examined to look for hyperemia, blurred vision, orbital ecchymosis, and swelling. For pupils, check to see if there is dilation, constriction, deformity, or asymmetricity. Bilateral direct and indirect light reflex should be also checked, as well as nystagmus. Otorrhea, rhinorrhea or throat hematoma are often indications of a fracture of the skull base. Patients with dislocation of the mandible have their mouths half-open and experience biting difficulty.

(II) Palpation

Palpation is the diagnostic method using one's hand to examine certain surface areas of the patient's body to distinguish cold, warm, moist, dryness, swollen, distention, and pain; and at the same time, to observe the patient's response to the pressure.

1. Fontanelle Examination on Infants From in front of the child's head, place the two palms on the left and right temples respectively, the thumb on the forehead, and use the middle and index fingers to check the fontanelle. A normal anterior fontanelle is one that can be reached with the beat consistent with the pulse, level with the skull, and exhibits a slight sense of tension. Bulging of the anterior fontanel is commonly seen in condition or diseases such as high fever, intracranial hemorrhage and increased intracranial pressure, except when the child is crying. The anterior fontanelle should close at 12 to 18 months after birth, and if the closure time is longer than that, it is considered delayed, seen in diseases such as rickets.

2. Measurement of Mouth Opening The distance between the superior and inferior teeth should be equivalent to the width of distal phalangeal joints of the index, middle, and ring fingers combined. With stiffness of the mandibular joint, the width decreases or the teeth are clenched.

3. Examination of Head Trauma Even if the appearance of a patient has no obvious change, it is still necessary to carefully examine them during palpation, with focus on depression of the skull, open wounds or avulsion of the scalp, and scalp bleeding or subcutaneous hematoma. In addition, it is necessary to pay extra attention to fractures underneath the surface if subcutaneous hematoma exists. In mandibular joint dislocation, the socket of the joint is empty, so that the condylar process can be palpated in the anterior position.

II. Examination of the Neck

(I) Observation

Patients should generally take the sitting position. For patients with serious condition restricting them from supporting their head, they should lie down. Since the majority of cervical diseases involve the sensory and motor activities of upper limbs, the patient would need to remove their shirt to expose the neck, shoulders, and upper limbs with shoulders relaxed, upper limbs hanging, and looking straight forward.

1. Examine to determine if there are any scars, sinuses, and cold abscess (most cold abscess are cervical tuberculosis) on the skin and soft tissue of the neck. Pay attention to lesions above the neck to look for abscess on the posterior pharyngeal wall, while edema is usually the problem on the neck. Moreover, check to see if either side of the neck has localized swelling or bulging.

2. Check to see if cervical lordosis is normal, straightened, and has limited kyphosis, scoliosis, or torsion. Other deformities such as angular kyphosis are often the result of cervical tuberculosis or fractures. In addition, pay attention to spasms or shrinking of neck muscles.

3. Look for neck deformity and asymmetricality of the face. In torticollis, or congenital pediatric muscle torticollis, the patient's neck tilts to one side, often with facial asymmetry, and bulging of the sternocleidomastoid muscle on one side. If the head is in a slightly forward position with forced posture, it mostly indicates stiff-neck, also known as *lào zhěn* or cervical spondylosis. Patients with cervical spine disorders or dislocation have symptoms including the mandibular deviated to one side, the head is not able to turn and has a sense of heaviness, and the need to be supported and protected with hands. People experiencing ankylosing spondylitis have cervical rigidity, hunchback, and limited head movement. In addition, due to difficulty turning the head to look at objects on either side, they would have to rotate their whole body for that purpose.

(II) Palpation

1. Palpation Method Ask the patient to flex their neck forward about 30° while the physician supports the patient's forehead with their left hand. Then, palpate spinous processes one by one from the occipital tuberosity down. Note that the processes of C7 and T1 is larger than others and easier to be felt. Palpate spinous processes, interspinous space and muscles on both sides. Check superficial lymph nodes below the surface of the the the neck simultaneously.

2. Major Items to Check Pay attention during the examination if any spinous process deviates from the midline, and whether tenderness is located in central area of the spinous process or on either side. Determine if the tender point is located at the superficial or deep level with palpating forces transitioning from light to heavy. In general, superficial tenderness usually indicates diseases of interspinous ligament, supraspinous ligament, or subcutaneous fascia. If the tender point is in the transverse process of cervical vertebra, it means that the facet joint may be inflammed or injured, as in facet joint disorder. In most cases, it is cervical spondylosis if the tenderness is next to the cervical spinous process, and multiple tenderness can be found at the upper corner of the scapula. Tenderness in the interspinous ligament or muscles of the neck are indications of sprain or "stiff-neck". If there is tenderness above the clavicle or the lateral triangle of the neck, then there may be cervical fasciitis. Patients with stiff-neck or cervical spondylosis often have tangible stiff muscles and spasm. For cases of cervical kyphosis, the palpating force should not be too heavy. If cervical tuberculosis is suspected, the examiner would need to check the posterior pharyngeal wall for the presence of abscess formation of the posterior pharynx. Along the line of cervical spinous processes, if there is palpable hard knots or bands, there may be calcification of the cervical ligament.

(III) Motion Examination

Examine the Motion of the Neck Ask the patient to be seated, head straight and shoulders stable. Keep the body still so it does not participate in cervical movement, and then move the neck in all directions (Figure 4-1).

1. Flexion and Extension Ask the patient to flex their head forward as much as possible. Normally the jaw can touch the chest with an anteversion angle of 35° to 45°. Then, ask the patient to extend their head backwards. A normal head extension should be 35° to 45°, making the patient look up right at the ceiling above them.

2. Rotation Ask the patient to turn their head to one side and lower it. Normally the jaw can almost touch the ipsilateral shoulder with a rotation angle of 60° to 80°. Then do the same for the contralateral side and make a comparison.

3. Lateral Bending Ask the patient to tilt their head towards the shoulder. Normally the angle should be 45°.

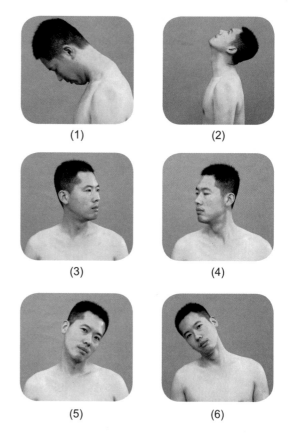

(1) (2) (3) (4) (5) (6)

Figure 4-1 Motion Examination of the Neck
(1) Anteflexion (2) Rear Extension (3) Left Rotation (4) Right Rotation (5) Left Lateral Bending (6) Right Lateral Bending

Caution: The focus of the examination is to observe if there is unrestricted movement, without movement disorders, and to exclude compensatory action. In the case of cervical spondylolisthesis dislocation, do not do exercise so as to prevent spinal cord injury.

(IV) Special Examination

1. Extrusion Test Also known as the Foraminal Compression or Spurling Test. With the patient in a seated position, place overlapped hands on top of the patient's head. Press the head downwards with the cervical spine at different angles, such as with the head extended to the back and tilted to the affected side. If neck pain or radiating pain on an upper extremity occurs, it is a positive reaction. The mechanism of a positive extrusion test is used to narrow down the foramen and aggravate the stimulation of the cervical nerve root, causing pain or radiating pain (Figure 4-2).

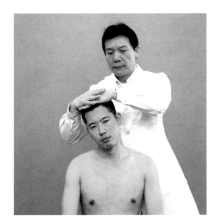

Figure 4-2 Extrusion Test

2. Separation Test Also known as the Foraminal Distraction Test. Have the patient in a seated position, and while supporting the patient's jaw and occipital area using two hands, respectively, pull upwards. It is positive if the patient feels relief of the pain in the neck and upper extremity. The mechanism of separation test is used to expand the narrowed intervertebral foramen and stretch the joint capsule of the neck, leading to reduced compression and stimulation of the nerve root, and relieved pain (Figure 4-3).

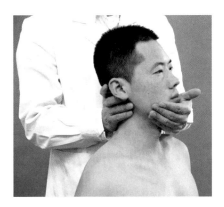

Figure 4-3 Separation Test

3. Brachial Plexus Traction Test With the

patient in a seated position and head slightly flexed away from the affected side, place one hand on the affected side of the head, the other hand holding the wrist and pulling it downward. Apply traction to the brachial plexus nerve. If there is radiating pain or numbness on the affected limb, then it is positive, suggesting brachial plexus compression, commonly seen in cervical spondylosis of nerve root type clinically (Figure 4-4).

4. Vertebral Artery Torsion Test Have the patient to be in a seated position with head slightly extended towards the back. Ask them to turn to the left and right. If the patient experiences symptoms including dizziness, headache, and blurred vision, and these symptoms disappear while they stop said movements, the test is positive, suggesting that the patient suffers cervical spondylosis of vertebral artery type (Figure 4-5)

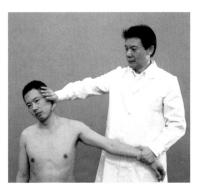

Figure 4-4 Brachial Plexus Traction Test

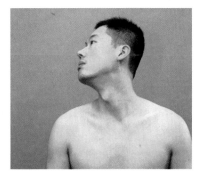

Figure 4-5 Cervical Torsion Test

Section 2　Examination of the Chest and Abdomen

I. Examination of the Chest

(I) Observation

1. Skin and Soft Tissue　This examination requires the patient to expose their chest area thoroughly, so be sure to be aware of gender-specific concerns and act accordingly. Pay attention to rashes, swelling, mass, and protrusion of subcutaneous veins. In patient with mastitis, the breasts are inflamed, become hard with tenderness spot, often accompanied by fever.

2. Thoracic Morphology　Check the shape of the thorax. Barrel chest is common in patients with emphysema and bronchial asthma with the entire thorax raised and especially expanded anteroposteriorly, shaped like a barrel. Pigeon breast is seen in rickets, with significant protrusion of the sternum, especially in the lower part, causing an expanded anteroposterior diameter, and a reduced transverse thoracic diameter. Any changes of the thoracic shape can also be caused by spinal deformity. For example, in patients suffering kyphosis caused by spinal tuberculosis and other diseases, one can observe decreased thoracic diameter, ribs are often closer to each other or even overlapped, and thorax forced closer to the spine. Developmental deformity, certain spine disorders, or muscle paralysis along one side of the spine causes scoliosis, resulting in bulging and widening of the intercostal spaces on one side of the thorax. At the same time, the other side of the thorax becomes flatter with narrower distance or even overlapped ribs, and uneven shoulders. When examining the costal cartilage through both observation and palpation, highly convex areas that are hard, immovable, and which exhibit no skin color change, indicate costochondritis. If cartilage in the superficial chest wall is soft to the touch and volatile, it is most probably a circumscribed abscess or thoracic tuberculosis.

3. Examination of Trauma Patients　Pay attention and observe the presence of chest breathing. Patients with chest trauma usually use abdominal breathing to reduce the pain. In addition, patients with multiple bilateral rib fractures may have a significantly collapsed chest, presenting a flail chest and abnormal breathing, and may exhibit discoloration and tenderness to the touch.

(II) Palpation

1. Tenderness Points　In general, visceral lesions present with pain, and tenderness can be found at the anatomical location of the organ, on its corresponding body surface. Ask the patient to point out the approximate location of pain to have a definite treatment target.

2. Examination of Trauma Patient　When applying pressure on the chest wall of a patient suffering from subcutaneous emphysema, crepitus or a sense of pressing on snow often indicates lung or tracheal rupture with air spilling out and accumulating under the skin owing to trauma on the chest. For examination of rib fracture, place the index and middle fingers of both hands on both sides of the ribs to gradually and carefully palpate along the path of ribs from the upper back towards the bottom front. If there is displacement on top of the fracture, then the broken ends and tenderness can be felt. If a fracture displacement is not obvious, the practitioner may only elicit a tenderness response and be unable to feel any dislocation.

(III) Special Examinations

Thoracic Compression Test　This test is used to diagnose rib fractures and thoracic rib dislocation. There are two steps in the test. The first step is to create pressure to the front and back while holding the back with one hand, with the other hand pushing the sternum from the front. Rib fractures can be determined by apparent pain or joint crepitus. The second step is to perform the lateral compression with both hands placed on both sides of the thorax respectively, and apply the force towards the middle. If there is a fracture or rib dislocation, pain occurs at the location of the injury (Figure 4-6).

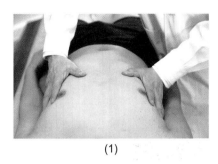

(1)

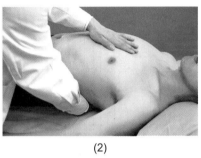

(2)

Figure 4-6　Thoracic Compression Test

II. Abdominal Examination

(I) Observation

1. Abdominal Diseases　When the patient stands, if the upper abdomen is sunken, and the umbilical area and lower abdomen are bulging, most likely the patient suffers from gastroptosis. The peristaltic waves cannot be seen if the abdomen is normal; however, they may be seen on emaciated individuals or those with a thin abdominal wall. On those with pyloric or intestinal obstruction, obvious gastric or intestinal motility waves can appear, often accompanied by a visible shape of the stomach or intestine. Superficial varicose veins on the abdominal area with ascites and an enlarged spleen are mostly the result of portal hypertension owing to liver disease. A thin child with a big bulging abdomen with blue veins exposed usually suffers from malnutrition and indigestion.

2. Examination of Patient with Traumatic Injury　While checking a patient with trauma, observe if the abdomen is bulging, and if there is localized mass, the presence of abdominal breathing, and congested blood. In addition, pay attention if the　injury is in the upper or lower abdomen, since pelvic fractures often causes hematoma and ecchymosis of the lower abdomen.

(II) Auscultation

Abdominal auscultation should be performed before palpation. Note the presence of bowel sounds during auscultation, and whether it is increased or weakened.

(III) Palpation

1. Tenderness Points　The rebound tenderness point of appendicitis, also known as the McBurney's point, is at one-third the distance from the anterior superior iliac spine to the umbilicus on right side of the abdomen. Upon appendicitis attack, obvious tenderness or soreness often be found on *làn wěi* (EX-LE 7, 阑尾), literally meaning appendix point, two *cun* straight down from *zú sān lǐ* (ST 36, 足三里), especially on the right side. The tenderness point indicating cholecystitis, called the gallbladder point, can be found at the crossing of the edge of the right hypochondrium and the right edge of the rectus abdominis. Use four fingers or the thumb to press the gallbladder point, and ask the patient to take a deep breath, which causes the gallbladder to move downwards. A positive sign is when the patient feels a sharp pain with the pressure of the fingers and suddenly stops breathing. The tenderness point of patients with biliary ascariasis is located two-finger widths below the the xiphoid and two-finger widths lateral to the midline, which is the same as the tenderness point of the choledochus. The tenderness area revealing gastric ulcer is in the middle of the upper abdomen or slightly to the left of it, which has a relatively wide range. The tenderness area indicating duodenal ulcer is at point slightly right from the upper abdomen. Patients with gastrointestinal perforation and other acute peritonitis have signs of peritoneal irritation, showing abdominal guarding, general abdominal tenderness, and rebound abdominal pain. During palpation, the tension of abdominal muscles are often as stiff as a hard woodboard.

2. Examination of Patient with Traumat-

ic Injury Focus on damage of any organs while performing palpation on the abdominal area. Whether the injury is of the liver, the spleen, or any hollow bowels, a patient with traumatic injury will have significant abdominal muscle tension. Start with the liver and spleen areas, checking for tenderness. Then note if the dull sound of the liver disappears. Thirdly, check if any shifting dull sound exists. For tenderness in other areas, be cautious of injuries of bladder, ureter, or renal parenchyma. Based on the overall situation of the patient, determine if there is any active bleeding as soon as possible. When a mass in the abdominal cavity is palpated, it could be a hematoma as a result of trauma, or lumbar tuberculosis, cold abscess, or vertebral tumors that are orthopedic problems. Also, pay attention to factors including the size, hardness of the boundaries, smoothness, fluctuation, mobility, and sensitivity of the tenderness of the tumor, in order to determine the nature of the injury.

(IV) Special Examination

Abdominal Reflex Have the patient be in the supine position with lower limb flexed and abdominal muscles relaxed. Use a blunt object, and scratch the skin gently and quickly on both hypochondrium, the area at the same level with the umbilicus and lower abdomen from the outer margin to the middle of the patient's body. Abdominal contraction can be seen on a normal person. The reflex center of the upper abdominal wall is the 7th and 8th thoracic spinal cords, while the center of the middle abdomen is the 9th to 10th thoracic cords, and the 11th and 12th thoracic cords are responsible for the lower abdomen. Absence of reflex on one side of the abdominal wall indicates damage of the pyramidal tract damage, while the missing reflex on a horizontal level of abdominal wall reveals lesions of peripheral nerve or spinal cord at the corresponding level (Figure 4-7).

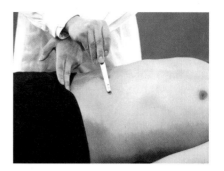

Figure 4-7 Abdominal Reflex

Section 3 Examination of the Back and Lower Back

I. Observation

1. Bony Landmarks and Physiological Curvature The patient needs to expose both iliac crests. Stand behind the patient. Have the patient stand in a upright position and look forward with their head and chest straight, upper limbs naturally hanging, and feet close together. Thoroughly observe the physical shape and physiological alignment and curvatures of the patient. First, check the bony landmarks of the lumbar and upper back area from the posterior aspect of the patient. Both shoulders should be even and symmetric, while the inner angles of the scapulae are at the same level with the third thoracic spinous process, and the inferior corners of both scapulas align with the seventh thoracic spinous process. All thoracolumbar spinous processes should be at the midpoint between the occipital tubercle to the first sacral spinous process. In addition, the line between the two iliac crests should align with the fourth lumbar spinous process. Then, observe physiological curvature of the back and lumbar areas of patient from the lateral aspect. Check if the physiological curvatures of the thoracic and lumbar vertebrae are normal. In general, the outward thoracic curve is relatively smaller, and the inward lumbar curve is greater among young adults compared to an elderly patient. Therefore, the examination must be performed carefully and the physian should pay attention to abnormal changes.

2. Abnormal Curves

(1) Kyphosis: There are two shapes of thoracic kyphosis, arc-shaped posterior convex, (i.e. round back deformity), and angular posterior convex (i.e. hunchback deformity). Due to the large individual differences, specific analysis should be done to determine whether it is pathological or not. Round back deformities occur when multiple vertebrae are affected, as in vertebral cartilage lesions among youth, rheumatoid spondylitis, and senile osteoporosis. Hunchback deformities commonly indicate lesions involving one, two or three vertebrae, such as vertebral compression fractures, dislocation, vertebral tuberculosis, and bone destruction due to tumor.

Clinically, increased lumbar lordosis are also commonly observed with significantly outward convex of the buttocks and upper body leaning backwards, mostly due to forward tilt of the pelvis, resulting from decreased lumbosacral angle, spondylolisthesis of the lower lumbar vertebrae, and bilateral congenital dislocation of the hip joint among children. With this posture, the deformity appears more obvious, resulting in saddleback dysmorphosis.

(2) Scoliosis: The spine of a normal person should form a straight line from the posterior view. If a sideways curvature appears, it is known as scoliosis. During the examination, pay attention to the primary scoliosis, whether it is in the thoracic or lumbar region, which side it bends to, if there is a chest deformity, or whether it forms a posterior convex. If the scoliosis is not obvious, ask the patient to bend forward with two upper limbs crossed and placed on the chest, with hands on the contralateral shoulders. This posture allows scoliosis to be fully revealed. Scoliosis can be result from a variety of causes, such as poor posture, varying leg length, shoulder deformities, lumbar disc herniation, polio sequelae, and chronic lesion of the thoracic cavity or thoracic wall. Scoliosis is therefore often the sign of another disease or sequelae, but not an independent disease. If the scoliosis oc-curs in lower lumbar, it is necessary to differentiate if it is primary or compensatory scoliosis. For instance, if there is thoracic scoliosis, the lower lumbar may have compensatory scoliosis. The primary lower lumbar scoliosis is more common in lumbar disc herniation.

According to whether there are anatomic changes on the spine, scoliosis is classified as being either functional or structural. There are no structural abnormalities in functional scoliosis, and most cases are reversible. There are several methods to identify functional scoliosis. While the patient is lying sideways, or is hanging with both hands on a horizontal bar, if the scoliosis disappears, then it is functional. Another diagnostic method is the spinal flexion test by asking the patient to bend forward to 80°. Functional scoliosis can disappear in this case, while structural scoliosis still exists.

The clinical significance of differentiating the two is that structural scoliosis is irreversible and cannot be corrected by changing posture or physical position, due to structural lesions of vertebrae, ligaments, intervertebral discs, nerves, or muscle tissue. Moveover, structural scoliosis is more severe, often accompanied by a thoracic wall deformity, having more fixed curvature, more prominent rotation of affected spine, and more pronounced deformity while the spine flexes.

3. Luster and Complexion of Skin　During the observation of the back and the lumbar areas, there is a need to pay attention to the complexion of the skin, hair, and swelling of the local soft tissue. Brown spots on the back with different shapes may suggest neurofibromatosis or fibrous dysplasia. Extra-long hair in the lumbosacral area with a deepened skin tone is often associated with congenital spina bifida of the sacrum. Soft tissue swelling along the midline of the lumbar area is mostly bulging out of dura matter, while swelling on one side of the lumbar triangle commonly indicates gravity abscess.

II. Motion Examination

Individual differences are significant in terms of the motion ranges of thoracic and lumbar vertebrae. Generally speaking, the range of motion decreases with aging. People with different occupations can have different motion ranges. For instance, the thoracic and lumbar vertebrae of gymnasts and acrobats have a wider range of motion compared to the normal population. Therefore, even if their motion is limited, they are still able to have a normal range of motion equivalent to that of an average person. Therefore, occupation and medical history are both factors to be considered. In different segments of the thoracic and lumbar spine, the mobility is different, mainly related to the directions of small joints. The small facets of the thoracic vertebrae, with coronal articular surfaces, have relatively longer protrusions. At the same time, they are restrained by the ribs; therefore, they have the least range of motion. Conversely, lumbar vertebrae have sagittal articular surfaces, so they have a greater range of motion. There are four types of thoracic and lumbar movements (Figure 4-8).

1. Forward Flexion   Ask the patient to stand in an upright position with their head flexed, then have them slowly bend forward. Observe the movement of each spinous process. Pay attention to whether the motion of the spine forms a gradual and even arc, or whether there is tension or spasm of the sacral spine muscle, compensatory anteversion of the pelvis, or obstacles during the flexion movement. A normal lumbar flexion is between 80° and 90°.

2. Extension   Hold the anterior side of the patient's pelvis with one hand, and the shoulders with another hand to prevent the pelvis from moving forward and lower limbs from bending. This way, the torso does not tilt backwards, which would partially compensating posterior extension of the spine. In assisting the patient to perform posterior extension of the spine by asking the patient to look upward, and slowly extend the spine backward. A normal person should reach a 30° angle. At the same time, carefully observe the changes of each spinal segment, and be cautious to the occurrence of pain and sites of dyskinesia in order to analyze the location of the lesion.

3. Lateral Bending   Have the patient stand in an upright position, and hold their pelvis steady with both hands to prevent the patient from leaning towards the left or right side. Then let the patient lean their head and chest together to the lateral sides. Observe whether there are any abnormal manifestations and note the degree of the disorder. In addition, compare the movement bilaterally. The range of lateral bending is normally 20° to 30°.

4. Rotation   Use both hands to stabilize both wings of ilium of the patient to maintain pelvic balance, instruct the patient to rotate their torso left and right, and observe the range of motion with bilateral comparison. The normal range is about 30°. Dyskinesia or pain are abnormal signs.

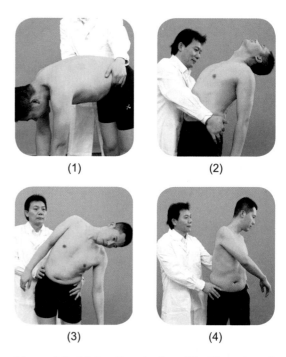

(1)   (2)

(3)   (4)

Figure 4-8   Motion Examination of the Thoracic and Lumbar Vertebrae
(1) Forward Flexion   (2) Backward Extension
(3) Lateral Bending   (4) Rotation

Limited motion due to lesions of the lumbar vertebrae may lead to a change in gait associated with an unnatural swinging of the upper extremities while walking. Observation of various abnormal gaits can help determine the presence of a lumbar lesion and its nature.

III. Palpation

Lower back palpation consists mainly of touch, tapping the lower back, and, through searching, analysis of tenderness to determine the lesion.

1. Palpation of Spinous Processes   Place the middle finger over the most prominent aspect of each spinous process, and the index and ring fingers on each side of the spinous process. Palpate with the fingers sliding from top to bottom and pay attention to unusual bulging or depression of each spinous process. Check to see whether the spaces between the spinous process are equal, and whether there is any thickening, swelling, and tenderness of spinous, supraspinous and interspinous ligaments. Examine whether all spinous processes are in a straight line, with or without scoliosis or deviation.

2. Searching for Tenderness   Search the spine from cervical to lumbar vertebrae by pressing each spinous process, interspinous ligament, lumbosacral joint, facet joint, transverse process, paraspinal muscle, and sacroiliac joint to discover the location and depth of tenderness points, and record them. Tenderness is often a hint of the lesion site. Superficial tenderness reveals that lesions are more towards the surface and may include damage of the supraspinous ligaments, interspinous ligaments, fascia, and muscles. A tenderness at a deeper level is often a sign of vertebral or appendage lesions or injuries. For example, patients suffering fracture of transverse process or laceration of transverse ligament experience deep and localized tenderness along the lateral edge of sacrospinalis. The third lumbar transverse process syndrome has obvious deep tenderness on the prominence of the process, and sometimes radiates along the superior gluteal nerve to the buttocks area. Patients with lumbar disc herniation between L4 and L5 can experience obvious deep tenderness in the interlaminar area, radiating to the affected side of the lower extremity and all the way down to the midline of the foot. Deep tenderness can also indicate vertebral tuberculosis or vertebral fractures.

3. Muscle Spasm   During the examination, have the patient lie in a prone position with the muscles of the whole body relaxed. Palpate to check for spasm of   paravertebral muscles. Muscle spasm often means injury of local soft tissue, bone fracture, or dislocation. Spasms might also be secondary in nature and occur as a protective spasm because of other lesions.

4. Percussion Examination   With the patient lying in the prone position, use a percussion hammer to tap on every spinous process gently from C7 to the sacral vertebra. Pay attention to deep percussion pain and its location.

IV. Special Examination

1. Straight Leg Raise Test (SLR) and Braggard's Test   SLR Test is also called Lasègue's Test. Ask the patient to lie supine and alternately raise each leg while holding the patient's foot using one hand, and keeping the patient's knee straight with the other hand. A normal range of motion for each leg would be 70° or better, depending upon level of flexibility, personal fitness and age. Except for a sense of tension in the popliteal fossa, no pain or other discomfort should be present. The test is positive if one or both legs have decreased angle of elevation accompanied by radiating pain, as is commonly seen in patients with lumbar disc herniation. If it causes radiating pain to the sciatic nerve on the affected leg while performing the test on the contralateral leg, it is also positive, as is found in a significant lumbar disc herniation, or central lumbar disc herniation.

When pain is elicited when the straight leg is raised to the maximum angle with dorsiflexion of the ankle, it is positive Braggard's test, which can be seen as the accentuated straight leg raise test. Braggard's test makes it possible to rule out limited range of motion as a function of tension in the iliotibial band, hamstring, or knee joint, since ankle dorsiflexion only aggravates the tension of the sciatic nerve and gastrocnemius with no effect on muscles above the calf (Figure 4-9).

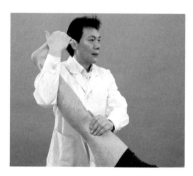

Figure 4-9   Straight Leg Raise Test and Accelerated Test

2. Neck Flexion Test (Lindner's Test)   Position the patient to supine with legs straight, causing tension to the sciatic nerve. Have their neck flex actively or passively. A positive result is when this causes pain on the affected lower limb, mainly seen in patients with lumbar disc herniation of the shoulder type (Figure 4-10).

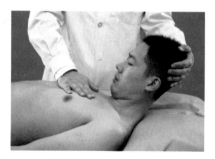

Figure 4-10   Neck Flexion Test

3. Femoral Nerve Stretch Test (FNST, Mackiewicz Sign)   Ask the patient to lie prone, while stabilizing the patient's pelvis using one hand and the lower end of affected lower limb using the other. With the knee straight or flexed, passively extend the thigh. The test is positive if the patient experiences anterior thigh pain, suggesting compression on the root of the femoral nerve (Figure 4-11).

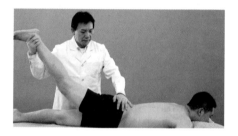

Figure 4-11   Femoral Nerve Stretch Test

Section 4   Examination of the Upper Extremities

I. Shoulder Examinations

Due to nerve conduction, some visceral diseases can manifest clinically as pain at a distal site on the body surface some distance from the affected organ. Pain under such circumstances is called "referred visceral pain". Therefore, when encountering patients suffering from pain on specific body areas, pay special attention to exclude the pain caused by visceral disease. Here are some typical examples: For left shoulder pain, rule out heart disease; and for right shoulder pain, lesions of the liver or gallbladder. In addition, some types of shoulder pain are caused by a type of cervical spondylosis known as cervicobrachial syndrome. Therefore, a thorough examination for shoulder pain is completely necessary and important.

(I) Observations

When observing the shoulders, both shoulders must be exposed at the same time, in order to compare during the examination.

1. Swelling   Pay attention to the following aspects if shoulder swelling is observed: Complexion of the skin, presence of fistula, lumps and engorgement of veins. Furthermore, compare the shape of the deltoid muscles on both sides to determine whether there is atrophy. Any kind of relatively severe shoulder injury, such as contusion, sprain, strain, rotator cuff rupture, and other tendon injuries, may cause varying degrees of shoulder swelling. The swelling is more serious in shoulder fracture or dislocation, such as surgical neck of the humerus fracture or tuberosity fracture. In acute suppurative shoulder arthritis, there will be swelling, heat sensation, and obvious tenderness of the shoulder. In dislocation of the acromioclavicular joint, the swelling appears on top of the shoulder (piano key sign). Swelling due to clavicle fracture appears on the anterior part of the shoulder, causing supraclavicular fossa to seem full.

2. Deformity Observe whether the shoulders are symmetric and level with each other. Check to see if the distance between medial border of the shoulder blades and the midline is equal. Where injuries include a clavicle fracture or shoulder dislocation, shoulders often incline to the affected side since the patient would need to ease the pain from muscle traction. In addition, shoulder muscle paralysis caused by brachial plexus injury or hemiplegia may also lead to vertical chord deformity. In shoulder joint dislocation, the acromion can be abnormally prominent and look more square. Shoulder muscle atrophy and axillary paralysis, causing subluxation of the shoulder, also cause the affected shoulder to appear more square. A congenital high scapula, also known as the Sprengel's deformity, causes a shoulder blade to be higher than normal; if both sides are higher, the neck would appear shortened. Serratus anterior paralysis or long thoracic nerve damage can cause weakening of the scapulothoracic joint and protrusion of the scapula, forming what is clinically called 'winged scapula'. Be careful, however, to distinguish between a winged scapula and a protrusion deformity of the scapula resulting from scoliosis.

3. Atrophy of the Shoulder Muscles Situation muscular atrophy   is more usually seen in the late stage of certain illnesses. For example, in shoulder fractures, long-term fixation will result in disuse atrophy. Nerve damage would cause muscle paralysis and loss of motor function, which can then lead to neuromuscular atrophy. Additionally, problems such as shoulder suppurative inflammation, tuberculosis, periarthritis of shoulder, and shoulder tumor also cause restricted shoulder mobility, further leading to muscle atrophy.

(II) Motion Examinations

The patient takes the standing position while standing on the lateral side of the patient (Figure 4-12).

1. Flexion The normal range of flexion is up to 90°. Use one hand to stabilize the ipsilateral shoulder, and ask them to lift the upper limb forward. The main muscles involved in flexion movement are the anterior fibers of the deltoid and coracobrachialis.

2. Extension The normal range of motion of extension is up to 45°. During the examination, instruct the patient to extend the upper limb backwards. Muscles involved in the extension movement are the latissimus dorsi, teres major, the great round muscle, and the posterior fibers of the deltoid muscle.

3. Abduction Movement The normal range of abduction is around 90°. Ask the patient to flex the elbow to 90°, and perform abduction movement. Main muscles involved in abduction are supraspinatus (0° to 15°) and deltoid (15° to 90°).

4. Adduction The normal adduction range is up to 45°. Ask the patient to flex the elbow being examined, position the upper arm in front of the chest, and move inward. The main muscle involved in adduction is the pectoralis major.

5. External Rotation The normal external rotation can reach 30°. Ask the patient to flex their elbow to 90°, then hold the elbow with one hand, and the other holding the patient's wrist to perform passive external rotation of the upper arm. The main muscles involved in this procedure are infraspinatus and teres minor.

6. Internal Rotation Normally, internal rotation can be as wide as 80°. The examination requires the patient to flex the elbow to 90°, and adduct forearm to reach the chest, or have the forearm touch the inferior angle of contralateral scapula angle. Major muscles involved in internal rotation are the subscapalaris and latissimus dorsi.

7. Arm Raise Arm raise is a shoulder-specific movement. To complete this movement, one can raise the upper arm in either the coronal plane or the sagittal plane. In the process of lifting up in the coronal plane, the humeral head must make an external rotation; and in the sagittal plane, an internal rotation occurs. Therefore, restricted external or internal rotation of the humeral head affects the completion of arm raise movement. Since this is a relatively sophisticated movement, ability to complete this action reveals normal shoulder function.

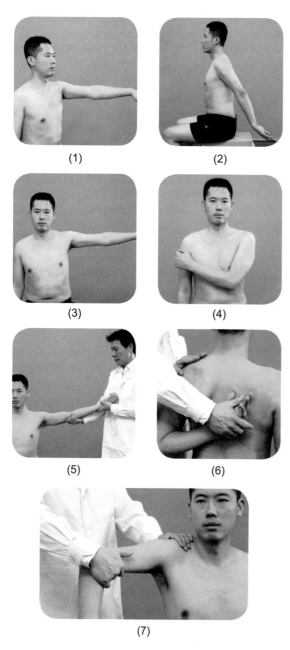

Figure 4-12 Motion Examinations of the Shoulder
(1) Forward Flexion (2) Backward Extenstion (3) Abduction (4) Adduction (5) External Rotation (6) Internal Rotation (7) Circumduction

8. Circumduction Circumduction causes the upper arm to trace a circle in the air with the glenohumeral joint as the center. This movement can be done in any one of the coronal, sagittal, and transverse planes.

(III) Palpation

1. Bony Landmarks The palpation examination of the shoulder should focus on the bony landmarks. First, the shoulder triangle is formed by the acromion, humeral tuberosity, and the three points of coracoid. The acromion is the highest bony prominence on the lateral side of the shoulder, with humeral tuberosity, another bony prominence immediately below. Second, the lateral end of the clavicle is located anterior to the acromion. Third, coracoid processes is at one-third the distance of, and one finger width, below the clavicle on its lateral edge, and above the medial side the humerus head.

2. Tenderness Point In clinical practice, bony landmarks are often common tender points. Take periarthritis of shoulder (frozen shoulder) as an example: the tenderness points are located in coracoid process, supraspinous fossa, and the intertubercular groove of the greater and lesser humerus tubercles, with dysfunction owing to extensive adhesion in later stages. For biceps tendinitis of the long-head tendon, the tenderness is more localized in the intertubercular groove, with tangible thickening of the long-head tendon. For biceps tendonitis short-head tendon, the tenderness is usually limited to the coracoid process. In deltoid bursitis, though, the tenderness is widespread, but mainly in the deltoid area. Tenderness areas for supraspinatus tendonitis or rupture of the supraspinatus tendon are on top of the greater humeral tuberosity, while in shoulder myofascitis, multiple tender points and nodules can be found around shoulder blades on the posterior side.

3. Examination of Patients with Trauma Palpation can be used for the diagnosis of fractures or dislocation. The subcutaneous fracture of clavicle, is easily felt; and when displacement of the fracture occurs, it is possible to detect bony crepitus and abnormal movement. Shoulder joint dislocation induces alteration of the shoulder triangle, and leads to distinctive depression and emptiness feeling, inferior to the acromion and palpable humeral head in the armpit or anterior of the shoulder. In dislocation of the acromioclavicular joint, the protruding lateral end of the clavicle is tangible. While pressing it, one can feel keyboard-like bouncing, and the patient has apparent tenderness.

(IV) Special Examinations

Dugas' Sign   With the patient's elbow flexed, place the patient's hand to their contralateral shoulder, and make their elbow touch their chest wall. If the patient is not able to position their palm on the contralateral shoulder, or when their hand is on the contralateral shoulder but the elbow cannot touch the chest wall simultaneously, it is a positive Dugas' sign, indicating shoulder dislocation (Figure 4-13).

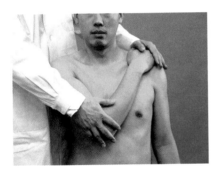

Figure 4-13   Dugas' Sign

II. Elbow Examinations

(I) Observation

Both condyles need to be exposed while examining the elbows, comparing both sides by observing whether there is swelling or deformation of the elbow outline on either side.

1. Elbow Swelling   Be very careful while examining the patient with evident elbow swelling to distinguish if it is intra-articular or extra-articular, and whether it affects the entire joint or is of limited location. The nature of the swelling must also be carefully analyzed, whether it involves a traumatic injury or is the result of another pathology such as purulent infection or tuberculosis. When intra-articular effusion is initially present, the normal physiological depressions on both olecranons disappear, and the joints appear to be plump. When a large amount of effusion is present, the swelling of the joint is most obvious while the joint is semi-flexed; since in this position, it holds the largest volume of fluid. For those who have intra-articular effusion, further examination is required to determine its nature.

If localized swelling appears in patients with trauma, it often indicates a limited injury. For example, if the medial aspect of the elbow swells, it may indicate a fracture of the medial condyle of humerus; likewise, if the lateral side swells, consider the possibility of a fracture on the humeral epicondyle or the radial head. If the swelling is mainly on the posterior side of the elbow, the fracture is probably at the olecranon process. In addition, local soft tissue contusion has more limited swelling.

2. Elbow Deformity

(1) Elbow Valgus: With the normal elbow fully extended, the upper arm and forearm form a physiological angle called the carrying angle, which is 5° to 10° in males and 10° to 15° in females. When the carrying angle is more than 15°, it is considered elbow valgus deformity, commonly seen in congenital dysplasia and poor alignment after lower humerus fracture. It may also be a gradual deformity during growth and development due to epiphyseal humerus injury. Patients with elbow valgus often suffer from ulnar neuritis or even neurological paralysis later in life because of frequent pulling or wearing of the ulnar nerve.

(2) Elbow Varus: A carrying angle of less than 5° is known as elbow varus. The most common clinical cause is growth and development disorders as an effect of poor diaplasis or epiphyseal damage after a supracondylar humeral fracture of the ulnar type.

(3) Flail Elbow: When the carrying angle is

greater than 10° with a fully extended elbow, it is called flail elbow, and is mostly due to poor dysplasia of the lower humerus fractures, causing the condyle stem angle to be too small.

(4) Boot-shaped Elbow: Clinically, this is seen in elbow dislocation or supracondylar fracture when the relative positions of the lower end of the humerus and upper end of the ulna change. Therefore, when the elbow is observed from its lateral aspect, the injured joint would be shaped like a boot, thereby giving its name: boot-shaped deformity. It is more common in children than in adults.

(5) Miner's Elbow: When a patient suffers olecranon bursitis, a ball-shaped cystic mass would form on the posterior side of the elbow. Since this condition was most commonly seen among miners, it is called miner's elbow.

(II) Motion Examinations (Figure 4-14)

1. Elbow Flexion Normally, the range of elbow flexion can reach 140°, and the main flexor muscle is the brachialis. When performing an examination, ask the patient to flex their elbow. If the patient's hand can reach the ipsilateral shoulder during flexion at the elbow, it is considered normal. The active movement is then followed by the passive movement as the second part of the examination. Common causes of elbow motion disorder are suppurative arthritis, rheumatic arthritis, synovial tuberculosis, fracture and dislocation near joints, and ossifying myositis.

2. Elbow Extension The normal angle is 0° to 5° when the elbow is extended with the main muscle as the triceps. First, instruct the patient to perform maximum flexion of elbow, and then to extend it to observe whether it can reach the normal range. Most common conditions affecting elbow extension include intercondylar fracture of the humerus, and olecranon fracture. Another cause is long-term fixation with the elbow flexed, resulting in fibrous tissue filling the olecranon fossa and further obstructing elbow extension. Furthermore, other factors restricting the elbow

from extending are scar tissue formation, skeletal obstruction, or tendon spasm and contraction of the anterior side of the elbow.

3. Forearm Rotation Forearm rotation is mainly achieved using the upper and lower distal radio-ulnar joint, and secondly with the brachioradialis joint. Therefore, when the forearm rotates, it is mainly achieved by the radius rotating around the ulna. The normal range of forearm rotation is between 80° to 90°, while the muscles for backwards rotation are the supinator and biceps. During the examination, the patient can be seated or standing with their elbow flexed to 90°, and perform passive supination. Then, compare both sides to determine whether dysfunction of forearm supination exists. At the same time, prevent the patient to substitute elbow adduction with forearm supination. Pronation movement is mainly completed by the pronator teres and pronator quadratus with a normal range of forearm pronation up to 90°. It is necessary to prevent the patient to substitute pronation with forearm abduction. The occurrence of rotational dysfunction is commonly seen in malunion after forearm fracture, distal radioulnar dislocation, and radial head fracture or dislocation.

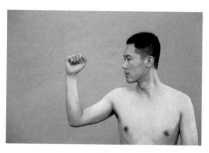

(1)

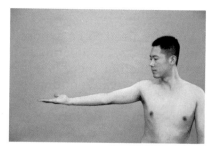

(2)

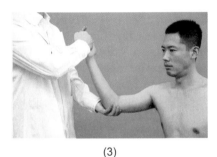

(3)

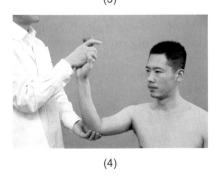

(4)

Figure 4-14   Motion Examination of the Elbow
(1) Elbow Flexion   (2) Elbow Extension   (3) Forearm Rotation (1)   (4) Forearm Rotation (2)

(III) Palpation

1. Palpation of the Posterior Triangle of the Elbow and the Clinical Significance   When the elbow is flexed to 90°, the lateral epicondyle, medial epicondyle, and olecranon process of the humerus form an isosceles triangle, which is referred to as the posterior triangle of the elbow. When the elbow is fully extended, the three points from a straight line. In clinical examinations, any position change of these three points can be used to determine elbow fracture or dislocation. In the case of supracondylar humerus fracture the isosceles triangle of the three points remains normal, whereas after an elbow dislocation, the triangle is altered. The shape of the triangle can therefore be used to distinguish between the two conditions. When an olecranon fracture occurs, the proximal triceps is pulled upward. Lastly, displacement owing to lateral or medial condyle fracture of humerus also causes the triangular relationship to alter.

2. Elbow Tenderness and Its Clinical Significance   The origin of the forearm extensor muscles is the humeral epicondyle, which is prone to traction injury or strain, further leading to the formation of humeral epicondylitis. In particular, the occurrence is frequent among tennis players; therefore, it is referred to as tennis elbow. Humeral epicondylitis with tenderness on the corresponding affected area is less common. Tenderness located in front of the radial head indicates a radial head subluxation in children, while tenderness on the anterior lateral side of the elbow among adults indicates radial head fracture. In addition, among patients suffering avulsion of the medial and lateral humerus, ulnar coracoid process and olecranon fracture, the tenderness is limited to the site of the fracture. If a cystic mass is palpated at posterior aspect of the elbow, it is most likely olecranon bursitis. When both sides of the olecranon have rigid, movable masses about the size of soybeans within the joints, it is most likely due to intra-articular free particles (or joint mice). During the later stages of an injury, if a relatively hard mass with an unclear border is felt on the anterior side of the elbow, it is usually ossifying myositis.

(IV) Special Examinations

1. Test of Forearm Extensors   Ask the patient to flex their elbow to 90°, with wrist and finger joints naturally bent, and perform forearm pronation. Then, place one hand on the dorsal side of the patient's fingers, apply pressure, and instruct the patient to extends the fingers and wrist. A positive sign is when pain occurs on the lateral epicondyle, suggesting lateral epicondyle of the humerus (Figure 4-15).

2. Biceps Tendon Reflex   Upon examination, the physician should support the patient's elbow with one hand, and place their thumb on the biceps tendon. Then, use the other hand to hold a reflex hammer and hit the thumb. The normal reaction is contraction of biceps, causing rapid flexion of the forearm (Figure 4-16).

3. Biceps Long Head Stability Test   This test is also known as the Yergason Sign Instruct the patient to flex their elbow, and perform passive external rotation of the forearm. If the patient experiences pain in the bicipital groove, the test is positive, indicating tendon tenosynovitis of the long head of the bicep. (Figure 4-17).

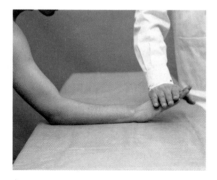

Figure 4-15   Extensors of the Forearm Test

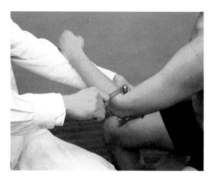

Figure 4-16   Biceps Tendon Reflex

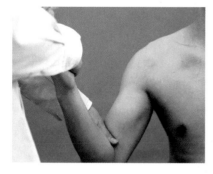

Figure 4-17   Biceps Long Head Stability Test

III. Examinations of the Wrist and Hand

(I) Observation

The natural resting posture of the hand is slight dorsiflexion of the wrist at about 15°,

thumb next to the index finger, other four fingers flexed, the flexion degrees of the second to fifth fingers gradually increased, and all fingertips pointing to the scaphoid. The status of the hand preparing for a handgrip should be wrist dorsiflexion at approximately 30° and inclination of 10° to the ulnar side. At the same time, the thumb is abducted, facing the palm, and flexed, with the remaining fingers flexed, as if the hand is ready to grab a cup. If the hand can quickly form a fist and fully extend all fingers, its function is normal.

1. Swelling of the Wrist and Hand   If the entire wrist appears swollen, the probable cause is an intra-articular injury or lesion, such as wrist fracture, dislocation, or ligament tear in the joint capsule. The occurrence of acute suppurative arthritis is less frequent, but there will be significant swelling of the entire wrist once it occurs. Swelling due to development of wrist tuberculosis develops slowly, showing joint deformity without redness or heat sensations. Conversely, swelling development due to rheumatoid arthritis is rapid, often symmetrical, and intermittent. In scaphoid fracture, swelling at the anatomical snuff box is obvious with disappearance of the normal physiological depression. Fusiform swelling of the second to fifth interphalangeal joints mostly indicates rheumatoid arthritis. Swelling along the tendon are usually signs of tenosynovitis or peri-tendinitis. Clubbed fingers mostly signify illnesses such as pulmonary heart disease, bronchiectasis, and cyanotic congenital heart disease. Lastly, most ganglion cysts are solitary and localized masses with clear boundaries.

2. Finger Tremor   Finger tremor is common in hyperthyroidism, Parkinson's disease, and chronic alcoholism. Patients with Parkinson's disease are characterized by a resting tremor that is reduced or even disappeared during exercise. If the tremor is mild, ask the patient to close their eyes and lift their hands to shoulder level. Then, place a piece of paper on the dorsal side of the hand, and note any shaking that occurs.

3. Infantile Finger Venule   The color of the superficial veins on the palmar side of the index finger among infants and young children under three years of age can be used as a reference to determine the severity of a disease. The proximal phalanx is called the wind pass, and the middle phalanx is named qi pass, while the distal phalanx is the life pass. The normal infantile finger venule should be light red that is indistinct within the wind pass. Bright red indicates an externally-contracted pathogen, purple reveals excessive heat, blue means infantile convulsions, and a paler color usually shows deficient cold. The disease is mild when the venule is visible only at the wind pass, and more severe as it reaches the qi pass, and critical while it goes through the life pass.

4. Wrist and Hand Deformity

(1) *Dinner Fork Deformity*: Also known as a bayonet deformity, it is found in displaced distal radial fracture of an outstretched hand. The distal fragment is dorsally displaced towards the radius, resulting in a fork-shaped deformity from the lateral view of the wrist.

(2) *Claw Hand*: The claw hand deformity is due to ischemic muscle contracture of the forearm characterized by hyperextension of the metacarpophalangeal joints, and flexion of the proximal interphalangeal joint. In ulnar nerve or brachial plexus injuries, the interphalangeal joints are semi-flexed, metacarpophalangeal joint hyperextended, the fourth and fifth digits are not able to move closer to the third, and muscle atrophy of hypothenar muscle occurs. A claw hand caused by burn damage has obvious scars and symphysodactylia deformity.

(3) Ape Hand (flat hands, shovel-shaped hands): An ape hand is caused by the concurrent damages of the median and ulnar nerve. The symptoms are atrophy of the thenar and hypothenar muscles, disappearance of both the transverse arches of the palm, making it flat, shaped as an ape hand.

- Thenar muscle atrophy if often due to muscle paralysis as the result of median nerve injury, or carpal tunnel syndrome caused by chronic compression of the median never.
- Hypothenar muscle atrophy is caused by ulnar nerve injury, cubital tunnel syndrome or ulnar nerve inflammation.

- Interosseous muscle atrophy is frequently the result of ulnar nerve paralysis, injury or compression. The atrophy of the metacarpal interosseous muscles does not have obvious symptoms since their anatomical location is deeper. Although, since the dorsal interosseous muscle is located on the back of the hand, the atrophy can be clearly observed, especially between the first and the second digits.

(4) *Dropped Wrist*: often caused by the radial nerve injury, which leads to forearm extensor paralysis, inability to extend the wrist, and the formation of a wrist-drop deformity. In addition, traumatic rupture of the forearm extensor tendon can result in wrist-drop.

(5) *Hammer Finger*: Also known as mallet finger, as the finger extensor tendon of the distal phalanx is ruptured, causing the distal interphalangeal joint unable to flex, and being shaped like a hammer.

(6) *Ulnar Head Displacement*: The ulnar head shifts to the dorsal side, which is commonly seen in distal radioulnar joint displacement and triangular cartilage damage. The displacement is more obvious when the forearm is in a pronation position.

(II) Motion diagnosis (Figure 4-18 and 4-19)

1. Wrist Extension Wrist extension is primarily done with the simultaneous coordination of the extensor carpi radialis longus, the extensor carpi radialis brevis, and the extensor carpi ulnaris working together. The normal range of this movement is up to 70°. Ask the patient to flex their elbow to 90° with the palm down, and the hand half-clenched to perform forearm pronation. Then hold the distal end of the forearm of the patient with one hand, instruct the patient to extend their wrist, and observe whether there is any restriction in motion.

2. Wrist Flexion The muscles involved in wrist flexion are mainly flexor carpi radialis and flexor carpi ulnaris with a normal range of 80° of flexion. Upon examination, instruct the patient to flex their elbow to 90° with the palm down, hand half-clenched, and forearm pronated. Then hold the distal end of the forearm of the patient with one hand, instruct the patient to perform wrist flexion, and observe whether there is dyskinesia or lack of strength.

3. Radial Deviation   Radial deviation, or radial flexion is achieved with the coordination of extensor carpi radialis and flexor carpi radialis with a normal range of up to 30°. The starting position is the same as in the previous tests. Ask the patient to move their wrist to the radial side, observe the range of motion, and determine whether or not the joint function is normal.

4. Ulnar Deviation   Ulnar deviation is a coordinated movement completed by the extensor carpi ulnaris and flexor carpi ulnaris with a normal range of motion of up to 45°. The starting position is the same as stated in the previous tests. Ask the patient to move their wrist to the ulnar side, and determine whether there is dyskinesia.

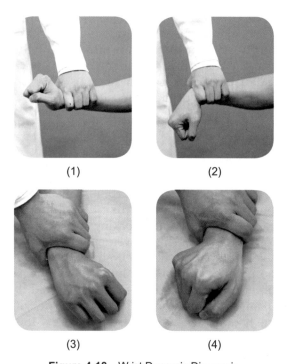

(1)   (2)

(3)   (4)

Figure 4-18   Wrist Dynamic Diagnosis
(1) Wrist Extension   (2) Wrist Flexion   (3) Radial Deviation   (4) Ulnar Deviation

5. Finger Extension   The primary finger extension muscles are extensor digitorum communis, extensor indicis proprius, and extensor digiti minimi. Upon examination, ask the patient to have their elbow flexed to 90°, forearm pronated, metacarpophalangeal joint extended, and proximal interphalangeal joint flexed. Then hold the patient's proximal phalanx, instruct the patient to extend their fingers, and observe whether there are any difficulties.

6. Finger Flexion   Flexion of each finger joint is completed by a single muscle respectively. Therefore, they must be checked separately. The flexion of the metacarpophalangeal joints is accomplished by fidicinales, normally up to 80°. The flexion of proximal interphalangeal joints is reached by the flexor digitorum superficialis at a normal range of up to 90°. The flexion of the distal interphalangeal joint is achieved by the perforans manus with a normal flexion range of 60°. During finger flexion examination, it is necessary to fix the proximal phalanx or metacarpal bone, and so, ask the patient to flex the interphalangeal or metacarpophalangeal joint, and observe the presence or absence of flexor dysfunction.

7. Finger Abduction   Finger abduction is mainly done by the dorsal interosseous muscles and the abductor digiti quinti. When the examination is being performed, instruct the patient to straighten their finger and move the other fingers away from the middle finger. Note that if the middle finger moves either way, it is considered abduction. Pay attention to the range, which normally can exceed 20°.

8. Finger Adduction   Finger adduction relies mainly on the palmar interosseous muscles. Upon examination, the fingers should start with abduction, then move closer together. If they are not able to move towards the middle finger and together, there is an adduction disability.

9. Dorsal Extension of the Thumb   Extension of the thumb is primarily completed by the extensor brevis pollicis and the extensor longus pollicis. Upon examination, tell the patient to perform dorsal extension with the thumb in an abduction state, and observe the movement of the metacarpophalangeal and interphalangeal joints of the thumb.

10. Flexion of the Thumb   Thumb flexion is mainly achieved by the flexor brevis pollicis and flexor longus pollicis. During examination, the patient's palm needs to face upward while holding the first metacarpal bone, and instruct the patient to flex their thumb. The normal range is up to 60°.

11. Abduction of the Thumb   Thumb abduction mainly relies on the abductor pollicis longus and abductor pollicis brevis. Radial (lateral) abduction and palmar abduction are the two types of thumb abduction. During radial abduction, the patient's palm needs to face upwards and with abduction parallel to the palmar plane. The normal lateral abduction is about 50°. While examining the palmar side of the abduction, the patient should extend their hand and move their thumb forward towards the palmar side, away from and perpendicular to the palmar plane. The range of movement is approximately 70°.

12. Adduction of the Thumb   Thumb adduction is achieve by use of the adductor pollicis. First ask the patient to abduct their thumb, then adduct the thumb back to the anatomical position. Or, make the thumb move from the anatomical position on the palmar plane. If the thumb can reach to the ulnar margin of the palm, it is considered normal, with the adduction angle at about 45°.

13. Thumb Opposition   The primary muscles for thumb opposition are opponens pollicis and opponens digiti quinti manus. During the examination, the thumb should start from the abduction position, and then move towards the other fingertips. Normally, the need to reach all other fingertips.

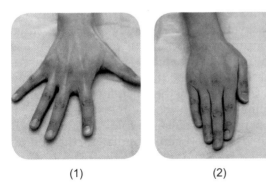

(1)   (2)

Figure 4-19   Finger Joint Dynamic Diagnosis
(1) Finger Abduction   (2) Finger Adduction

(III) Palpation

1. Masses of the Wrist and Hand   In semilunare dislocation, the bone can be palpated in the central part of the palmar side of the wrist. In patients with tendon sheath cysts, the examiner should feel palpable isolated cystic masses with clear borders and different sizes and shapes. Localized convexity can be palpated with ease during acute inflammation of stenosing tenosynovitis at the radial styloid process. Enchondrosis occurs mostly in the phalanx as an enlarged, hard, fusiform immobile   protruding bone body with a distinct border.

2. Wrist and Hand Tenderness   If there is tenderness on the radial styloid process, it is possible that there is tenosynovitis of the extensor pollicis longus or extensor pollicis brevis tendon. When the tenderness is at the snuff box, it indicates wrist injury, especially scaphoid fracture. While the tenderness is at the center of the wrist on the palmar side, it is probably due to a semilunare dislocation or fracture. Tenderness at the center of the wrist on the dorsal, though, is usually extensor digitorum tenosynovitis. If the tenderness is at the distal radioulnar interarticular joint and inferior to the capitulum ulna, it is wrist injury of the triangular fibrocartilage in most situations, or possibly a dislocation of the distal radio-ulnar joint. In carpal tunnel syndrome, the tenderness is usually at the middle of the lateral crease of the wrist on the palmar side, between the thenar eminence and the hypothenar eminence, often accompanied with radiating pain and numbness of the fingers. Lastly, in flexor tenosynovitis, tenderness can be found at the palmar side of the metacarpophalangeal joint (i.e., the head of the metacarpal).

(IV) Special Examinations

1. Ulnar Deviation Test   Hold the patient's thumb and deviate it to the ulnar side passively and quickly. If the patient feels obvious pain at the styloid process of the radius, the test is positive. Pain is mainly elicited in stenosing tenosynovitis of radial styloid process (i.e., de Quervain's tenosynovitis), or tenosynovitis of abductor pollicis longus or abductor pollicis brevis. The test is also called Finkelstein's Test.

2. Wrist Flexion Test   Ask the patient to sit upright with both elbows placed on the table, forearm perpendicular to the table, and the two wrists naturally flexed. In this position, the median nerve is pressed on the proximal end of the transverse carpal ligament. If pain occurs, it is positive, especially in patients with carpal tunnel syndrome (Figure 4-20).

3. Hoffmann's Sign   Hold the palm of the patient with one hand, and flick the patient's middle finger or tap on it with a percussion hammer. If this causes flexion of the patient's thumb and other fingers, the test is positive, found in pyramidal tract damage (Figure 4-21).

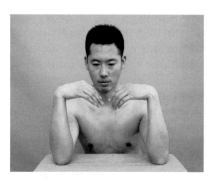

Figure 4-20   Wrist Flexion Test

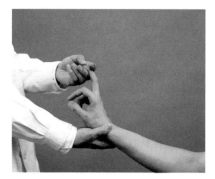

Figure 4-21   Hoffmann's sign

Section 5   Examination of the Lower Extremities

I. Hip Examinations

(I) Observation

1. Observation of the Front   To complete this examination, the patient should be in a standing position. First, observe from the front to check if both sides of the anterior superior iliac spine are level with each other, and if there is pelvic inclination. Also, determine whether both sides of the groin are symmetrical, and if there is any bulging, fullness, or vacuity. Bulging is mostly hip joint swelling, while the vacuity often indicates serious damage to the femoral head.

2. Lateral Observation   If the lumbar lordosis is greater than the physiologic range, so that buttocks kyphosis becomes more obvious and the hip is flexed, it indicates an old hip posterior dislocation or congenital dislocation of the hip and hip flexion rigidity among children.

3. Posterior Observation   Pelvic inclination can be caused by lumbar scoliosis, displacement from old pelvic fractures, hip pain, and unequal length of the lower extremities. Careful observation is required. In addition, pelvic ring fractures can also result in severe hematoma and ecchymosis. When observing from the back, pay attention to the iliac spines to see if they are level. If there is an upward shift or a backward prominence on one side, it is most likely sacroiliac joint dislocation. Also, pay attention to gluteal muscle atrophy. In chronic hip disease, muscle atrophy can occur due to insufficient use of muscles or dyskinesia, while neuromuscular atrophy can be the result of polio sequelae. Compare whether the gluteal creases are symmetrical, and check if there are increased, deepened, and elevated folds on one side. If so, it is likely congenital unilateral dislocation of the hip. Conversely, if both sides of the greater trochanter protrudes with widened perineum, it indicates congenital bilateral dislocation of the hip.

In unilateral hip varus deformity, there is often femoral contracture. Whereas in hip valgus deformity, the ipsilateral limb is in abduction status, which is unable to adduct, and appears to be slightly longer than the contralateral limb.

(II) Motion Examinations (Figure 4-22)

1. Forward Flexion   Forward flexion of the hip is mainly supported by the iliopsoas with a normal range of 140° and the anterior surface of the thigh should touch the abdominal wall. The ability to perform hip flexion can be determined by the angle of the flexion. Have the patient lie in a supine position, with the lower extremities in a neutral position. Place one hand under the lower lumbar area with another hand pinning the pelvis in place, and ask the patient to flex the affected hip. When the flexion reaches a certain angle, if dyskinesia occurs, then posterior inclination of the pelvis would be apparent, resulting in the physiological curvature of the lumbar to disappear. In this case, the physician can feel the waist drop and pelvis rotation.

2. Posterior Extension   Posterior extension is achieved mainly by the gluteus maximus with a normal range of 30°. Have the patient lie in prone with both legs straight. Perform active extension first, and observe the angle of it. Then hold the sacral area using one hand to fix the pelvis in place, support the lower thigh with the other hand, raise the thigh to extend the hip, and observe whether the pelvis leaves the treatment table.

3. Abduction   Abduction of the hip is mainly accomplished by the gluteus medius, and the normal range is up to 45°. Upon examination, ask the patient to take the supine position with their lower extremities extended and close together. Hold the ilium to fix the pelvis in place using one hand, and slowly move the affected leg outwards with the other hand holding at the ankle. When the leg reaches, or is close to, the maximum angle, the pelvis begins to move. Next, examine the contralateral limb as a control check.

4. Adduction   Adduction of the hip is accomplished by the coordination of adductors of the thigh, having a normal range of up to 30°. Ask   the patient to take a supine position with lower limbs in a neutral status. Hold the pelvis using one hand and the ankle of the ipsilateral limb with the other hand. Next, continue passive adduction by holding the affected limb and pass over the lower part of the contralateral limb anterolaterally, towards the midline of the body until the pelvis shifts at the maximum limit of adduction. Be aware that among obese patients, the adduction ability is hindered.

5. External Rotation   External rotation of the hip is achieved through external rotators mainly including: piriformis, gemellus superior, gemellus inferior, quadratus femoris, and obturator internus, with the normal range of external rotation up to 45° while the lower extremities are fully extended, and 80° while the knee is flexed to 90°. The examination for fully extended legs requires the patient to be in the supine position with legs close together and straight. Support the patient's foot with one hand, and instruct the patient to perform external rotation of the affected lower limb. Then ask the patient to do the same movement with the contralateral limb, so that a comparison can be made. When the examination is performed with the knee in a 90° flexed position, the same position is taken and the hip flexion should be 90° as well. Support the knee using one hand with the other hand holding the foot, adduct the the calf and feet passively, use the lower leg as a lever, and have the thigh rotate externally along the longitudinal axis (i.e. half of cross-legged action). Observe the adduction angle of the calf, which is also the external rotation angle of the hip.

6. Internal Rotation   Internal rotation of the hip rely on the function of gluteus medius and minimus, and vaginiglutaeus. Normally, internal rotation of the hip is between 35° to 45°. Upon examination, with the patient's legs extended, have the patient lie in the supine position, rotate the limb inward to observe the movement angle, and pay attention to any difficulties. During the examination with legs flexed, have the patient take the same position, push the foot outwards to make an inward rotation of the thigh. At the same time, observe the rotation angle to determine whether the hip suffers from internal rotation disorders.

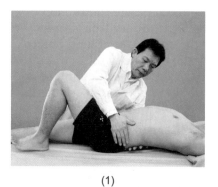

(1)

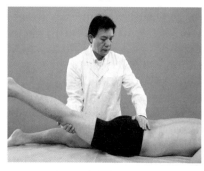

(2)

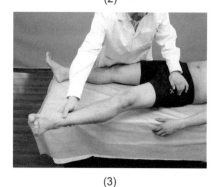

(3)

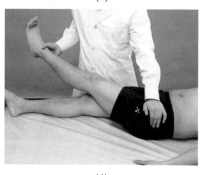

(4)

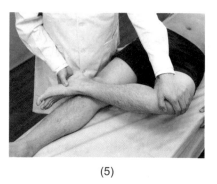

(5)

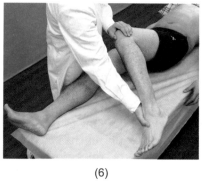

(6)

Figure 4-22 Motion Examination of the Hip
(1) Forward Flexion (2) Posterior Extension (3) Abduction (4) Adduction (5) External Rotation (6) Internal Rotation

(III) Palpation

1. The Bony Landmarks Hip examinations generally require the patient to be in the supine position. The first step is to palpate both anterior superior iliac spines and use them as the bony landmark for other areas of the body; this is especially important when working with obese patients, so this landmark should be clearly identified.

2. Tenderness and Its Clinical Significance Pay attention to swelling of the lymph nodes, localized bulging, puffiness, and tenderness while performing palpation of the groin. Puffiness and tenderness in the groin can indicate acute suppurative arthritis, hip tuberculosis, or a hip fracture. Tenderness in the pubic area among trauma patients is often the result of fractures. Where a fracture is not present, bone tumors and other bone diseases should be considered a possibility. Tenderness in the traumatic pubic symphysis with wider-than-normal gap indicats the separation of the pubic symphysis. Tenderness in the same area but with no trauma, on the other hand, is a sign of chondritis or tuberculosis of the pubic symphysis. During palpation of the lateral side of the hip, the major landmark is the greater trochanter; thus, pay attention to the top of the trochanter on both sides to observe whether there is a upward shift. Upward displacement of the greater trochanter is more common in femoral neck fracture, intertrochanteric fracture, and superior posterior hip dislocation.

Regarding greater trochanter bursitis, soft, movable, and cystic masses can be palpated around the trochanter. The sound of 'snapping' indicates the sliding back and forth of the iliotibial band across the greater trochanter when the hip is flexed and extended alternately. While palpating the posterior aspect of the hip joint, pay attention to the tensile force of gluteus maximus and tenderness in the buttock area. Since the exit of the sciatic nerve is at the lower edge of the piriformis, tenderness on the corresponding body surface often reflects lesions of the sciatic nerve. Tenderness on the lateral edge of the iliac crest, on the other hand, is mostly a sign indicating fasciitis of the buttock, or neuralgia of nervi clunium superiores. If widespread tenderness exists on the posterior aspect of the sacrum, suspect fascial damage at the base of the sacrospinalis. Tenderness at the sacroiliac joint is common in sacroiliitis, sacroiliac joint sprain, tuberculosis, loosening, or early rheumatoid arthritis. Palpable fiber cords in the gluteus maximus is a sign of fiber contracture or gluteal fasciitis, while tenderness at the ischial tuberosity is often a sign of ischial bursitis or ischial tuberculosis. Sacrococcygeal tenderness mostly reveals sacrococcygeal contusion, lower sacral fracture, coccyx fracture, or dislocation. In summary, all tender points need to be analyzed in combination with the patient's clinical history to make a clear diagnosis.

(IV) Special Examinations

1. Figure Four Test (Patrick's / Faber Test, Figure 4-23) Have the patient in the supine position, and place the affected ankle over and proximal to the patella of the healthy leg while one hand holds the contralateral anterior superior iliac spine in place. Then, use the other hand to push the ipsilateral knee downwards to touch the treatment table, so that the upper part of ilium moves towards the lateral side. At this point, if there is sacroiliac pain, the test is positive, revealing sacroiliac joint lesion. The immediate step is to rule out that the sacroiliac joint itself is diseased.

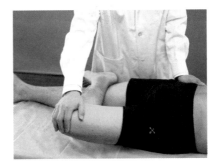

Figure 4-23   Figure Four Test

2. Thomas' sign Have the patient in the supine position on the treatment table with the affected lower limb extended and flex their unaffected leg to their chest. If the affected lower limb cannot stay on the surface of the table and compensatory lumbar lordosis appears, the test is positive, suggesting hip joint contracture. Thomas's sign (Figure 4-24) is also known as the hip flexion contracture test.

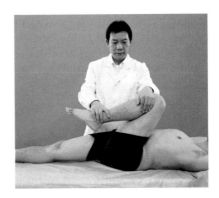

Figure 4-24   Thomas' Sign

3. Lower Limb Extension Test Have the patient lie in the prone position, with both lower extremities fully extended. Hold the back of the sacrum using one hand, support one side of the thigh, and perform passive extension of the hip to the patient. If sacroiliac joint pain occurs, the test is positive, indicating sacroiliac joint lesion. The lower limb extension test (Figure 4-25) is also known as the single hip extension test.

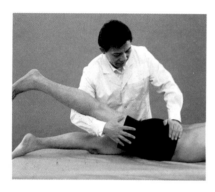

Figure 4-25 Lower Limb Extension Test

II. Knee Examinations

(I) Observations

1. Knee Swelling When there is mild swelling of the knee, both infra-patellar eyes of the knee disappear. In severe swelling, the suprapatellar capsule would be affected, and sometimes even the entire knee appears swollen. The most common cause of swelling is trauma, such as knee contusion, fracture of the patellar, the medial or lateral condyle tibia, or the intercondylar spine of tibia. If there is acute suppurative infection, the joint swelling will be accompanied by red skin, burning, and severe pain. In addition, diseases such as knee joint synovitis, rheumatoid arthritis, knee tuberculosis, and tumor can cause the knee to swell.

2. Localized Swelling Around the Knee Patella bursitis, tuberculosis, and tumor can lead to localized swelling, and epiphysitis of the tibial tuberosity to a significant high convex deformity. A circular mass at the posterior side of the knee is usually a popliteal cyst.

Cystic mass and osteochondroma can occur in the femur or tibia at the medial or lateral top, and a protuberance can be visible in the local area.

3. Quadriceps Atrophy Quadriceps atrophy is commonly a symptom of knee meniscus injury, lumbar disc herniation, or lower extremity fracture after long-term fixation. Examinations need to record the degree of muscle atrophy in combination with the analysis of medical history.

4. Knee Deformity A normal knee joint has a 5° to 10° physiological valgus angle. Over 15° is what is known as knee valgus deformity. Unilateral knee valgus is referred to as K-shaped legs; bilateral knee valgus referred to as X-shaped legs. Conversely, when the normal physiological valgus disappears, if there is a formation of bilateral calf varus deformity, it is referred to as O-shaped legs. Normal knee extension has a 0° angle, thought it can hyperextend up to 5°. However, if the extension exceeds 15°, then it would be known as genu recurvatum (back knee). The deformity is common in rickets, fracture malunion, epiphyseal dysplasia, or polio sequelae.

(II) Motion Examination (Figure 4-26)

1. Knee Extension When a normal knee joint is extended, the angle is 0°, while adolescents or some women may have a hyperextension angle of 5° to 10°. Knee extension is mainly achieved with the quadriceps. During examination, the patient should sit at the edge of the bed, have both legs hanging, and straighten their legs. Observe whether there is limited movement.

2. Knee Flexion The normal knee flexion can reach a maximum angle of 140°, and is mainly accomplished by the hamstrings. Upon examination, have the patient lie in the prone position with legs close together, and hold the lower thigh with one hand and the feet with the other hand, ask the patient to perform knee movements, and observe.

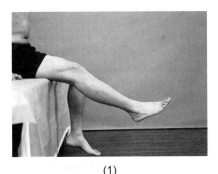

(1)

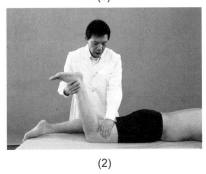

(2)

Figure 4-26 Motion Examination of the Knees
(1) Knee Extension   (2) Knee Flexion

(III) Palpation

Ask the patient to lie in the supine position, legs straight. When suprapatellar bursitis occurs, cystic masses with a sense of volatility and mild tenderness can be palpated above the patella. In transverse patellar fracture, a cleft and obvious groove-like depression can be felt at the front of the patella, and there exists a sensitive tenderness. For patients with chondromalacia patella, the patella will move while being pressed gently, and there may be an obvious pain response. For patients with inflammation of tibial tubercle epiphysis, a protruding hard mass with significant tenderness can be felt at the local area. For patients with infrapatellar fat pad hypertrophy, a swelling, flexible, and ductile masses can be felt on either side of the patellar ligament. Knee joint tenderness is a sign of probable meniscus injury. Palpable masses at the popliteal fossa are most likely cystic masses, and sometimes there can be tenderness. Tenderness points on the knee are common.

(IV) Special Examinations

1. Patellar Tap Test (Figure 4-27)   Have the patient straighten their lower extremities, press the suprapatellar bursa with one hand, and squeeze it downward to move the joint effusion flow into the articular cavity. The thumb and the middle finger of the other hand should hold lateral and medial aspects of the patella respectively. Simultaneously, press the patella with the index finger. If the index finger feels that it is floating, the test is positive, indicating effusion in the knee cavity.

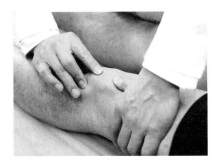

Figure 4-27 Patella Tap Test

2. Apley's Grind and Distraction Tests (Figure 4-28)   Ask the patient to lie in the prone position with the affected knee flexed to 90°. Use one hand to hold the distal side of the thigh, the other hand to hold the ankle of the affected leg, lift the leg away from the treatment table, which checks the integrity of medial and lateral collateral ligaments. Then, perform passive abduction and external rotation, or adduction and internal rotation. If there is pain on the lateral or medial side of the knee, then the test is positive, indicating that the collateral ligament of the lateral or medial side of the knee is injured.

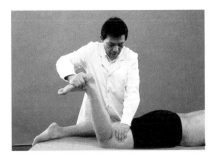

Figure 4-28 Apley's Grind and Distraction Tests

3. McMurray Circumduction Test   Ask the patient to lie in a supine position with the hip and knee flexed at 90°. Use one hand to hold the distal side of the thigh, the other hand to hold the ankle of the affected leg, lift the leg away from the treatment table. Hold the ankle with both hands, apply pressure and create friction at different angles to the knee, and at the same time performing abduction and external rotation, or adduction and internal rotation. If there is pain or snapping sound, then the test is considered positive, indicating medial or lateral meniscus injury.

4. Single Leg Half Squat Test (Figure 4-29)   Have the patient stand on the affected lower extremity and gradually bend the knee. If there is weakness of the leg, pain of the knee, or friction sound, the test is considered positive. It is mainly used to identify chondromalacia patellae (runner's knee).

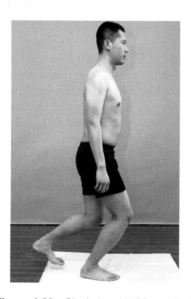

Figure 4-29   Single Leg Half Squat Test

5. Patellar Clonus (Figure 4-30)   Have the patient in the supine position, with lower extremities straight. Hold the patella with the thumb and index finger, then suddenly push the patella down, and keep the patella in this position. If it results in a continuous up and down vibration of the patella, the test is positive, suggesting pyramidal tract damage.

6. Patellar Grind Test (Figure 4-31)   Dur-ing the examination, with the knee extended, squeeze the patella against its corresponding femoral intercondylar articular, or, slide the petella up and down, left and right while it is squeezed against the femur. If there is friction, pain or discomfort, the test is positive, indicating the patella femoral syndrome. It is also known as the Clarke's test.

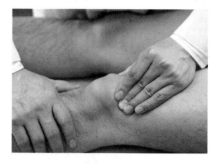

Figure 4-30   Patellar Clonus

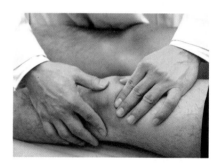

Figure 4-31   Patellar Grind Test

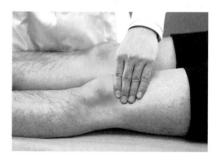

Figure 4-32   Zohlen's Sign

7. Zohlen's Sign (Figure 4-32)   Ask the patient to lie in the supine position with knees extended during examination, and use the thumb and pointer fingers to press the patella. Ask the patient to tense the quadriceps femoris, causing the patella to slide across the top of the femur. If it results in significant pain, the test is positive. A positive test indicates chondromalacia patella, or other patellar joint degeneration pathology. Be aware, that normal people may also have pain during the test. If the test is negative, patellar joint diseases such as chonromalacia can be ruled out.

III. Examination of the Ankles and Feet

(I) Observations

1. Swelling of the Ankle   Trauma is the most usual cause of ankle swelling, of which ankle ligament injury is the most common. If there exists fracture of the medial or lateral malleolus or of the lower tibia, the swelling is more pronounced. If there exists ankle tuberculosis or arthritis, the formation of swelling is slow. The disappearance of ankle depression, widening of the calcaneus, pain at the beginning and end of the Achilles tendon may indicate fracture of the calcaneus. The disappearance of normal recesses below the medial and lateral malleolus and both sides of the Achilles tendon in combination with fluctuations, may indicate intra-articular effusion or hematoma. Swelling limited to one side is more common in collateral ligament injury, while foot swelling is more common in tendon inflammation, bursitis, and hyperostosis.

2. Foot and Ankle Deformities

(1) Clubfoot: Also known as talipes equinus. When walking, the front part of the feet bear the most weight, the ankle joint is kept in plantar flexion with heels dangling.

(2) Talipes calcaneus: The deformity is observed when the foot is excessively dorsiflexed with valgus.

When walking, the heel of the affected foot bears the most weight, the ankle keeps dorsiflexed, and the front of the foot is away from the ground.

(3) Varus foot: The bottom of the foot has an inward angle, so that when walking, the dorsal lateral margin touches the ground.

(4) Valgus foot: The bottom of the foot has an outward angle, so that when walking, the medial side of the foot touches the ground.

(5) Flat foot: Flat footedness is also called pes planus or fallen arches. The arch of the foot collapses and become flat with valgus of the heels. The scaphoid becomes low and flat, and in serious cases may even make contact with the ground.

(6) High-arched foot: An abnormally high longitudinal arch is also known as cavus foot. In this condition the heel and the head of the metatarsal bones come to contact with the ground while the patient walks.

(II) Motion Examinations (Figure 4-33)

1. Dorsiflexion   The normal range of dorsiflexion of the ankle is up to 35°, which is accomplished mainly by the anterior tibialis and extensor longus digitorum. During the examination, have the patient take the sitting position with lower extremities straight and close together, and then have them perform dorsiflexion for both feet. Observe and compare to check any limitations of this movement. If necessary, perform passive dorsiflexion.

2. Plantar flexion   Plantar flexion is normally up to 45°, and depends mainly on the gastrocnemius. During the examination, Instruct the patient to perform plantar flexion. Observe, compare, and check if there is any limitations for the patient to complete this movement. If necessary, perform passive plantar flexion.

3. Varus of the subtalar joint (talocalcaneal joint)   Normally, varus of the foot depends on the movement of the subtalar joint and the posterior tibialis muscle, with the normal varus range of up to 45°. In an examination, have the patient to sit on the edge of the treatment table with both legs hanging, instruct the patient to perform a foot varus movement, observe whether there are obstacles preventing the patient from this movement, and perform passive examination.

4. Valgus of the subtalar joint   This movement depends mainly on the musculi peronaeus longus and musculi peronaeus brevis, with a normal range of up to 20°. During a checkup, have the patient to sit on the edge of the treatment table, ask the patient to perform foot valgus, and observe whether there is any limitation. If necessary, perform a passive valgus examination, and compare with the contralateral side.

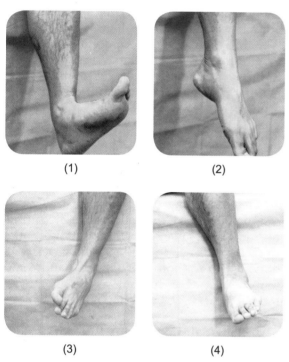

(1)　　　　　　　　(2)

(3)　　　　　　　　(4)

Figure 4-33　Motion Examination of the Foot and Ankle
(1) Dorsiflexion　(2) Plantar flexion　(3) Varus of the subtalar joint　(4) Valgus of the subtalar joint

(III) Palpation

Swelling of the entire ankle joint is mostly caused by serious intra-articular fractures, dislocation, tuberculosis, or tumor. When effusion exists, a floating sense can be felt, as well as tenderness around the joint. Limited swelling around the foot and ankle area is more common in ligament injuries and joint fractures. If there is extensor tenosynovitis of the big toe, there will be long strip-shaped swelling at the back of the foot and obvious tenderness. If there is metatarsal fracture, there may be swelling at the parapharyngeal axis, and fracture and tenderness can be felt. Tenderness can be felt at the proximal meta-

tarsophalangeal joint of the second toe when there is aseptic necrosis of the second metatarsal head. When the medial malleolus is fractured, tenderness points can manifest antero-inferiorly to, and at the tip of the medial malleolus. The existence of inward protrusion on the medial aspect of the scaphoid may indicate deformity of the accessory scaphoid bone or aseptic necrosis of the sclerotin at the end of the posterior tibial muscle; and both have tenderness. Tenderness at the calcaneus joint space may indicate arthritis. If there is a subcutaneous cystic mass and obvious tenderness on the medial head of the first metatarsal bone, it is often hallux valgus bursitis. If there is lateral malleolus fracture, there will be obvious local swelling and tenderness on the lateral malleolus. If there is lateral collateral ligament injury, swelling and tenderness will be on the anterior inferior aspect of the lateral malleolus. If there is fracture of the fifth metatarsal base, tenderness and swelling will be on the fifth proximal metatarsal joint. Heel tenderness with swelling is more common in situations such as fractures, tuberculosis, and osteomyelitis of the calcaneal bone. If there is pain at the tuberosity of the calcaneus with no swelling, then it is most likely Achilles tendonitis. If the pain is at the base of the calcaneus, and the patient cannot walk or carry weight, it is often fat pad hypertrophy, a bone spur, or bursitis of the calcaneus. If young people have pain at the back of their heel, most commonly it is calcaneal epiphysis inflammation.

(IV) Special Examinations

1. Ankle Clonus (Figure 4-34)　Ask the patient to lie in the supine position, hold the patient's foot with one hand and the popliteal fossa with the other, and flex the knee and hip. Next, push the foot with pressure causing dorsiflexion of the ankle, and relax. If the ankle has rhythmic plantar flexion and dorsiflexion, then the test is positive, suggesting pyramidal tract damage.

2. Babinski's Sign (Figure 4-35)　Use the edge of a reflex hammer to gently stroke the lateral metatarsal from the heel to the toe. Normally, there will be plantar reflex and plantar flexion of the five toes. If the action causes hallux dorsiflexion, with the rest of the toes separating into a fan-shape, the test is positive, suggesting pyramidal tract damage.

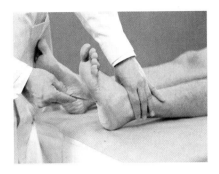

Figure 4-35   Babinski's Sign

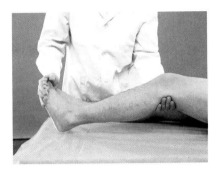

Figure 4-34   Ankle Clonus

Chapter **Five**

Preparation Prior to Applying the *Tuina* Therapy

I. The Preparation of the Setting

1. Set the room temperature to 72 ~ 79 ℉, which is optimal for *tuina* operations.
2. The setting for performing *tuina* therapy should be cozy, comfortable, clean, tidy, and quiet, so that patients can relax both mentally and physically.
3. Soothing music should be played according to the patient's personal interests. It is appropriate to add gentle and quiet music to calm the patient's mood.

II. Doctor's Preparation

1. Frequently trim nails to prevent scratching the patient.
2. Avoid wearing jewelry such as watches and rings to avoid scratching the patient.
3. Wash hands under warm water prior to treatment to ensure that the physician's hands are warm.
4. Avoid the use of strong fragrances such as perfumes and colognes
5. Before the first treatment, inform the patient in advance that *tuina* may cause some pain, and ask the patient to have an empty stomach, or have had a meal more than one hour before accepting *tuina* therapy. Have the patient sign the consent form.
6. The physician should turn off the phone before starting treatment.

III. Preparation of the Patient

1. Before treatment, the patients should be in good mood, relaxed, and free of any distractions.
2. Before treatment, the patient should turn off the phone.
3. The patient should be wearing comfortable, preferably easy-to-wear and light-weight clothes, so that it is easier for the therapist to work.
4. Patients should take a reasonable and appropriate posture to ensure both the patient's own comfort and the convenience of the physician to work.

Chapter **Six**

Contraindications of *Tuina* and Exception Handling

Section 1   Contraindications of *Tuina*

As a natural remedy, *tuina* has a good curative effect for many medical conditions of trauma, internal medicine, gynecology, and pediatrics. *Tuina* can sometimes causes side effects. Therefore, during the treatment, the doctor must understand clearly the contraindications of *tuina* treatment listed below:

1. Having skin damage, such as an open wound trauma or skin disease.

2. Patients with blood diseases and bleeding disorders of various diseases.

3. Infectious diseases in patients, such as hematosepsis or pyemia, and abscess caused by infection.

4. Patients with tumors.

5. The patient is pregnant or having their menstrual period.

6. Patients with muscular rupture, fracture, dislocation, spinal cord injury, etc.

Section 2   Handling Special Situations During *Tuina*

Tuina in general is a safe and effective physical medical procedure that has almost no side effects, but some abnormal conditions can occur if techniques are not used properly, the patient is in an uncomfortable position, or is too nervous. When an abnormal condition occurs, the *tuina* doctor must make the correct judgment immediately and deal with it promptly and effectively.

I. Ecchymosis

Ecchymosis refers to the subcutaneous hemorrhage, local skin bruising, and ecchymosis phenomenon of the treatment site of the patient during the treatment of *tuina* manipulation or after treatment.

(I) Causes

1. There is excessive stimulation during the treatment, or the treatment time is excessively long.

2. The patient has thrombocytopenia.

3. The patient is a senior with capillary fragility.

(II) Handling methods

1. For localized ecchymosis in a small area, generally there is no need to handle it specially. Bruising is usually absorbed naturally and disappear after about three days.

2. For a severe, localized bruise, first thing is to apply cold compress to it. After the bleeding stops, gently use techniques such as pressing, kneading and rubbing, and apply wet-heating pack to decrease swelling, relieve pain, and promote dissipation and absorption of blood stasis in that area.

(III) Prevention

1. Unless necessary, strong and overly stimulative *tuina* maneuvers should not be used in treatment.

2. For elderly patients, techniques used must be gentle, and the session should not be overly long.

3. For patients with acute soft tissue injury, techniques should only be applied after subcutaneous bleeding stops.

II. Fainting

Fainting (syncope) refers to sudden dizziness, chest tightness, nausea, palpitation, or shortness of breath, while a patient is in the process of receiving certain therapy. In severe cases, there will be coldness of the limbs, cold sweat, and even a short period of losing conscious.

(I) Causes

1. The patient is overly stressed.
2. The patient's physique is particularly weak.
3. The patient is hungry, overworked, having profuse sweat, or blood glucose being relatively low.
4. During treatment, physician has used too much force.
5. During treatment, the patient's position is improper.

(II) Handling methods

1. Terminate the treatment immediately.
2. Have the patient lie in an area with adequate air circulation, take the Trendelenburg position, allow patients to relax, and take deep breaths. For patients with mild symptoms, have them lie in a quiet setting for a moment, and drink warm or sugared water so they can revive. In severe cases, help the patient to revive using a combination of press-kneading *nèi guān* (PC 6, 内关) and *hé gǔ* (LI 4, 合谷), pinching *shuǐ gōu* (DU 26, 水沟) and *shí xuān* (EX-UE 11, 十宣), and grasping *jiān jǐng* (GB 21, 肩井).
3. When necessary, take other emergency measures as well.

(III) Prevention

1. Always pay attention to the patient's physical condition, mental status, and the tolerance to treatment techniques.
2. Choose a correct and comfortable position that supports long treatment sessions. Generally, the supine position is better.
3. Stimulation of *tuina* techniques should not be excessively strong, and the treatment time should not be excessively long.
4. Hungry and exhausted patients should eat something and rested prior to *tuina* treatment.
5. For first-time patients receiving *tuina* and those that are mentally stressed, the physician should explain the process to eliminate the patient's concerns.
6. Pay attention to maintaining adequate air circulation in the room.

III. Fracture

Fracture happens while the physician uses improper techniques, especially techniques of passive joint movement or that are strongly stimulating.

(I) Causes

1. When performing *tuina*, the maneuver is carried out improperly, such as using excessive pressure, stimulation, range of motion, or being harsh.
2. The position of the patient is not appropriate when receiving treatment.
3. Patient has osteoporosis, bone disease, or incomplete fracture healing.

(II) Handling methods

1. Terminate the treatment immediately.
2. Refer patient for an X-ray, CT, or MRI scan to confirm the diagnosis.
3. Consult with an orthopedist, perform the necessary targeted treatments, and have the fracture fixed and reduced immediately.

(III) Prevention

1. Before treatment, carefully examine and assess the patient's bone condition to rule out fractures and bone lesions. If in doubt, refer patient for X-ray first.
2. Techniques such as passive joint movement must be conducted within the normal range of physiological activities, and should not use violence or brute force.
3. For elderly patients, the maneuvers should not be forceful, and the session should not be too long.
4. The patient's position must be correct and comfortable, so that it is convenient for the physician to work.

IV. Pain

Pain may occur in areas receiving *tuina* treatment, and the pain may be aggravated while being pressed or durng the night, especially the first-time patients.

(I) Causes

1. The physician's maneuvers were not standardized.
2. The time spent on *tuina* operation was too long, or the maneuver was too extensive or too forceful.

(II) Handling methods

1. Generally, there is no special handling measures, since one to two days after the *tuina* session, pain wll normally fade on its own.
2. If the pain is intense, infrared therapy, gentle kneading or wet-heat patch can be used to ease the discomfort.

(III) Prevention

For the first-time patients receiving *tuina* treatment, the techniques used must be gentle, and session should not be excessively long.

V. Skin Injury

Skin damage may occur. Typical skin damage can include but not be limited to redness, pain, blisters, scratches, and/or bleeding.

(I) Causes

The maneuvers were not performed properly. For example, if the scrubbing method is carried out for excessively long time, it will cause excessive heat and skin burns. In applying one-finger pushing maneuver, if the finger is not firmly adhering to the surface of the skin with some force, it would cause abnormal frictional movement. When applying press-kneading method, excessive force or extended range of movement will lead to repetitive rolling of the skin.

(II) Handling methods

1. Immediately stop treatment at the damaged site.
2. Disinfect the skin of the operating area, and consult a dermatologist if necessary.

(III) Prevention

1. During treatment, the essentials and requirements of various techniques must be carefully and exactly mastered.
2. When using the scrubbing and press-kneading methods, apply lotion or massage oil to prevent damaging the skin. In addition, pay attention to controlling the heat produced by these maneuvers.

Part **Two**

Tuina for Adults

Chapter Seven

Tuina Maneuvers for Adults

Section 1 Maneuvers with Swinging Motions

I. Thumb Pushing

Thumb-pushing uses the tip or pulp of the thumb as the surfacing applying *tuina* force, and through the swinging back and forth of the wrist, it reaches the result of continuous force on the operation site or acupuncture point through the thumb.

Essentials of the Maneuver

1. Thumb-tip Pushing   Straighten up the thumb, the rest of the fingers in their natural flexion. The end of the thumb is used to apply the physical force to the operation site, with it interphalangeal crease of the thumb closely touching the radial margin of the index finger. At the same time, relax the shoulder, elbow and wrist, and use them as the fulcrum of the maneuver. Swing the forearm rhythmically, flex and extend the interphalangeal joint of the thumb passively through the turning of the wrist, while the force of the continuous pushing at the treatment site alternates between light and heavy. The swinging frequency of the forearm should be controlled at about 120 to 160 times per minute (Figure 7-1).

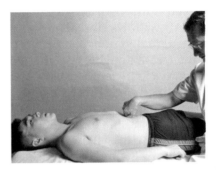

(2)

Figure 7-1   Thumb-tip Pushing

2. Pushing with the Radial Side of the Thumb   The thumb should be extended and relaxed and use the radial side of the thumb as the origin of force against the operating site. The rest of the fingers should be slightly bent and relaxed, with shoulder, elbow, and wrist relaxed serving as the fulcrum for the maneuver. Rhythmically swing the forearm and the wrist, causing the metacarpophalangeal and interphalangeal joints of the thumb passively flexing and extending, so that the radial side of the thumb performs continuous pushing at the treatment site, with the force alternating between light and heavy. The swinging frequency of the forearm and wrist should be controlled at about 120 to 160 times per minute (Figure 7-2).

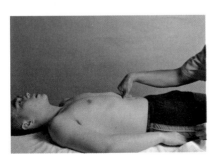

(1)

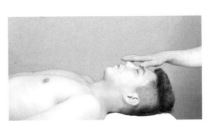

(1)

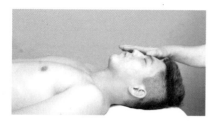

(2)

Figure 7-2 Pushing with the Radial Side of the Thumb

3. Flexed Thumb-pushing Keep the thumb bent, with its dorsal radial margin of the interdigital joint as the origin of force against the treatment site, and the other fingers bent into a half-clenched fist. Next, press the pulp of the thumb firmly against the radial aspect of the index finger on its first interphalangeal joint, have the shoulders, and wrist relaxed, use the elbow as the fulcrum, and rhythmically swing the forearm. By rolling back and forth, this maneuver passes the force from the wrist to the interphalangeal joint at dorsal radial aspect of the thumb, and applies it to the treatment site. The swinging frequency of the forearm is controlled at 120 to 160 times per minute (Figure 7-3).

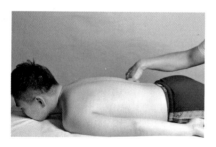

(1)

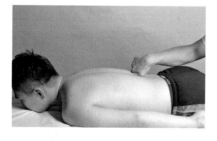

(2)

Figure 7-3 Flexed Thumb-pushing

Requirements and Precautions

1. Basic Requirements During the execution of the thumb techniques, it is necessary to have the body in upright position and keep the mind calm. The shoulders, elbows, and wrists must be relaxed, and keep the intention on the thumb, so that maneuver are strong yet gentle, uniting body and spirit.

2. Relax Shoulders Keep the shoulder relaxed in a slightly abducted position, scapula naturally sunken, and do not shrug to make the shoulder stiff.

3. Relax the Elbow Allow the elbow hang naturally, slightly lower than the wrist. Do not prop the elbow outwards, nor tighten it inwards.

4. Hanging Wrist Keep the wrists raised, and flexed as much as possible. During outward swinging of the wrist, the ulnar side must be below the radial side, and when swinging back to its maximum capacity, the ulnar side should level with the radial side.

5. Focus on the Thumb with the Palm Relaxed The thumb tip or pulp naturally press a treatment point with firm force, while the other four fingers and palm are relaxed.

6. Quick Transition and Slow Advancing After each thumb pushing move is completed, the next cycle should follow instantly, while the essentials of the maneuver and the swinging frequency remain the same. As a consequence, the hand movement trajectories interlock, and the movement of the maneuver should advance slowly.

7. There cannot be sliding or friction while applying thumb-pushing maneuver. When pushing along a meridian, there is a need to slowly advance on the basis of firm pressing.

8. The *tuina* physician needs to coordinate active and passive movements. During the operation, the forearm is the origin of the force transferring to the hand, while forearm swinging is an active action. At the same time, flexion-extension at the interphalangeal joint are passive, and they have the role of cushioning and distributing hand force. There should not be deliberate flexion and extension, as it could result in the formation of a sense of pause and shock.

9. The forearm swinging drives the thumb, and produces alternating light and forceful pressure on the body surface. The ratio of swinging out to swinging back pressures should be 3:1, that is, "pushing three, retreating one".

Applicable Areas: Meridians and acupoints across the whole body. The thumb-pushing maneuver that uses the tip or the pulp of the thumb is most appropriate to use along the meridians and acupoints. For facial area, the therapist usually uses the radial side of the thumb. Lastly, flexed thumb-pushing is mostly used in the neck area and intra-articular spaces.

Effects and Indications: Thumb pushing maneuvers can be used to relax the sinews, activate the collaterals, promote qi to invigorate blood, sedate and soothe the mind, dissolve spasm, fortify the spleen, harmonize the stomach, unblock the vessels, and relieve pain. Thumb pushing is mainly used for different internal and gynecological diseases, such as headache, insomnia, facial paralysis, myopia, neck pain and stiffness, coronary heart disease, back pain, stomach pain, diarrhea, constipation, irregular menstruation, and joint pain.

II. Rolling

The rolling maneuver employs the dorsal side of the fifth metacarpophalangeal joint at the treatment site. Rolling is achieved by performing flexion and extension movements of the wrist by push-rolling of the forearm, so that the dorsal-ulnar side of the hand and the hypothenar eminence continuously roll back and forth against the treatment site.

Essentials of the Maneuver:

The thumb should be naturally extended, while the metacarpophalangeal and interphalangeal joints of the little and ring finger flexed for 90°. Simultaneously, the index and middle fingers are in their natural flexion status as the metacarpophalangeal joint flexed, and interphalangeal joint slightly flexed. Simultaneously, tighten the dorsal side of the hand to make it arc-shaped, have the dorsal

side of the 5th metacarpophalangeal joint placed on the treatment site. Using the elbow as a fulcrum, actively perform push-rolling with the forearm, causing the wrist to perform relatively large scale flexion and extension actions, so that the ulnar side of the dorsum and the hypothenar eminence roll back and forth continuously on the treatment site, with a frequency of 120 to 160 times per minute (Figure 7-4).

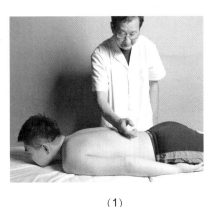

(1)

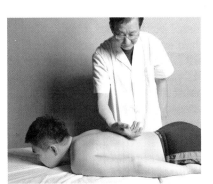

(2)

Figure 7-4 Rolling

It is important to note that there are different parts of the hand such as the metacarpophalangeal joints, the hypothenar eminence, and the top of fist that are in contact with the body surface during the treatment. Therefore, in accordance with the basic rolling maneuver, can be divided into metacarpophalangeal joint rolling, hypothenar eminence rolling, and fist rolling.

Metacarpophalangeal Joint Rolling: Keep

the thumb relaxed, having the rest of the fingers' metacarpophalangeal joints flexed to 90° and use the dorsal aspect of these joints as the origin of the force. The wrist should slightly bent toward the ulnar side. The rest maneuver essentials and the operating procedures are the same as those of the rolling maneuver (Figure 7-5).

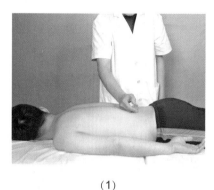

(1)

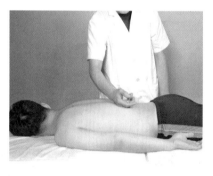

(2)

Figure 7-5 Metacarpophalangeal Joint Rolling

Hypothenar Rolling: Relax the thumb, have the remaining four fingers naturally flexed, apply force onto the treatment area through the hypothenar eminence using the elbow as a fulcrum. Perform an active push-rolling with the forearm, as the force is transferred through the wrist with a wide range of flexion and extension to reach the hypothenar eminence and part of the dorsum of the hand. Roll back and forth continuously on the treatment site at a frequency of 120 to 160 times per minute (Figure 7-6).

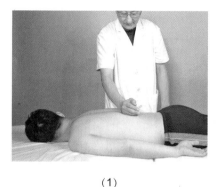

(1)

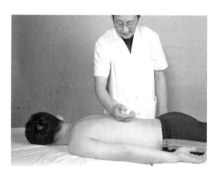

(2)

Figure 7-6 Hypothenar Rolling

Fist Rolling: In first rolling, the thumb is relaxed, the remaining fingers half-clenched into a hollow fist, and the dorsal side of the first phalangeal joints of the four fingers is used as the origin of force at the treatment site. Flex the elbow to about 140° to 160°. Actively apply force with the forearm, and simply perform pushing, pulling, and swinging without rotation, causing the wrist to perform ulnar and radial flexion and extension. Consequently, there will be continuously rolling on the treatment site performed by the first phalangeal, metacarpophalangeal, and interphalangeal joints of the dorsal side of the four fingers (Figure 7-7).

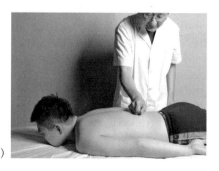

(1)

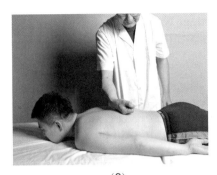

(2)

Figure 7-7 Fist Rolling

Requirements and Precautions:

1. Relax the shoulders and wrist, and keep elbow flexion at about 140° and then keep the middle of the upper arm about a fist-width from the chest.

2. During treatment, the metacarpophalangeal joints of the four fingers should always maintain a state of flexion, while the interphalangeal joint tends be straight during forward rolling, and naturally flexed during backward rolling.

3. During treatment, the wrist flexion and extension range should be about 120°. When forward rolling is at its maximum, the wrist flexion is around 80°. While backward rolling is at its maximum, the wrist extension is around 40°, causing nearly half of the ulnar side of the dorsal side of the hand to be in contact with the treatment site.

4. During treatment, be careful not to cause grinding, drag-scrubbing, and bumping. it is important to maintiain a firm rolling contact. The rolling method should produce alternating light and heavy stimulus, the forward rolling and backward rolling having a force ratio of three to one, respectively; that is, "rolling three, retreating one". When performing the rolling, the movement speed should moderate and constant, moving slowly forward on the treatment site from the beginning point to the end.

5. When used clinically, rolling often consolidates the passive movements of limbs and joints, and there is a need to pay attention to the coordination of two hands.

Applicable Areas: Neck, shoulder, waist, buttocks, limbs, and other muscular parts of the body.

Effects and Indications: The rolling method can relax meridians, unblock collaterals, invigorate blood, dissolve stasis, relax muscles and tendons, resolve spasm, relieving pain, soothe and relax joints, and release adhesions. The rolling method is mainly used for cervical spondylosis, frozen shoulder, lumbar disc herniation, various sports injuries, cerebrovascular accident sequelae, hypertension, diabetes, dysmenorrhea, and irregular menstruation.

III. Kneading

The kneading maneuver uses the palm, the fingers, limbs or other parts of the body as the origin of force, make firm contact with the surface of the treatment site, and perform gentle and mild movements such as up and down, left to right, or circular motions. The kneading maneuver can be performed in different ways such as palmar kneading, finger kneading, arm kneading, and elbow kneading based on the respective origin of the force.

Essentials of the Maneuver

1. Palmar Kneading   The palm kneading maneuver can be further divided into whole palm kneading, thenar kneading, and palm root kneading.

(1) Whole Palm Kneading: Use the palm surface as the origin of force. Actively press the forearm and move it in a circular motion, and drive the entire palm through the wrist to perform circular kneading on the treatment site, while keeping the shoulder, elbow, and wrist relaxed. The action causes the subcutaneous tissue at the treatment site to move along with it with a frequency of 120 to 160 times per minute (Figure 7-8).

(2) Thenar Kneading: Have the wrist slightly flexed or in its natural extension, the thumb adducted, and the other fingers naturally straight, the thenar eminence connected to the treatment site. Using the elbow as a fulcrum, perform an active motion with the forearm, which drives the wrist to swing or to perform a circular motion. As the result,

the thenar eminence performs the kneading maneuver in up and down, left to right, or circular motions gently on the treatment site, causing the subcutaneous tissue of the site to move along with the action at a frequency of 120 to 160 beats per minute (Figure 7-9).

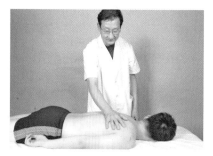

Figure 7-8 Whole Palm Kneading

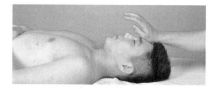

Figure 7-9 Thenar Kneading

(3) Palm Root Kneading: The root of the palm should be in contact with the treatment site, with elbow slightly flexed, wrist relaxed and its dorsal side slightly extended, the fingers naturally bent. Actively press the forearm and move in a circular motion, and drive the palm root to perform small-scaled gyratory kneading through the wrist, and at the same time causing the subcutaneous tissue of the treatment site to move along with motion of the palm root, at a frequency of 120 to 160 times per minute (Figure 7-10).

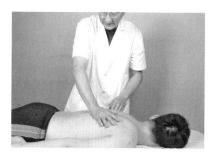

Figure 7-10 Palm Root Kneading

2. Finger Kneading

(1) Thumb Kneading: The pulp of the thumb is used as the origin of force against the treatment site, with the rest of the fingers lightly placed in the appropriate position so that they provide support. The wrist should be slightly flexed or extended, the forearm should be the main source of force, which causes the wrist along with the thumb to move in a circular motion on the treatment site, as well as driving the subcutaneous tissue of the site to move together with the movements at a frequency of 120 to 160 times per minute. (Figure 7-11).

(2) Middle Finger Kneading: Extend the middle finger, and place the index finger on the dorsal side of the tip of the middle finger. Slightly bend the wrist, and use the pulp of the middle finger as the origin of force against the treatment site or acupoint. Actively move the forearm, have the force pass through the wrist, and cause the pulp of the middle finger to make small-range circular, up and down, or side to side movement at a frequency of 120 to 160 times per minute (Figure 7-12).

(3) Three-finger Kneading: Use the index, middle and ring fingers closed together and use the pulps of them to apply force on the operation site. During treatment, the movement is essentially the same as the middle finger kneading (Figure 7-13).

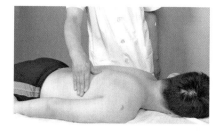

Figure 7-11 Thumb Kneading

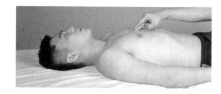

Figure 7-12 Middle Finger Kneading

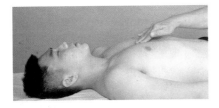

Figure 7-13 Three-finger Kneading

3. Forearm Kneading Lean forward, and use the back one-third of the dorsal or ulnar side of the forearm as the origin of force against the treatment site. Have the elbow in flexion and the shoulder flexed and abducted. Actively press and move the upper arm in circular motion, causing the forearm to knead in the same manner, with the frequency at 80 to 120 times per minute (Figure 7-14).

4. Elbow Kneading Lean forward, using the olecranon as the origin of force against the treatment site. The elbow should have an extreme flexion, and the shoulder should be flexed and abducted. Actively press and move the upper arm in a circular motion, bringing the forearm to knead along with it, with a frequency of 80 to 120 times per minute (Figure 7-15).

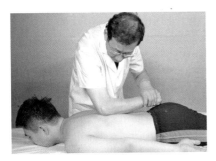

Figure 7-14 Forearm Kneading

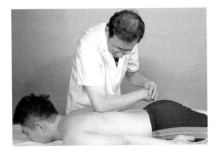

Figure 7-15 Elbow Kneading

Requirements and Precautions

1. The pressure exerted should be moderate and with the consideration of the patient tolerance.

2. The movement of the physician need to be flexible yet rhythmic.

3. Kneading can be fixed at one point, or knead and migrate at the same time, and kneading in a back and forth manner should proceed while maintaining a firm attachment to the treatment surface. Sometimes friction movement can be used, forming circular friction movement, making the technique more fluent.

4. In thenar kneading, the forearm has a push-gyrating action, as the wrist is relaxed. Conversely, the wrist needs to be kept tense to a certain degree in finger kneading. In palm root kneading, the wrist should have slight backward extension and appropriately moderate tension.

5. In the kneading maneuver, the part of the limb applying the force should be firmly attached to the treatment site. The attachment to the treatment site causes the subcutaneous tissue to move simultaneously with the action, and prevents the occurrence of friction on the body surface.

Applicable Areas: Palmar kneading is applicable to the abdomen, while thenar kneading is mainly applied to the head, chest, abdomen, and limbs. The palm root kneading maneuver is suitable for the back and limbs, while the middle finger and thumb kneading methods are appropriate for acupoints on all parts of the body, and commonly used in pediatric *tuina*. Furthermore, three finger kneading is usually used on a child's neck. The forearm and elbow kneading are normally used in the back, waist, and buttocks. Moreover, elbow kneading is relatively forceful, making it suitable for muscular areas and robust patients.

Effects and Indications: The kneading method can soothe and unblock the meridians and collaterals, move qi, invigorate blood, strengthen the spleen, harmonize the stomach, dissolve swelling, and relieve pain. Kneading is mainly applicable for abdominal pain, chest tightness, rib pain, constipation, diarrhea, headache, dizziness, pediatric disorders, soft tissue injury, and cervical spondylosis. In addition, it can also be used for head, face, and abdominal health maintenance.

Section 2   Frictional Maneuvers

I. Rubbing

Utilizing the fingers or palm to perform circular or linear back and forth friction movements is known as the rubbing maneuver. There are two types of rubbing maneuvers, finger rubbing and palmar rubbing.

Essentials of the Maneuver

1. Finger Rubbing   Extend the thumb with the rest of the fingers close together and naturally extended. Slightly bend the wrist, use the pads of the four fingers as the origin of the force against the treatment site. Actively move the forearm, causing the pulps of the four fingers to move along with the wrist and perform circular or linear rubbing back and forth (Figure 7-16).

2. Palmar Rubbing   Naturally extend the palm, relax and slightly extend the wrist. Place the palm flat against the treatment site. Actively move the forearm, causing the palm to rub along with the wrist in a circular or linear back and forth motion (Figure 7-17).

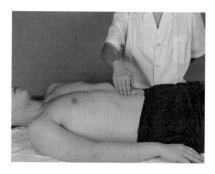

Figure 7-16   Finger Rubbing

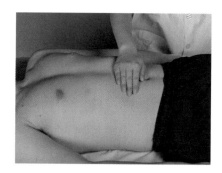

Figure 7-17   Palmar Rubbing

Requirements and Precautions

1. Relax the shoulder and the upper arm with the wrist flexed at an angle of about 120° to 140°. During rubbing, the hand and arm should maintain a stable and light pressure.

2. When using the finger rubbing method in a linear and back and forth fashion, the wrist needs to maintain a fixed tension; when using the method in a circular manner the wrist almost never moves. When using the palmar rubbing method in a linear and back and forth fashion, the wrist needs to be relaxed; when in a circular manner, the wrist needs to perform passive swinging in the direction of rubbing.

3. The speed of rubbing and applied pressure should be uniform. Normally, finger rubbing should be quick, at a frequency of 120 times per minute; and the palmar rubbing method should be slightly slower, at a frequency of 100 times per minute.

4. The direction of rubbing needs to be in accordance with the state of the illness. Clinically, the circular type is used more often, while the linear back and forth type is used relatively less often.

Applicable Areas: All body areas, especially the chest and abdomen.

Effect and Indications: Rubbing has many effects such as harmonizing the stomach, rectifying qi, promoting digestion, guiding out food stagnation, diffusing the lung, relieving cough, warming the uterus, regulating menstruation, astringing essence, and preventing enuresis, warming the kidney, strengthening yang, moving qi, invigorating blood, scattering stasis and reducing swelling. Rubbing is used for abdominal fullness and distention, indigestion, diarrhea, constipation, coughing, shortness of breath, distended pain on the chest sides, irregular menstruation, menstrual pain, impotence, spermatorrhea, and traumatic pain and swelling.

Appendix: *Gāo Mó* (Ointment Rubbing, 膏摩)

During *tuina*, in order to decrease skin damage due to friction, or to draw on the aid of certain medicinals, *tuina* physicians often apply medicinal liquid, ointment, or powder onto the treatment site, then proceed to perform *tuina* techniques. The type of *tuina*, in which the techniques and medicinals complement each other, is called *gāo mó* (ointment rubbing). The liquids or ointments applied at the treatment site are collectively referred to as the *tuina* media.

Types of *Tuina* Medias: *Tuina* medias can be not only lubricating materials, but also liniments, ointments, or powders that have medicinal properties in their own right. Commonly used lubricating media include talc, talcum powder, moisturizing oil, et cetera. At present, the properties of lubricants and medicinals are generally combined, creating forms such as powder, pills, vinum, tincture, ointment, decoction and other different forms. Each form has its own distinct characteristics. Clinically, the commonly used *tuina* medium can be either a single ingredient or multi-ingredient compound.

1. Commonly Used Single Ingredient Media Talcum powder, onion juice, ginger juice, spirit, sesame oil, peppermint tincture, egg white, common aucklandia root water, et cetera.

2. Commonly-used Compound Media Wintergreen oil, safflower oil, Chen Yuan poultice, Major Supplementing Rubbing Cream, Waist Rubbing Cream, Aconite Molasses Rubbing Cream, et cetera.

Media Selection:

1. Selection Based on Pattern Differentiation Ointment rubbing is a modality that pertains to the scope of external treatment, but works in the same way as internal treatment, because it is based on Chinese medicine pattern differentiation theory. When choosing media, it is necessary to choose specific media for specific patterns, generally using the general principle of differentiating heat and cold, and deficiency and excess. For cold patterns, use media with properties such as warming and scattering cold, such as onion juice, ginger juice or wintergreen cream. For heat pattern, media with properties such as cooling and scattering heat is appropriate, such as cool water or medical alcohol. In cases of deficient pattern, nourishing media such as medicinal liquor can be applied, while in excess patterns, media with heat clearing property, such as egg whites, and safflower oil, or *Chuan Dao* (conductive) oil.

2. Selection Based on Disease Differentiation Different media should be chosen according to the different conditions and specific location of illnesses. For soft tissue damage, such as joint sprains or tendonsynovitis, choose a medium such as safflower oil, or wintergreen cream, which have properties of invigorating blood, dissolving stasis, reducing inflammation, relieving pain, and venting heat. For pediatric muscular torticollis, use a medium with strong lubricating effect, such as talcum powder. For children with fever, apply a medium with strong heat clearing properties, such as cold water, ethyl alcohol, or mint water.

3. Selection Based on Age For young to mid-aged patients, water, oil, or powder can be used . For the elderly, use oil or alcohol. For children, because they have delicate skin, the medium should not have strong stimulating properties, and therefore talc, talcum powder, ethyl alcohol, mint water, onion ginger juice, or egg whites, are suitable.

Requirements and Precautions

When performing *tuina* with medium, no matter if it is single or multiple compound, or its form, they need to follow three basic principles: One, they need to ease the application of techniques; two, they cannot damage the skin; and three, they need to ensure efficacy. The specifics are stated as the following.

1. Patients should choose the appropriate body position, first of all, to ease the application of techniques, and secondly, to help patients feel comfortable. The treatment site should be fully exposed. If there is skin damage, or severe skin disease, do not apply *tuina* medium.

2. Apply appropriate amounts of *tuina* medium evenly across the treatment site. Too much medium makes the site overly wet, so the maneuvers can not be applied firmly. On the other hand, if the amount is too little, then the technique will be too sluggish owing to dryness of the skin, and it would easily damage the skin.

3. Clinically, *tuina* maneuvers using medium are usually rubbing, scrubbing, pushing, kneading, and smearing. No matter what type of techniques are used, they should follow the principles of being light and gentle, stable and firm, and not using brute force.

4. After *tuina* treatment, be sure the local area is kept warm, prevent pathogenic factors entering through weak points, causing the illness to aggravate.

II. Scrubbing

In applying the scrubbing maneuvers, apply the fingers or the palm to a certain part of the body surface, and perform quick linear back-and-forth movements to generate heat through friction. The maneuver can be divided into finger scrubbing and palmar scrubbing, while palmar scrubbing is further divided into whole palm scrubbing, thenar eminence scrubbing, and hypothenar eminence scrubbing.

Essentials of the Maneuver

Apply frictional force at the treatment site using the palm, the thenar eminence, the hypothenar eminence, or the four finger pads except the thumb. Extend the wrist and have the forearm and palm at the same level. Use the elbow or shoulder joint as the fulcrum and perform active movement using the forearm or upper arm, causing the origin of force of the hand to make linear back-and-forth rub-scrubbing evenly, in up and down

or side to side directions, until the treatment area appears light red and warm. If the four finger pads are used as the origin of force, the technique is called the finger scrubbing maneuver (Figure 7-18). Similarly, if the palm, the thenar eminence or the hypothenar eminence is used as the origins of force, it is respectively known as the palmar scrubbing (Figure 7-19), thenar eminence scrubbing (Figure 7-20), and the hypothenar eminence scrubbing (Figure 7-21) maneuver.

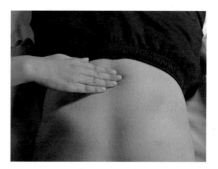

Figure 7-18 Finger Scrubbing

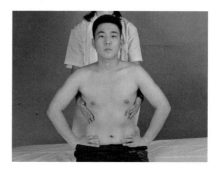

Figure 7-19 Palmar Scrubbing

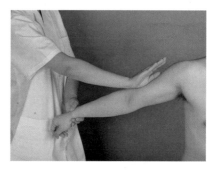

Figure 7-20 Thenar Eminence Scrubbing

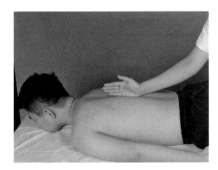

Figure 7-21 Hypothenar Eminence Scrubbing

Requirements and Precautions

1. The origin of the force should firmly applied to the body surface, the pressure applied should be moderate, and the path of the scrubbing maneuver should remain a straight line. At the same time, the length of the scrubbing line should be as long as possible in general, while the movement should be continuous like dragging a saw. The physician should not hold the breath during operation, but rather breathe naturally. The movement of scrubbing should be continuous, uniform, stable, and rhythmic, at the frequency of 120 to 160 times per minute.

2. In finger scrubbing, use the elbow as the fulcrum, and forearm as the power source, while the distance of the move should be short, making it a special case among scrubbing maneuvers. Conversely, scrubbing using the palm, thenar eminence or hypothenar eminence use the shoulder as the fulcrum and the upper arm as the power source, while the moving distance of the maneuver should be long.

3. When the area being treated using the scrubbing maneuver is thoroughly warm, it indicates that it is the time to cease treatment at that site .

4. The scrubbing pressure applied should be moderate, because excess pressure will be heavy and sluggish movements that can easily damage the skin. If the pressure is too mild, however, it is not easy to generate the frictional heat necessary for an effective treatment.

5. In addition to mastering the essentials of the scrubbing maneuver to avoid abrasions and grazes, the physician can also apply lubricants, such as wintergreen cream, and safflower oil to prevent the skin from being damaged. Moreover, with the aid of these media, the heat generated from the scrubbing can penetrate deeper and more thorough, so that the treatment effect can be enhanced.

6. When the scrubbing technique is completed, and the resulting blush of the skin is evident, do not continue, so as to avoid breaking the skin.

7. Perform the technique in direct with the skin at the treatment site.

Applicable Areas: Scrubbing is applicable in all areas of the body. Since the contact surface of finger scrubbing is small, it is suitable for areas such as the neck and intercostal spaces. In contrast, the contact surface of palmar scrubbing is bigger, and therefore appropriate for shoulders, back, chest, abdomen, and hypochondria. The thenar eminence scrubbing method is great for the extremities, especially in the upper limbs, while the hypothenar eminence scrubbing maneuver is suitable for shoulder, both sides of the spine and the lumbosacral region.

Effects and Indications: The effects of scrubbing include loosening the chest, rectifying qi, relieving cough, calming asthma, fortifying the spleen, harmonizing the stomach, warming the kidney, promoting kidney yang, moving qi, invigorating blood, dissolving swelling, and relieving pain. The maneuver is mainly used for cough, asthma, chest tightness, chronic bronchitis, emphysema, chronic gastritis, indigestion, female infertility, impotence, tendon injury of the limbs, soft tissue swelling and pain, and rheumatic *bi* pattern.

III. Pushing

Applying the fingers, palm, fist or elbow to a certain part of the body surface, and pushing forward in a one-way linear manner or following a curved route, is known as the pushing. In adults, pushing is mainly performed along imaginary straight line, and is known as flat pushing.

Essentials of the Maneuver

1. Finger Pushing Including thumb tip pushing, flat thumb pushing, and three-finger pushing.

(1) *Thumb tip pushing*: Keep the thumb in extension and apply force using the tip of the thumb on the treatment area or certain acupoints, while the other fingers are together and firmly placed on the treatment site or opposite to the treatment side. The wrist should be in flexion position and slightly facing the ulnar side. The thumb and wrist provide the active source of the power and push towards the tip of the thumb with a short one-way linear route (Figure 7-22) .

(2) *Flat thumb pushing*: Keep the thumb in extension, and use the pad of the thumb as the contact surface for the force at the treatment site or an acupoint. The other fingers should be closed together and placed anteriorly and exteriorly to the thumb as supplementing source of the force. Have the wrist slightly flexed, use the forearm and wrist as the active force, so that the thumb can move towards the direction of the index finger, and perform pushing straight forward, one-way and in a short distance. During the movement the pad of the thumb, should gradually turn to the radial aspect as it moves, while the wrist should gradually straighten (Figure 7-23).

(3) *Three-finger pushing*: Extend and straighten the index, middle and ring fingers, keeping them close together, and use the finger pads as the contact surface for the force at the treatment site. The forearm actively initiates the power, and transfers the force through the wrist and palm to reach the pads of the three fingers. Perform one-way and straight forward pushing to the direction of the fingertips (Figure 7-24) .

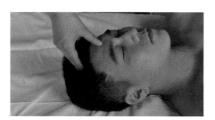

Figure 7-22 Thumb Tip Pushing

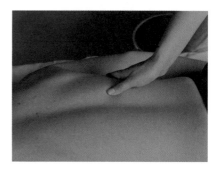

Figure 7-23 Flat Thumb Pushing

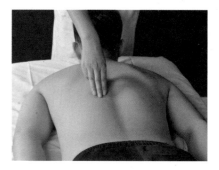

Figure 7-24 Three-finger Pushing

2. Palmar Pushing The root of the palm is the contact surface applying the force at the treatment site. The wrist should be slightly extended and the shoulder joint is used as the fulcrum. The upper arm part is used to exert force, through the elbow joint, the forearm and the wrist joint to the palm root. The pushing is a linear forward motion, in one direction only (Figure 7-25) .

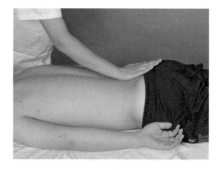

Figure 7-25 Palmar Pushing

3. Fist Pushing Make a fist and use the proximal interphalangeal joints of the four fingers as the contact surface at the treatment area. The wrist should be fully extended, elbow slightly flexed. The forearm actively applies the physical force, pushing forward along a straight line only (Figure 7-26).

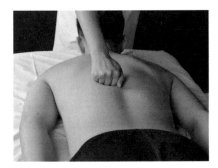

Figure 7-26   Fist Pushing

4. Elbow Pushing   Keep the elbow flexed, with the olecranon process as the contact surface at the treatment site, and the shoulder as the fulcrum. The upper arm actively applies the force, slowly pushing straightly forward in one direction. The opposite hand can be used to hold on the top of the pushing fist as additional help (Figure 7-27).

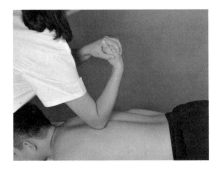

Figure 7-27   Elbow Pushing

Requirements and Precautions

1. The contact area applying physical force needs to be applied firmly to the body surface. Push straight forward in a slow and even manner, with the pressure to be stable and moderate .

2. The fist and elbow pushing should move along the direction of muscle fibers.

3. The operation distance should be short while applying the thumb tip and flat thumb pushing.

4. To prevent skin damage, apply a *tuina* media such as vaseline or talcum powder.

5. The pushing technique should be applied in the direction of muscle fibers at the treatment site. The only exception to the rule is in the intercostal spaces, when the pushing should follow the direction of the ribs.

Applicable Areas: Pushing can be applied to all regions of the body. Finger pushing is suitable to the head, neck, hands and feet, while palmar pushing is applicable to the chest, abdomen, back and four limbs. Fist pushing can be applied to the back, waist and four limbs. Lastly, elbow pushing is suitable to both sides of spine of the back and waist region, and the posterior aspect of the lower extremities.

Effect and Indications: The effects of pushing include regulating the organs, calming the liver, subduing the liver yang, unblocking the meridians, invigorating blood, dissolving blood stasis, relieving pain, soothing the tendons, quickening the collaterals, dispelling wind, dissipating cold, dissolving distention, eliminating fullness, promoting defecation and resolving digestive accumulation. Pushing is mainly used for hypertension, headache, dizziness, insomnia, low back and leg pain, stiffness of the back and the lumbar region, pain due to arthritic *bi* pattern, feeling insensitive, soft tissue injury, localized swelling and pain, chest oppression, hypochondriac distention, irritability, bloating, constipation, and food accumulation.

IV. Foulage

The foulage maneuver can be divided into clamping foulage and pushing foulage.

Essentials of the Maneuver

1. Clamping Foulage   Both palms hold the patient's upper limb or hypochondria simultaneously, use the arms to actively initiate physical force so that the operation site is firmly clamped, and perform foulage with the palms moving in opposite directions quickly. Migrate from one spot to another gradually, as twisting a rope (Figure 7-28).

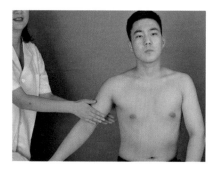

Figure 7-28 Clamping Foulage

2. Pushing Foulage Ask the patient to lie in a prone position, and use one or both palms at a treatment site, such as the lower back or lower limbs. Apply the force parallel to the treatment table and use the palm or both palms as the contact surface. Use the forearm to provide active force, quickly perform pushing foulage, which is to push forward and rub backward, while the palm or palms migrate from one spot to another following a particular direction. If the treatment site is a limb, then this maneuver should make the limb roll back and forth on the treatment table (Figure 7-29).

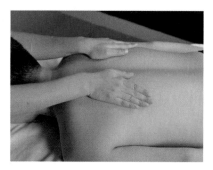

Figure 7-29 Pushing Foulage Method

Requirements and Precautions

1. The movements of the technique need to be coordinated and continuous.

2. The speed of foulage should be fast, while the migration of the palm or palms should be slow.

3. The force of both palms should be equal while applying clamping foulage.

4. Do not overly apply the physical force. When the clamping is too tight, or the push is to hard, the maneuver would be sluggish.

Applicable Areas: Clamping foulage is suitable for the four limbs and the hypochondria, while pushing foulage is more applicable to the back, lumbar region and the posterior aspect of the lower extremities.

Effects and Indications: Clamping foulage has many effects such as soothing and relaxing muscles and tendons, harmonizing qi and blood, resolving spasm, relieving pain, soothing the liver and rectifying qi. Clamping foulage is mainly used in diseases with aching, limited range of motion of the joints, and injury and sudden hypochondriac pain.

Section 3   Vibrating Maneuvers

I. Shaking

Hold the distal end of a limb with one or both hands, pull it slightly, and shake it continuously with a small range up and down or left to right. There is a variety of shaking maneuvers, according to the body part being treated, the position of the patient and the posture of the physician. Some common ones are upper limb shaking, lower limb shaking and waist shaking.

Essentials of the Maneuver

1. Upper Limb Shaking Let the patient sit upright or be in the supine position, and relax shoulders, elbows, and wrist relax. The doctor uses both hands to hold the patient's thenar eminence and hypothenar eminence respectively. Slowly pull the patient's upper limb anterior-laterally to about 60°, and shake it continuously. Initially, the shaking should be slow and with a smaller amplitude, and later, faster and with a larger amplitude. The wave generated by the shaking is continuously transmitted to the shoulder. When this maneuver is performed using one hand, the doctor should hold the patient's entire palm as if the two are about to make a hand-shake, and perform continuous shaking up and down or left to right, with a small range of motion (Figure 7-30).

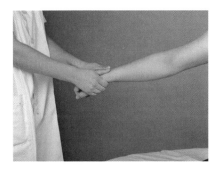

Figure 7-30   Upper Limb Shaking

2. Lower Limb Shaking   Ask the patient to lie in the supine position and relax the lower extremities as the physician stands to the side of the patient's foot, holding the patient's ankle receiving the treatment with both hands. Then, slowly pull and lift the lower extremity to leave the treatment table for about 30 cm. Next, the physician uses both arms to initiate continuous up and down shaking with a small amplitude. The other alternative is to have the patient be in the prone position. The procedure is the same, except that the range of the shaking can be slightly larger (Figure 7-31).

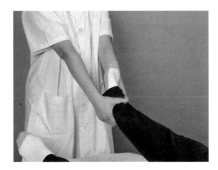

Figure 7-31   Lower Limb Shaking

3. Waist Shaking   Ask the patient to lie in the prone position with two hands grasping one end of the treatment table, or have an assistant to hold the patient's hypochondria. The physician holds both ankles of the patient with both hands with arms straight and the body leaning backwards. Next, pull the patient's waist, making his abdomen leave the treatment table. Once the patient adapts to the traction and relaxes his waist, the physician leans the upper body slightly forward, draws physical support from his back and abdomen to coordinate with the upper limbs, and then pulls and shakes at the same time. Using the inertia from the previous pulling and shaking, perform pulling-shaking with a larger amplitude several times, so that the patient's waist is passively extended and recoiled, resulting in wave-like movement (Figure 7-32).

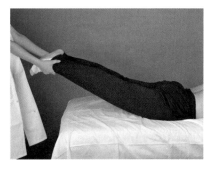

(1)

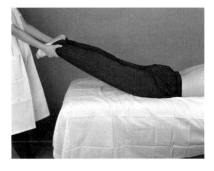

(2)
Figure 7-32 Waist Shaking

Requirements and Precautions

1. Ask the patient to relax and naturally extend the body area being shaken completely, and not to resist with counter-force.

2. Note that the amplitude of the shaking should start small, and the speed should be slow. Then, gradually increase both the range and speed, so that the wave from the shaking should be transmitted from the distal end of the limb being treated to the proximal end.

3. Generally, the amplitude of upper limb shaking is small with a slightly greater frequency of about 250 times per minute, while in the prone position, lower limb shaking should have a relatively larger amplitude with a lower frequency of around 100 times a minute.

4. Waist shaking is a composite maneuver combining pulling, traction and shaking with a large amplitude. Therefore, it is important for the physician to master the timing, while the physical force is accumulated in the back, lower back and abdomen. As a result, the upper limbs are actually depending on the inertial force to accomplish the shaking maneuver.

5. The technique is prohibited in patients suffering habitual dislocation of the shoulders, elbows, and wrists.

6. Shaking is prohibited in patients with severe lumbar pain, limited lumbar mobility, and those who are unable to relax their lumbar muscles.

Applicable Areas: The four limbs and the waist.

Effects and Indications: Shaking maneuver has effects such as dredging the meridians and collaterals, lubricating and benefiting joints, loosening and dissolving adhesion, and recovering dislocations. It is mainly used as a complemantary therapy for illness of the neck, shoulder, arms, waist, and leg, such as shoulder periarthritis, cervical spondylopathy, tendon injury of the hip, lumbar disc herniation, neck, shoulder, arm, waist and leg pain.

II. Vibration

Using the palm or a finger on the body surface to generate a rapid pulsing action is known as the maneuver of vibration. It can be categorized as either palmar vibration or finger vibration.

Essentials of the Maneuver

Place the pads of the index and middle fingers or one palm on the treatment area or the acupoints, and focus on the palm or fingers. Use the wrist extensors and flexors to apply force on and off with high frequency, so that a vibrational action can be created that is transmitted through the palm or the fingers to the treatment site. Usually, this maneuver will make the treatment area warm or generate a feeling of loosening up (Figure 7-33, Figure 7-34).

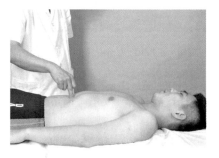

Figure 7-33   Finger Vibration

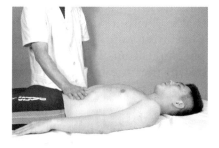

Figure 7-34   Palmar Vibration

Requirements and Precautions

1. The forearm and hand should remain stationary while applying the force. The motion creates a static force, which is achieved by tensing the forearm and hand muscles without active movement.

2. Focus your mind on the fingers or palm. It is generally believed that the maneuver of vibration pertains to the school of internal *qi*

gong tuina, which relies on the combination of intentions and the static force to accomplish the result. As a consequence, there is not much to show externally.

3. The frequency of vibration should be high. Due to the fact that the static force is generated by the muscles of the arm, making the hand involuntary movements very subtle, and forming a vibration similar to that of a factory machine during operation.

4. The pressure of the palm or fingers needs to be natural.

5. The arm should not have active movement during the operation. Except for the static force generated by the arm, the physician should not deliberately swing, tremble, or exert pressure on the treatment site.

6. After applying vibration on patients, it is easy for the physician to feel tired. It is important to pay attention to prevent over working.

Applicable Areas: Finger vibration is applicable to all parts of the body or acupoints, while palmar vibration is suitable for the head, chest, abdomen, back, and waist.

Effect and Indications: Finger vibration has many effect including calming the mind, improving vision, boosting brain power, warm the center, rectifying qi, dispersing accumulation, guiding out food stagnation, and regulating gastrointestinal motility. Finger vibration is mainly used for headaches, insomnia, gastroptosis, stomach pain, cough, asthma, dysmenorrhea, and irregular menstruation.

Clinical Applications: For headache and insomnia, apply vibration on acupoints such as *yìn táng* (EX-HN 3, 印堂), *tài yáng* (EX-HN 5, 太阳), and *bǎi huì* (DU 20, 百会), in combination with press-kneading. For gastroptosis and stomachache, use finger or palmar vibration on the upper abdomen, often combining with press-kneading the same region. For cough and asthma, apply finger vibration on *dàn zhōng* (RN 17, 膻中), and combine with press-kneading on both sides of the spine along the line of the bladder meridian. Lastly, for dysmenorrhea and irregular menstruation, use palmar vibration on the lower abdomen and lumbosacral region and often combine with application of other maneuvers such as kneading the lower abdomen and scrubbing the lumbosacral region.

Section 4 Maneuvers of Squeezing and Pressing Types

I. Pressing

The maneuver of using the fingers or the palm to press on the surface of the body is called pressing, which can be further divided into finger pressing and palmar pressing.

Essentials of the Maneuver

1. Thumb Pressing Use the pad of the thumb as the contact surface of the force and keep the other fingers open and placed naturally in support of the thumb. The thumb actively applies the force squarely with gradually increasing pressure. Once the force reaches the necessary level, stop for a moment, which is called "pressing and retaining". Relax and repeat. The action should be stable and rhythmic. If the power with one thumb is not enough, use both thumbs, one on top of the other (Figure 7-35).

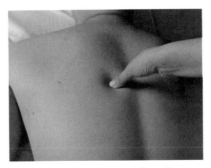

Figure 7-35 Thumb Pressing

2. Palmar Pressing Have one palm or both palms overlapped on the treatment site. Utilize the weight of the upper body, use the upper arm and forearm to transmit the pressure to the palm, and perform pressing squarely. The other instructions remain the same as the thumb pressing maneuver (Figure 7-36).

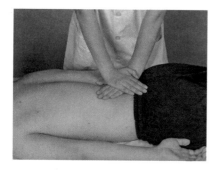

Figure 7-36   Palmar Pressing

Requirements and Precautions

1. During finger pressing, the wrist should be flexed at 120° to 140°, because it makes it easier for the thumb to apply power, and other fingers to support the action.

2. Use the shoulder as the fulcrum in performing palmar pressing, so that the weight of the upper body would be easily transferred to the palm through the arm. When performed correctly, the *tuina* physician is not prone to be tired, and the physical power applied is steady, deep, and stable.

3. The direction of the physical pressure applied should be downwards and squarely to the treatment area.

4. The pressure should start light, and gradually increase and be both stable and continuous, so that the stimulation can reach a deep level of the body.

5. During technique, the pressure should follow the pattern of light, powerful, and light.

6. The contact surface of thumb pressing is narrow, and the stimulation is strong. Therefore, each strong thumb pressing is often followed by three gentle kneading maneuvers.

7. Avoid violent force during the operation. Whether it is thumb pressing or palmar pressing, the principle of applying the power is from light to strong, then returning to light again. Never apply sudden and fierce force. Also, to avoid fractures, pay attention to the bone strength of the patient, and make

a clear diagnosis to see if there is any risk of conditions like osteoporosis that weaken the bones.

Applicable Areas: Thumb pressing is applicable to any body area, especially on meridians, acupoints and tenderness points, while palmar pressing is suitable for back, waist, posterior aspect of the lower limbs, and chest where there is a large flat surface and the muscles are thick.

Effect and Indications: The effects of pressing include moving qi, invigorating blood, opening up blockages, unblocking congestion, dredging the meridians, relieving pain, scattering wind, dissipating cold, warming the meridians and unblocking the vessels. Pressing is often applied in treating headache, cervical spondylopathy, back pain, lower back pain, fasciitis of the back and lower back, pain of the lower limbs, and common cold.

II. Precision Pressing

Applying continuous pressure on the site of operation or acupoints with the tip of the finger or the process of an interphalangeal joint at its flexion is known as precision pressing or "finger acupuncture". Precision pressing mainly includes thumb tip precision-pressing, flexed thumb precision-pressing, and flexed index finger precision-pressing.

Essentials of the Maneuver

1. Thumb Tip Precision Pressing   Make a hollow fist with thumb extended and closely attached to the middle phalanx of the index finger. Use the thumb tip as the contact surface at the treatment site or acupoint, while the forearm actively serves as the origin of the force, passing it to the tip of the thumb. The pressure needs to be vertical and continuous. Another method   is similar to that of the thumb pressing, but only use the tip of the thumb to apply the pressure (Figure 7-37).

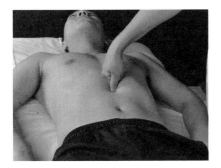

Figure 7-37 Thumb Tip Precision Pressing

2. Flexed Thumb Precision Pressing Make a half fist with thumb flexed, and use the radial or dorsal aspect of the interphalangeal joint of the thumb on the treatment area or the acupoint, with the thumb tip placed firmly against the radial aspect of the middle phalanx of the index finger to gain more power. Have the forearm, wrist and thumb actively provide physical force, and perform precision pressing with continuous vertical pressure (Figure 7-38).

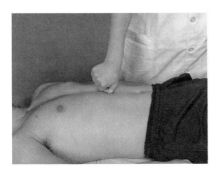

Figure 7-38 Flexed Thumb Precision Pressing

3. Flexed Index Finger Precision Pressing Use the interphalangeal joints of the index finger in flexion position and other fingers to make a fist. Use the proximal interphalangeal joint of the index finger as the contact surface placed on the site or acupoint to be operated on, and have the distal phalanx of the thumb tightly press the nail of the index finger to add more pressure. The forearm and index finger apply active force to perform continuous vertical precision pressing (Figure 7-39).

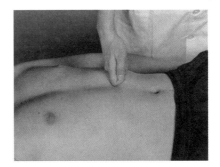

Figure 7-39 Flexed Index Finger Precision Pressing

Requirements and Precautions

1. When applying thumb tip precision pressing, the thumb should make an empty fist with the pad of the thumb tightly attached to the radial side of the middle phalanx of the index finger, so as to avoid possible injury of the interphalangeal joint of the thumb when a hefty amount of force is applied.

2. While using flexed thumb precision pressing, the tip of the thumb should firmly attach the middle phalanx of the index finger on the radial aspect for extra power and stability.

3. In using flexed index finger precision pressing, make a solid fist with the distal phalanx of the thumb tightly pressing against the nail of the index finger to stabilize and support it.

4. In precision pressing, it is important to accurately find the acupoint, while applying a steady force. Te pressure of the technique needs to be gentle to start with and gradually increased, while remaining stable and continuous. The intent is for the stimulation to reach the deep level of the body, which causes the "*de qi*" sensation to a degree that the patient can tolerate.

5. The direction of the force of precision pressing should be perpendicular to the treatment area.

6. Never use violent power. Equally, never start or end the technique suddenly.

7. Using precision pressing on elderly and patients with chronic disease that have frail constitution, especially among patients with

impaired heart function is contraindicated in all cases.

8. After precision pressing, it is appropriate to perform kneading to avoid accumulation of qi and blood at the treatment site, which may result in an effort to prevent soft tissue injury of the treatment site or the acupoint.

9. The characteristics of precision pressing are small contact surface, strong stimulation, and saving physical energy.

Applicable Areas: Precision pressing can be applied to all areas of the body, especially acupoints of all yang meridians and *ashi* points.

Effects and Indications: This technique can be used for regulating *zang-fu* organs, supplementing the deficient and draining the excess, and dredging the meridians and relieving pain. Precision pressing is therefore used mainly for a variety of pain disorders and medical diseases.

III. Grasping

The grasping maneuver uses the thumb opposite of the rest of the fingers to lift and hold or knead and pinch the soft tissue of the treatment region. There is a saying that "pinch and lift is grasping". According to the thumb and number of fingers, the grasping maneuver can be divided into the three-finger grasping and five-finger grasping methods. It can be carried out with one or both hands.

Essentials of the Maneuver

Using the thumb opposite of the rest of the fingers, pinch and hold the soft tissue of the treatment area. Use the force of the forearm to lift the soft tissues with the fingers and the palm, while actively applying force, gradually tighten up the pinch, so that the muscles and subcutaneous tissue along with the skin of the treatment site are lifted up collectively. Finally, loosen the grasp. Repeat the steps. The technique can be applied to one area repetitively, or, the physician can perform grasping on one area and gradually migrate to another (Figure 7-40).

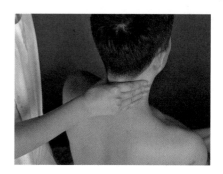

Figure 7-40 Grasping

Requirements and Precautions

1. Fingers should be straight, and use the palmar interphalangeal joint of the thumb and the fingers to operate, rather than having the fingertips flexed and facing inward.

2. As a composite *tuina* maneuver, grasping in fact combines lifting, pinching, and kneading and integrates them organically.

3. When the thumb and other fingers work together, the force should be symmetrical, the wrist should be relaxed, the action is soft and flexible, continuous and rhythmic.

4. While applying the grasping maneuver, pay attention to the coordination of the fingers, and avoid rigid movements. For novice clinicians, do not grasp forcefully for a long time, relax fingers while the patient feels a little pain and avoid damage to the patient's skin or the wrist, flexor tendon, and tendon sheath of the clinician.

Applicable Areas: Grasping is appropriate for the neck, shoulders, limbs and head.

Effects and Indications: The effects of grasping include moving qi, invigorating blood, dredging the meridians, unblocking the collaterals, relaxing muscles, soothing tendons, relieving pain, eliminating soreness, dispelling wind, and dissipating cold. The maneuver is commonly used in cervical spondylopathy, frozen shoulder, lumbar disc herniation, pain and soreness of the four limbs, headache, and chills.

Section 5 Maneuvers of Tapping Types

I. Patting

Using the cupped palm to pat on the body surface is the patting maneuver. The action can be perfomred with one hand or both hands alternately.

Essentials of the Maneuver

Have the five fingers naturally closed together with the metacarpophalangeal joints slightly flexed to make a cupped palm. Relax the wrist, perform active up and down movement with the forearm to have the cupped palm pat on the operating area rhythmically. When both cupped palms are performing the patting maneuver, use the palms alternatively (Figure 7-41).

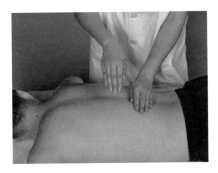

Figure 7-41 Patting

Requirements and Precautions

1. Use a cupped palm to carry out patting steadily, while the entire edge of the palm should be in contact with the body surface, making a loud crisp sound without causing pain.

2. Moderately relax the wrist. The force of patting is transmitted to the palm through the relaxed wrist while swinging the arm up and down, making the maneuver powerful yet gentle.

3. By making direct contact with the skin, patting should cause the skin to look slightly red, due to an increase in blood flow to the capillaries.

4. The action of patting should be steady and rhythmic. It cannot be chaotic. The power should be deep, thorough and even, to avoid slapping pain.

5. Be aware of the important indications of this maneuver. Patting is contraindicated in patients with diseases such as tuberculosis, cancer, coronary heart disease, and severe osteoporosis.

Applicable Areas: Patting is applicable for shoulders, back, lumbosacral area and the posterior aspect of the lower extremities. Mild patting can also be used on the chest, abdomen and head.

Effects and Indications: The treatment effects of patting include dredging the meridians, unblocking the collaterals, diffusing qi, invigorating blood, and promoting yang qi. Patting is applied in a variety of problems such as back fascia strain, lumbar disc herniation, hypertension, and diabetes. It is also commonly used in treating various pain owing to wind-damp *bi* pattern, strain due to injury in the past, blood stasis because of recent trauma, muscle atrophy, hypoesthesia, intestinal paralysis, chest tightness and pain, and dizziness, et cetera.

II. Striking

Striking is a *tuina* maneuver that makes use of physician's body area, such as the back of the fist, root of the palm, palmar side of the hypothenar eminence, and finger tips, or certain tools like mulberry sticks patting on specific body areas. According to the different means or ways, striking can be divided into fist striking, palm-root striking, lateral striking, finger-tip striking and mulberry striking.

Essentials of the Maneuver

1. Fist Striking Make a hollow fist, use the back, surface or radial aspect of the fist as the striking surface, the elbow as the fulcrum, the forearm as the source of active force, and pat rhythmicaly at the treatment site (Figure 7-42) .

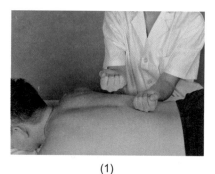

(1)

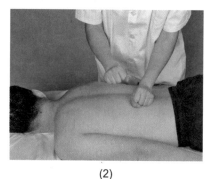

(2)

Figure 7-42   Fist striking
(1) Fist-back Striking   (2) Fist-surface Striking

The way to make the fist is also different according to the body area to be treated. When striking with the back of the fist, hold an empty fist or have the fingers flexed with the wrist in flexion position as much as possible, so that the back of the fist forms an arc. At the same time, the striking should be controlled and rhythmic. While using the fist surface to perform the striking, the four interphalangeal joints needs to be in flexion position and closed together, and the thumb should be firmly attached to the radial aspect of the index finger, so that the dorsal side of the second interphalangeal joints of the index finger, and little fingers, together the root of the palm, can form a hollow fist as a contacting surface. During striking, relax the wrist. If the radial aspect of the empty fist is used the contacting surfacing for the striking, the wrist should be in dorsiflexion position. In general, when the fist surface or radial aspect of the fist are used, both hands are performing the strike alternately.

2. Palm-root Striking   Use the root of the palm as the striking surface, have the wrist relaxed and natural flexed, and the elbow as a fulcrum, and use the forearm to control the force and the rhythm of the strike. At the moment that the wrist hits the target, the wrist should be in dorsiflexion position as much as possible. The rapidly applied force on the treatment area is combined with the forearm power and the power generated by the active dorsiflexion of the wrist. The fist should be lifted immediately after the strike with the wrist natural flexed at the time, before performing the next strike. Therefore, the maneuver should be repeated with a distinct rhythm (Figure 7-43).

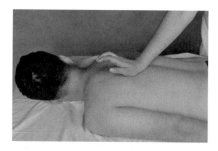

Figure 7-43   Palm-root Striking

3. Lateral Striking of the Palm   Keep the fingers and palm in extension position with the wrist slightly dorsiflexed. Use the ulnar side of both palms as the striking surface, have both forearms actively alternating the force, so that the ulnar aspect of the palms can strike on the treatment surface rhythmically and alternately (Figure 7-44).

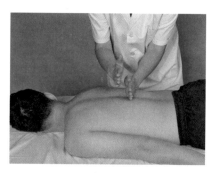

Figure 7-44   Lateral Striking of the Palm

4. Finger-tip Striking   Slightly flex all the fingers of one or both hands, and·separate the fingers to make them look like claws. Use the tip of the fingers as the contact surface. Relax the wrist and use active forearm force to gently and rhythmically strike on the head (Figure 7-45).

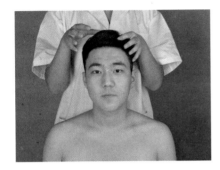

Figure 7-45 Finger-tip Striking

5. Stick Striking   Use dried mulberry or willow branches as the tool. Hold one end and use the other end as the striking surface. Allow the forearm actively control the force and frequency of the strike to strike the treatment area in a short and rhythmic manner.

Requirements and Precautions

1. Control force of the strike so that it is moderate. Strike and stop freely.

2. For different people, disease and body areas, use different level of striking force, but avoid violent power.

3. There needs be a sense of quick bounce while striking with no pause or delay.

4. The striking maneuver need to be continuous, rhythmic, and with moderate speed.

5. While applying various striking maneuvers, adhere to the strict guidelines of indications, applicable body areas and contraindications.

Applicable Areas: Since fist striking is heavy and solid, it is appropriate for the shoulder, back, and lumbosacral region. Palm striking though, has a strong penetrating power, so that it is suitable for *dà zhuī* (DU 14), the medial edge of the scapula, and the buttocks. Lateral striking is more soothing, applicable to areas such as the shoulders, four limbs, and along the spine. Finger strike is light and rapid and suitable to the head. Stick striking is powerful; therefore, it is suitable for the back, waist, buttocks and the posterior aspects of the lower extremities.

Effects and Indications: The effects of striking include unblocking the collaterals, relieving pain, diffusing qi and blood, dispelling wind, eliminating dampness, engendering muscle, and improving atrophy. Fist striking is mainly used for problems such as soreness, pain, and numbness caused by cervical and lumbar disorders, pain owing to wind-damp *bi* pattern, muscle soreness due to fatigue, and muscle atrophy.

Section 6   Passive Joint Movements

Maneuvers of joint movements are *tuina* techniques that perform passive joint movements within their physiological range of motions, such as flexion, extension, adduction, abduction and traction. Joint movement techniques include rotation, spontaneous torquing, and traction, and are effective in loosening up adhesion or reducing dislocation of the affected joints.

I. Rotation

Rotation is the technique to perform passive circular movement, commonly used on the neck, waist and limbs.

Essentials of the Maneuver

1. Neck Rotation   Ask the the patient to remain a sitting position with neck relaxed. The physician stands on the posterior or posterior-lateral aspect of the patient, hold the head of the patient with one hand, and put the other hand under the patient's chin. Therefore, the palm centers of the physician should be opposite of each other. Both arms coordinate to apply some force and move to the opposite direction, so that the head and neck are passively rotated clockwise or counterclockwise. Repeat this procedure several times (Figure 7-46).

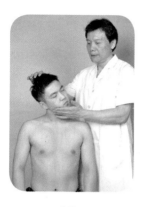 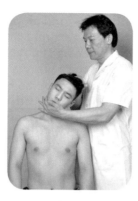

(1)   (2)

Figure 7-46   Neck Rotation

2. Shoulder Rotation   The types of shoulder rotation include elbow- holding shoulder rotation, hand-holding shoulder rotation and wide-range shoulder rotation.

(1) *Elbow-holding Shoulder Rotation*   Ask the patient to remain in a sitting position with shoulders relaxed and elbow in flexed. Stand laterally to the patient with the upper body slightly leaning forward, and use one hand to hold the upper part of the patient's shoulder and the other hand to lift and hold his elbow, so that the patient's forearm is placed on the forearm of the physician. Then, use the power of the forearm to make the patient's shoulder perform passive rotation with moderate range clockwise or counterclockwise (Figure 7-47).

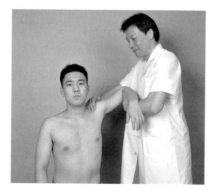

Figure 7-47   Elbow-holding Shoulder Rotation

(2) *Hand-holding Shoulder Rotation*   The patient should be in a sitting position with

both shoulders relaxed. Stand laterally to the patient with one hand holding the affected shoulder and the other hand holding the patient's hand. Then, use moderate power to perform traction to the arm of the affected side. When the arm is straightened, the physician uses the force of his or her own arm to perform clockwise or counterclockwise shoulder rotation with small range (Figure 7-48).

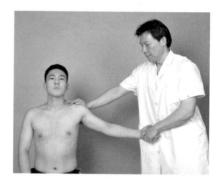

Figure 7-48   Hand-holding Shoulder Rotation

(3) *Wide-range Shoulder Rotation*   Ask the patient to remain in a sitting position with both upper limbs naturally hanging and relaxed. Make a T-stance at the anterolateral aspect of the patient. Put the palms together to lock the patient's wrist of the affected upper limb in between, pull and raise it to about 45° anterolaterally, and continue to gradually lift up the patient's upper limbs. During the process, turn the palm below the wrist until the patient's arm is 160° from the hanging position and grab the wrist with the upper thenar space facing down. At the same time, the other hand slides to the upper shoulder along the forearm and then the upper arm. After a brief stop, both hands should coordinate, so that the hand on the patient's shoulder slightly presses it down to make it stable, and the hand holding the patient's wrist lift up a bit to have the shoulder in extension position. Then the hand holding the wrist rotates to the posterior-inferior aspect, and circles back to its starting spot. At this point, the hand on the shoulder has moved back to the wrist by passing the upper arm and forearm. There-

fore, both hands are back to their original position. The wide-range shoulder rotation can be repeated several times (Fig. 7-49).

It is necessary to adjust the body's center of the gravity by moving the feet around while applying this maneuver. That is, when the patient's shoulder is lifted and rotated posterolaterally, the physician's front foot steps forward a little with the body's center of gravity shifting to the front. When the patient's shoulder is rotated downward and anterolaterally, the physician's front foot should step back with the center of gravity moving to the back.

clockwise (Figure 7-51). A third method of performing the wrist rotation is to hold the patient's five fingers together with the wrist in flexion status. Hold the upper part of the patient's wrist in one hand and the fingers in the other hand, and perform rotation to the wrist clockwise or counterclockwise.

5. Metacarpophalangeal Joint Rotation Use one hand to hold the lateral side of the patient's palm, and the other one hold one of the patient's five fingers. Pull with moderate force and perform passive rotation to the metacarpophalangeal joint clockwise or counterclockwise (Figure 7-52).

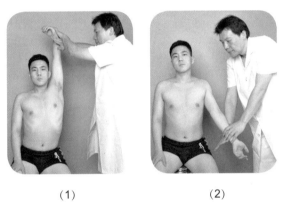

(1)   (2)

Figure 7-49 Wide-range Shoulder Rotation

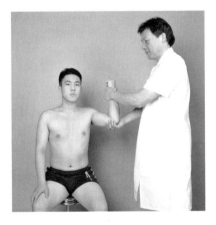

Figure 7-50 Elbow Rotation

3. Elbow Rotation Ask the patient to be seated, elbow flexion of about 45°. Hold the back of his elbow in one hand and the wrist in the other hand, and perform elbow rotation clockwise or counterclockwise (Figure 7-50).

4. Wrist Rotation Ask the patient to remain in a sitting position with palms facing down. Hold the patient's palm using both hands with two thumbs on the dorsal aspect of the wrist and the other fingers holding the thenar eminence and the hypothenar eminence. Coordinate the force of both arms, slightly pull the wrist and perform clockwise and counterclockwise rotation. Alternatively, keep the patient's four fingers close together with the palm facing down. Hold the upper part of the patient's wrist in one hand and the four fingers in the other hand, pull it slightly, and perform rotation clockwise and counter-

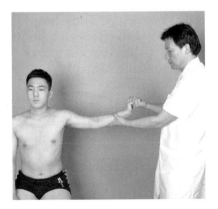

Figure 7-51 Wrist Rotation

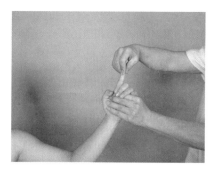

Figure 7-52   Metacarpophalangeal Joint Rotation

6. Lumbar Rotation   There are various forms of the lumbar rotation methods, including supine lumbar rotation, prone lumbar rotation, and rolling lumbar rotation. The first two types of lumbar rotation are introduced as the follows.

(1) *Supine Lumbar Rotation*: Ask the patient to lie in a supine position with both legs together, knees and hip in flexion position. Use each hand to hold one knee, or one hand hold the knees and the other hand press the ankle, coordinate the force and perform clockwise or counterclockwise rotation (Figure 7-53).

(2) *Prone Lumbar Rotation*: Ask the patient to lie prone with both lower extremities straight. Press the patient's lumbar area with one hand, hold both the lower limbs with the other arm to lift them up, and perform clockwise or counterclockwise lumbar rotation (Figure 7-54). When rotating both the lower limbs, apply some pressure to the hand holding on the patient's waist to facilitate the range of the lumbar rotation.

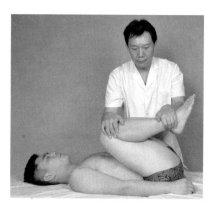

Figure 7-53   Supine Lumbar Rotation

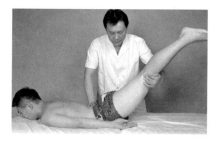

Figure 7-54   Prone Lumbar Rotation

7. Hip Rotation   Ask the patient to lie supine with the hip and knees in flexion position. Hold and press the patient's knee with one hand, and the ankle or heel with the other hand, and adjust the flexion angle of the hip and knees to about 90°. Then, with the coordination of both hands, perform hip joint rotation clockwise or counterclockwise (Figure 7-55).

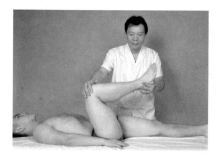

Figure 7-55   Hip Rotation

8. Knee Rotation   Ask the patient to lie supine with one side of lower extremity straight and relaxed, and the other side of the hip and knee in flexion position. Support the popliteal fossa of the flexed leg with one hand, hold the ankle or heel of the same leg, and perform clockwise or counterclockwise rotation to the knee (Figure 7-56).

9. Ankle Rotation   Ask the patient to lie supine with the lower limbs being naturally straight. The physician should sit on the side of the patient's feet, hold the affected heel securely with one hand, and the toes with the other hand, and rotate it clockwise or counterclockwise while slight pulling (Figure 7-57). Alternatively, with the patient in the prone position and the ipsilateral knee in flexion position, use one hand to hold firmly on the heel, the other hand to hold the toes, and perform clockwise or counterclockwise ankle rotation. The alternate methodis actually easier to perform and generates a wider range of the rotation.

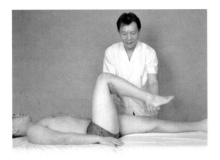

Figure 7-56 Knee Rotation

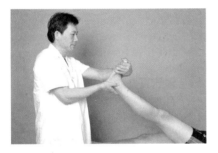

Figure 7-57 Ankle Rotation

Requirements and Precautions

1. The rotation maneuver should be performed within the normal physiological range of motion, starting with a small range and gradually increasing, without exceeding the normal range. Since each joint is different, therefore, the rotation of each joint also varies.

2. The speed of the rotation should be slow, especially at the beginning. Sudden and rapid rotation should be avoided. Speed can be increased with the increased number of rotations, as the patient gradually adapts to the motion.

3. The power used in rotation should be coordinated and stable. In addition, the motion should be isolated to the joint or limb being rotated, other body parts should not involved in the action.

4. For patients who are susceptible to habitual articular dislocation, rotation should be used with caution. Furthermore, neck rotation is contraindicated for patients suffering from disorders including cervical spondylopathy of vertebral artery and sympathetic types, neck trauma, and cervical spine fractures.

Applicable Areas: Passive rotation is applicable to all joints of the body.

Effects and Indications: Treatment effects of rotation include soothing the tendons, unblocking collaterals, smoothing joints, and resolving adhesion. It is mainly applicable to all kinds of soft tissue injury and motor dysfunction disorders.

II. Spontaneous Torquing

The performance of passive torquing on certain joints is called the spontaneous torquing maneuver.

Essentials of the Maneuver

1. Spontaneous Neck Torquing Types of this technique include oblique spontaneous neck torquing, cervical rotation with positioned spontaneous torquing, atlantoaxial joint rotation with spontaneous torquing, and lateral cervical spontaneous torquing. For the purpose of this book, only the first two techniques will be introduced.

(1) Oblique Spontaneous Neck Torquing:Ask the patient to be in a sitting position, neck relaxed, and head slightly leaning forward or in neutral position. Stand to the posterolateral aspect of the patient, place one hand firmly on the patient's posterior of the vertex, the other hand under the chin. Coordinate the movement of both hands, rotate the head to the lateral side. When there is the sense of resistance, pause a moment, then use "dexterous force and agile strength" to perform a sudden, rapid, yet controlled spontaneous torquing. A snapping sound can often be heard. Perform the same procedure to the other side (Figure 7-58).

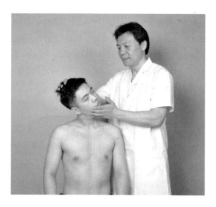

Figure 7-58 Oblique Spontaneous Neck Torquing

(2) Cervical Rotation with Positioned Spontaneous Torquing: Ask the patient to sit and relax their neck. The physician should stand on the rear lateral side of the patient. Use one thumb to press firmly on the cervical spinous process where the lesion is located, and the other hand supporting the contralateral chin. Ask the patient to flex his neck. When the thumb can feel the movement of the spinous process and the enlargement of the joint space, instruct the patient to flex his neck to the ipsilateral aspect until its limit. Then, slowly rotate the patient's head until there is resistance, pause for a moment, then use "dexterous force and agile strength" to perform a controlled and rapid spontaneous torquing. At this point, a snapping sound can often be heard, while the thumb can experience a bouncing-like feeling of the spinous process (Figure 7-59).

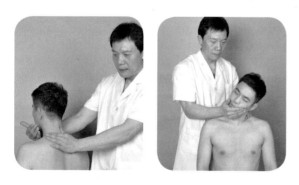

(1)   (2)

Figure 7-59 Cervical Rotation with Positioned Spontaneous Torquing

2. Thoracodorsal Spontaneous Torquing The thoracodorsal torquing maneuver includes chest expansion traction spontaneous torquing, opposing thoracic reduction spontaneous torquing, shoulder spontaneous torquing for the thoracic spine, and elbow-pressing thoracic reduction in the supine position. Of these, the first two methods are more commonly used.

(1) Chest Expansion Traction Spontaneous Torquing: The patient takes sitting position with fingers crossed and holding the occipital area of the head. The physician stands behind the patient, with one side of the knee against the back of the patient on where the lesion is, both hands each holding an elbow. First, instruct the patient to bend forward with deep inhale and backward with thorough exhale. After a few times, when the patient's body bends back to the maximum, use the "dexterous force and agile strength" to suddenly pull both elbows towards the back. At the same time, use the knee to push the patient's body forward. A clear snapping sound can often be heard (Figure 7-60).

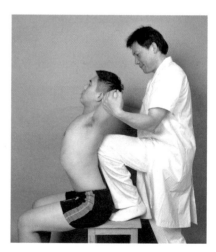

Figure 7-60 Chest Expansion Traction Spontaneous Torquing

(2) Opposing Thoracic Reduction Spontaneous Torquing:The patient is in a sitting position with hands crossed and holding the occipital region. The physician stands behind him, arms reaching the patient's lower fore-

arm by passing under the armpits, and one knee against the thoracic vertebra to be treated. Then, apply pressure to both hands holding the forearms, while lifting the two forearms, so that the spine of the patient is being pulled posterosuperiorly. At the same time, the knee against the affected vertebra should push anteroinferiorly, providing an opposing force to that of the forearms. Continue the traction for a moment, with both hands, arms and the knee in coordination, use the "dexterous force and agile strength" to perform a sudden, controlled, and rapid torquing, and a snapping sound can often be heard (Figure 7-61).

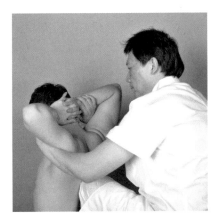

Figure 7-61 Opposing Thoracic Reduction Spontaneous Torquing

3. Spontaneous Lumbar Torquing Spontaneous oblique lumbar torquing, lumbar rotation reduction, and lumbar extension with spontaneous torquing are commonly used maneuvers in clinical practice.

(1) Spontaneous Oblique Lumbar Torquing: Ask the patient to lay on the non-affected side, hip and the affected knee in flexion position, and the healthy leg naturally straight facing the practitioner. Use one elbow or hand to hold against the front part of the patient's shoulder, another elbow or hand against the buttocks. Both elbows or both hands should coordinate, apply power to perform passive lumbar torsion for the patient. That is, the elbow or hand on the shoulder pushes the shoulder anteroinferior-

ly, while the elbow or hand on the buttocks pushes the buttock posteroinferiorly, both with moderate pressure, so that it forms a twisting effect with small range. When the patient's waist is completely relaxed, increase the range until a significant resistance is felt. After a short pause, use "agile force" to make a sudden, and rapid torquing with increase range, which often causes a snapping sound (Figure 7-62)

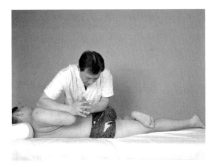

Figure 7-62 Spontaneous Oblique Lumbar Torquing

(2) *Lumbar Rotation Reduction*: Ask the patient to sit with waist relaxed and arms naturally hanging. For the sake of example, assume a right side lesion, therefore the treatment should be rotating to the right for the reduction. Have an assistant standing to the front left of the patient, hold the patient's left calf with his lower extremities, press the patient's upper part of the left leg with both hands, and stabilize the patient's lower half of his body. The physician stands on the posterior right of the patient, use the pad of the left thumb to press against the side of the displaced lumbar spinous process, with the right palm passing through the right armpit and placing against the back of the patient's neck. Slow apply pressure through the right palm, and instruct the patient to do waist flexion. The physician should feel the activities of the spinous process under the left thumb, when the gap of the spinous process can be felt, ask the patient to stop further flexion and maintain that position. Next, slowly apply force with the right arm, press the skewed lumbar spinous process firmly with the left thumb, making the waist forward flexion to

a certain extent, and then rotate the waist to the right until its limit. After pausing for a moment, further press the neck with the right palm, lift the right elbow, push the skewed spinous process to the opposite side with the left thumb. By coordinating the power of both hands, use the "dexterous force and agile strength" to perform a rapid spontaneous torquing with an increased range. At this time, a snapping sound can often be heard (Figure 7-63).

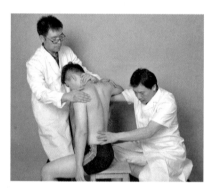

(1)

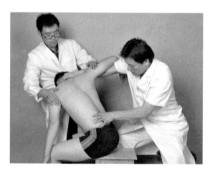

(2)

Figure 7-63   Lumbar Rotation Reduction

(3) *Straight Lumbar Rotation with Spontaneous Torquing:* Ask the patient to sit with two lower extremities separated at shoulder width and waist relaxed. Take the example of performing the maneuver to the right side. The physician clamps the patient's left thigh with both lower extremities for fixation. Use the left hand to press against the back of the patient's left shoulder, the right arm to pass under the patient's right armpit to use the

right hand pressing against the anterior aspect of the shoulder. Then use both hands to coordinate the force, with the left hand pushing the back of patient's left shoulder, the right hand to pull the right shoulder, and the right arm lifting the patient's body upwards at the same time, so that the waist is rotated to the right. While the resistance is felt, use the "dexterous force and agile strength" to make a sudden and rapid spontaneous torquing with increased range, and a snapping sound can often be heard (Figure 7-64).

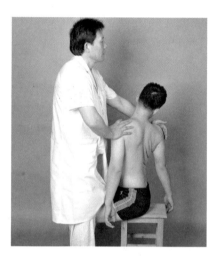

Figure 7-64   Straight Lumbar Rotation with Spontaneous Torquing

An alternative method for performing the straight lumbar rotation with spontaneous torquing: ask the patient to sit with two lower limbs close together. Stand opposite the patient. Clamp the patient's lower extremities with both legs. Keep one hand on the front side of the patient's shoulder, the other hand on the back of the other shoulder. Coordinate the force of both hands, perform pushing and pulling respectively, so that the lumbar spine rotates slightly a few times. When the waist is fully relaxed, rotate the lumbar spine until resistance can be felt, pause for a moment, and perform spontaneous torquing with "dexterous force and agile strength" rapidly with an increase range. Usually, a snapping sound can often be heard.

(4) *Lumbar Extension Spontaneous Torquing:*

Ask the patient to lie in the prone position with two lower limbs closed together. The physician presses the waist with one hand, holds the patient's legs above the knees with the other arm, and slowly lifts them to induce a passive back extension. When the extension reaches the maximum limit, have both hands coordinated, use "dexterous force and agile strength", perform a torquing with pressing the waist down and lifting the lower limbs up with increased range (Figure 7-65).

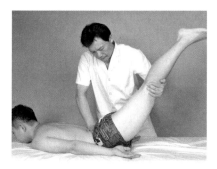

Figure 7-65 Lumbar Extension Spontaneous Torquing

4. Spontaneous Shoulder Torquing The subtypes of this maneuver include spontaneous flexion torquing, spontaneous abduction torquing, spontaneous adduction torquing, and spontaneous intorsion torquing, and spontaneous lifting torquing of the shoulder joint.

(1) *Spontaneous Shoulder Flexion Torquing*: Ask the patient to sit down, with the affected shoulder in flexion position at 30° to 50°. The physician makes a half squat anteriolaterally to the affected shoulder of the patient. Use both hands to hold tightly from the front and back of the same shoulder, and place the affected upper arm of the patient on the adjacent forearm of the physician. First, flex the shoulder several times or perform several rotation to make the shoulder relaxed as much as possible. Coordinate the force of both arms, slowly lift the patient's shoulder up. When the passive shoulder flexion encounters resistance, use "dexterous force and agile strength" to perform rapid spontaneous torquing with increased range (Figure 7-66).

An alternative way to perform spontaneous flexion torquing to the shoulder is to let the patient sit with arms hanging naturally, and shoulder relaxed. Stand behind the patient, hold the contralateral shoulder with one hand, and above the elbow of the ipsilateral arm with another hand. Slowly lift the affected arm to have the shoulder in maximum flexion position until resistance can be felt, and use the "dexterous force and agile strength" to perform a quick spontaneous torquing with increased range.

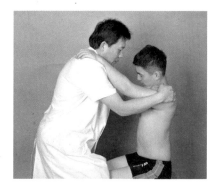

Figure 7-66 Spontaneous Shoulder Flexion Torquing

(2) *Spontaneous Shoulder Abduction Torquing*: Ask the patient to sit with the affected arm abducted at about 45°. The physician should be in half squat position lateral to the affected shoulder of the patient. Put the affected arm above the elbow of the patient on the physician's shoulder, grab the affected shoulder with both hands and lock it tightly. Slowly stand up, so make the patient's shoulder perform passive abduction. When resistance is felt, pause for a moment. Then, both hands, the body and shoulders of the physician should work coordinately, and use the "dexterous force and agile strength" to perform rapid spontaneous torquing with increased range. If adhesion is separated, a hissing or snapping sound can be heard (Figure 7-67).

(3) *Spontaneous Shoulder Adduction Torquing*: Allow the patient to sit, and place the elbow of the affected upper limb in flexion position in front of his/her chest with the hand on the contralateral shoulder. The physician stands behind the patient. Hold the patient's ipsilateral shoulder firmly with one hand. Support

the elbow of the affected side with the other hand, and slowly lift it up towards the contralateral chest. When resistance is encountered, perform rapid spontaneous torquing with "dexterous force and agile strength" with an increased range (Figure 7-68).

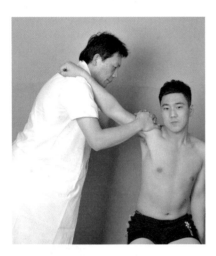

Figure 7-67   Spontaneous Shoulder Abduction Torquing

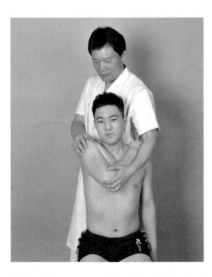

Figure 7-68   Spontaneous Shoulder Adduction Torquing

(4) *Spontaneous Shoulder Intorsion Torquing* (1): Ask the patient to sit, and place the affected hand and forearm behind the back. Stand at the posterolateral aspect of the affected limb, hold the affected shoulder firmly with one hand, and grab the wrist with the other hand. Next, slowly lift the affected forearm to

make gradual internal rotation of the shoulder until resistance is felt. Then, perform a fast and controlled lift of its forearm with "dexterous force and agile strength" to make the shoulder rotate to its limit. If adhesion is separated, a hissing sound can be heard (Figure 7-69).

Spontaneous Shoulder Intorsion Torquing (2): Ask the patient to sit. The doctor should stand opposite the patient with the body slightly squatting, and center of gravity stabilized. Hold the patient's contralateral shoulder firmly with one hand and press the chin on the ipsilateral shoulder to enhance the stability. Use the other arm to hold up the patient's ipsilateral arm, and slowly lift up. The actual spontaneous torquing is the same as stated in the previous example.

(5) *Spontaneous Shoulder Lifting Torquing* (1): Ask the patient to sit with arms naturally hanging. The physician stands behind the patient, holds the distal end of the affected upper arm with one hand and slowly lifts it up to 120° to 140° from the flexion or abduction position. Then, hold the forearm near the wrist with the other hand. Coordinate the force of both hands, gradually pull the patient's arm up. When there is resistance, make a quick and controlled pulling and torquing with "dexterous force and agile strength" (Figure 7-70).

Spontaneous Shoulder Lifting Torquing (2): Ask the patient to lay on his/her side with the affected shoulder facing the physician. The physician should sit beside of the patient's head. Ask the patient to lift his/her affected arm to about 120° to 140° from its flexion position, hold the patient's forearm with one hand, and the upper arm with the other hand. Next, the physician applies power with both upper limbs, pull the patient's arm upwards slowly until there is resistance, and the rest procedure is the same as stated previously.

5. Spontaneous Elbow Torquing   Ask the patient to lie in the supine position with the affected limb being flat and the physician sitting to the side of the elbow. Hold the upper part of the elbow with one hand, and the distal end of the forearm with the other hand. The type of spontaneous torquing to be selected is dependent upon the specific dysfunction of the elbow. If elbow flexion is limited, place the elbow in a flexed position after passive flexion and extension, and apply gradual pressure to allow it to slowly reach the functional position. When obvious resistance is encountered, use the hand holding the patient's forearm to apply continuous pressure making the elbow stay in flexion position. After a moment, both hands will coordinate their efforts to perform a rapid and pressurized spontaneous torquing with increased range and "dexterous force and agile strength" (Figure 7-71). In restricted elbow extension, the maneuver should be performed in the opposite direction. For flexion or extension limitations of the wrist, hip, knees and ankles, take the operation procedure for the elbow as a reference.

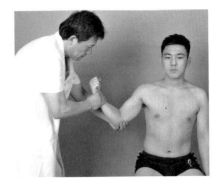

Figure 7-71 Spontaneous Elbow Torquing

Requirements and Precautions

1. All maneuvers must comply with the normal physiological function of each joint being treated. Each joint has its own characteristics in terms of structure, while the physiological functions of each is very different. Therefore, it is necessary to remember clearly the structural features, range of motion, the direction and characteristics of the movements of each joint. As the result, the operation of spontaneous torquing should be adapted to fit the characteristics of various joints.

2. Never exceed the physiological range of motion of each joint while performing spontaneous torquing. Otherwise, it is easy to cause damage to the joints, their associated muscles, ligaments and other soft tissues. Pay particular attention to the neck and chest when applying any torquing technique.

3. The procedure is to be perfromed in several steps. The first step is to relax the joints with small range of movements accordingly, such rotation, extension, or flexion. The second step is to extend or flex the joints to a greater extent to further prepare the actual implementation of the third step, which is the spontaneous torquing.

4. The physical force used at the moment of spontaneous torquing is in particular the "dexterous force and agile strength". The "dexterous force (*qiǎo lì*, 巧力)" refers to the skillful use of the physical power, while "agile strength (*cùn jìn*, 寸劲)" refers to the quick force and fully controlled torquing amplification. The force stops immediately after the

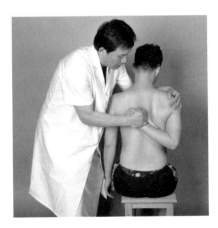

Figure 7-69 Spontaneous Shoulder Intorsion Torquing

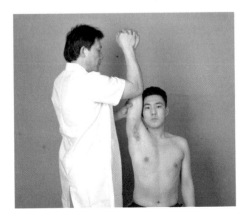

Figure 7-70 Spontaneous Shoulder Lifting Torquing

treatment effect is accomplished in less than a second.

5. Never apply careless force or blunt power. The former refers to using inadequately trained technique without preparation, not following appropriate stages, and starting spontaneous torquing at the beginning of the operation. In early stages of training, a practitioner may not be aware of the power level being applied and/or lacks the ability to effectively control the power. The latter means that the power is more than enough but lacks of dexterity while performing spontaneous torquing. In short, in either case the practitioner has not mastered the key element of this maneuver and does not understand the meaning of "dexterous force and agile strength". The consequences can be as mild as causing discomfort, or as severe as resulting in serious injury to patients, leading to *tuina* induced medical accidents.

6. The timing of spontaneous torquing needs to be precise, and the level of power used appropriate. If it is too early, the joint is not yet relaxed, so the effect will not as great. If the maneuver is performed later than the ideal timing while the joint has been in the state of extreme extension or flexion, or rotation for too long, it is easy for the joint to become tense, making the movement more difficult. Moreover, if the power applied is too low, it cannot reach the therapeutic effect. On the other hand, if it is too much, it is easy to cause adverse reactions.

7. Do not force to have a snapping sound of the joint. A snapping sound can often be heard while applying spontaneous torquing on the neck, chest or waist as the result of the joint bouncing or torsion friction. Generally, the sound is considered a sign of successful joint reposition. In the actual execution of the technique, however, if the sound does not appear, it should not be overly pursued. If the maneuver is repeatedly performed, it is easy to increase the joint tension, causing adverse consequences.

8. The spontaneous torquing is contraindicated where the diagnosis is unclear for a patient with spine trauma and of spinal cord signs and symptoms. Additionally torquing techniques must be applied with caution among elderly patients, especially those who suffers severe bone hyperplasia, and osteoporosis. Lastly, for those with joint tuberculosis and bone tumors, torquing techniques are prohibited.

Applicable Areas: Spontaneous torquing applies to all joints of the body.

Effects and Indications: Spontaneous torquing can benefit joints slip joint, fix dislocations, loosen adhesions, soothe tendons, unblocking collaterals, resolve spasm, and relieve pain. The method is mainly used for cervical spondylopathy, stiff neck, atlanto-axial instability, periarthritis of the shoulder, lumbar disc herniation, spine facet joint disorders, and dysfunction of the joints of four limbs as the result of trauma.

III. Traction

Pulling along the longitudinal axis of a joint or one end of a limb so that the use of confrontational forces will make the joint or limb to stretch, is known as the traction maneuver.

Essentials of the Maneuver

1. Cervical Vertebra Traction   The three types of cervical vertebra traction are palm lifting traction, elbow lifting traction and supine traction.

(1) *Palm Lifting Traction*: Ask the patient to be in a sitting position. The physician stands behind the patient, attach the ulnar aspect of his/her forearms on each side of the patient's neck over the shoulder, with the pads of both thumbs pressing both *fēng chí* (GB 20, 风池), palms under each side of the mandibular region. Next, with the power of arms, palms and fingers coordinated, the thumbs push up, and palms lift the neck, so that the neck is slowly being stretched upwards for one to three minutes, and the traction of the cervical spine is sustained for a short period of time (Figure 7-72).

(2) *Elbow Lifting Traction*: Ask the patient to sit. The physician stands behind the patient. Support the chin with elbow flexed, hold the contralateral side face with the palm to

enhance the stability, and support the occipital area of the patient to help enhance the application of power. Then, use both hands to coordinate the physical power, pull the patient's head slowly upward to maintain continuous traction to the cervical vertebra for between one to three minutes (Figure 7-73).

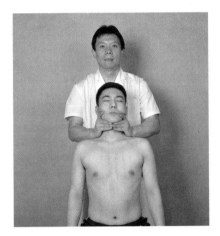

Figure 7-72 Palm Lifting Traction

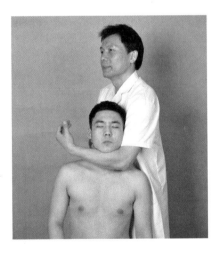

Figure 7-73 Elbow Lifting Traction

(3) *Supine Traction*: Ask the patient to lie supine. The physician sits beside of the patient's head. Support the occiput with one hand and the chin with the other. Coordinate the power of both arms, and pull the patient's head slowly. The traction time to the cervical spine can be determined according to the condition of the disease (Figure 7-74).

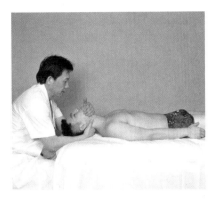

Figure 7-74 Supine Traction

2. Shoulder Traction There are three styles of arm raising traction, confrontational traction, hand-pulling and foot-pushing traction for shoulders.

(1) Arm Raising Shoulder Traction: Ask the patient to sit with arms naturally hanging. The physician stands on posterolateral side of the affected limb, holds the forearm using one hand, and raises the arm to the maximum extent. Then, with both hands holding the distal forearm, coordinate the effort of both hands and pull the patient's arm up slowly, continue the traction of the shoulder (Figure 7-75).

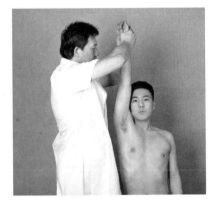

Figure 7-75 Arm Raising Shoulder Traction

(2) Confrontational Shoulder Traction: Ask the patient to sit with the upper limb relaxed. The physician stands or sits facing the affected side of the patient. First guide the affected side to be at abduction position at about 90°, hold his/her wrist or elbow with

both hands, and pull it with gradually increased force. At the same time, instruct the patient to tilt to the opposite side, or ask an assistant to help stabilize the patient's body, so that the force is against the traction (Figure 7-76).

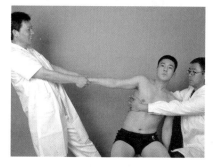

Figure 7-76   Confrontational Shoulder Traction

(3) Hand-Pulling and Foot-Pushing Shoulder Traction: The patient is in the supine position. The physician stands or sits on the affected side facing the patient's head, uses a heel or flexed knee under the armpit of the patient to stabilize the patient's body, and holds the wrist or forearm of the affected side with both hands. Then, pull it downwards slowly, while the heel or pushes hard against the armpit to confront the pulling power. Thus, the hand and leg coordinate to maintain continuous traction for one to two minutes. Then gradually perform passive adduction and internal rotation of the upper limb (Figure 7-77).

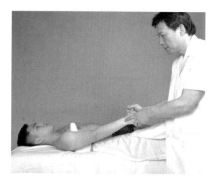

Figure 7-77   Hand-Pulling and Foot-Pushing Shoulder Traction

3. Wrist Traction   Instruct the patient to sit. Stand or sit anterolateral to the patient's affected side. Hold the lower end of the patient's forearm with one hand, and the palm with the other hand. Pull in the opposite direction with both hands at the same time (Figure 7-78). Alternatively, ask the patient to sit with the upper limb relaxed. Sit beside the patient, with both hands holding the patient's affected palm, lift the limb to perform passive abduction to about 60°, and stabilize the patient with the heel under his armpit and apply pressure. At the same time, have both hands pull the patient's wrist. A third method is to ask the patient to sit. Stand anterolateral to the patient's affected side with both hands holding the patient's palm, instruct the body to lean to the other side, or ask an assistant to help stabilize the patient's upper body for sustained traction.

4. Metacarpophalangeal and Interphalangeal Traction   Hold the distal and proximal metacarpophalangeal joint of the patient, slowly apply power, and pull towards both ends (Figure 7-79). If the same method is used to both ends of the interphalangeal joints, then it is called interphalangeal traction.

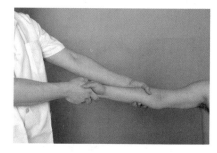

Figure 7-78   Wrist Traction

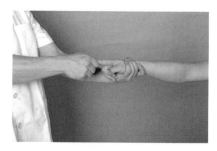

Figure 7-79   Metacarpophalangeal and Interphalangeal Traction

5. Lumbar Traction   Ask the patient to lie in the prone position, and hold the end of the treatment table tightly. Ask an assistant to stand beside the patient's head, with both hands clamping each armpit to stabilize the patient's body. The physician stands at the patient's feet, uses both hands to hold the patient's ankles, gradually pull them backwards, and continues the traction for one to three minutes (Figure 7-80). During the operation, the physician's torso should be leaning backwards to enhance the power of traction.

6. Ankle Traction   Ask the patient to lie supine with lower extremities in natural extension position. The doctor stands at the aspect of the patient's feet with one hand holding the sole of the affected side, the other hand holding his heel. Apply the power of both hands together to perform traction to the affected lower limb (Figure 7-81). It can also be performed with an assistant's hand holding the lower calf of the patient to create pulling opposite of that of the doctor. During the process, coordinate with passive ankle flexion and extension.

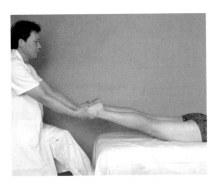

Figure 7-80   Lumbar Traction

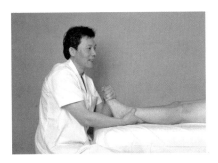

Figure 7-81   Ankle Traction

Requirements and Precautions

1. The power of traction should start gently and gradually increase. The traction should remain steady for a period of time.

2. Traction should be performed using proper strength and with appropriate direction according to the patient's specific physical and disease condition.

3. The action of traction should be steady and slow, the strength applied should be even and sustained. Avoid sudden and violent traction.

4. While performing joint reduction, traction should be avoided when there is severe joint pain and spasm, so that failure of the maneuver and increased pain can be avoided.

Applicable Areas: Traction is applicable to all body joints.

Effects and Indications: Traction has many benefits, including soothing tendons, invigorating blood, resolving spasm, relieving pain, releasing adhesions, rectifying tendons, joint reduction, and benefiting the joints.

Chapter **Eight**

Practice of *Tuina* Maneuvers for Adults

It is important to master *tuina* maneuvers in terms of sophisticated manual technique and continuous strength through diligent study in addition to clinical practice. In particular, some maneuvers that are more complex with high degree of difficulty, such as the thumb pushing and rolling, will take a long time and repeated practice to reach a level of therapeutic effect. The practice includes the training of the technique itself, and strength of the finger, wrist, and arm. The focus is how sophisticated the clinician is mastering each *tuina* technique. Therefore, the preclinical training is divided into two stages in order to making gradual, yet steady progress. The first stage is to use sandbags for basic training. Next, when a foundation of understanding has been developed, one can start operating on human body. In addition, strength exercise, including gentle power, sustaining power and strong power, can be achieved through a variety of internal practicing exercises, such as the classic sinew transformation exercise (*Yì Jīn Jīng*, 易筋经), Shaolin internal breathing exercise, grabbing jars, grasping sandbags, and pushing balls in water.

I. Practice Using Sandbags

Prepare a cloth bag that is about 26cm long, and 16cm wide, and fill it with sand or rice. Add some pieces of broken sponge, since the sponge pieces add some elasticity. It is also a good idea to have a slightly bigger bag as the cover, which makes it easier to replace the outside bag, rather than bag itself. At the initial stage, the bag can be tied tightly, and gradually loosened according to

the essentials of each action and level of difficulty, focusing on maneuvers such as thumb pushing, rolling, kneading, and rubbing. The posture for practicing can be sitting or standing. Thumb pushing, kneading and rubbing can be practiced while sitting, and rolling can be practiced while standing. Except that thumb pushing should be practiced for both thumbs, other maneuvers such as kneading and rubbing should be practiced with the right hand. The practice of rolling requires the use of left and right hands alternately, and the same level of proficiency to satisfy clinical needs. Only when the students have mastered the essentials of these maneuvers can they turn to practice on the human body.

II. Practice on Human Body

Practicing on the human body sets the foundation for clinical application. Therefore, the students should try their best to follow the general operational standards with a clinical mindset, while practicing on different body areas. Students need to pay attention not only to practicing the maneuvers single-handed, but also the coordination and cooperation of both hands when applying different maneuvers. At the same time, passive movements should often be combined while taking body's shape, structure and the functional action of joints into consideration. The following describes the practicing method while operating on human body.

1. Head and face

(1) *Thumb Pushing* (in the supine or sitting position)

① *Yìn táng* (EX-HN 3, 印堂) to *shén tíng* (DU 24, 神庭): Use the pad or lateral side of the thumb to perform thumb pushing from *yìn táng* (EX-HN 3) to *shén tíng* (DU 24), back and forth 3 times.

② *Cuán zhú* (BL 2, 攒竹) to *tóu wéi* (ST 8, 头维): Use the lateral side of thumb to push from *cuán zhú* (BL 2), move to *yáng bái* (GB 14, 阳白) and *tài yáng* (EX-HN 5, 太阳), and reach *tóu wéi* (ST 8). Perform this procedure back and forth three times.

③ *Jīng míng* (BL 1, 睛明): Start from the left *jīng míng* (BL 1), push along the superior orbit from the inner canthus to the outer canthus. Then, push along the inferior orbit from the outer canthus to the inner canthus, and continue to the right *jīng míng* (BL 1). The route of thumb pushing is "∞" shaped, and it should be performed for three times.

④ *Jīng míng* (BL 1) to *chéng jiāng* (RN 24, 承浆): Use the lateral side or the pulp of the thumb, push from *jīng míng* (BL 1), move to *yíng xiāng* (LI 20, 迎香), *dì cāng* (ST 4, 地仓) and *xià guān* (ST 7, 下关), push down to *jiá chē* (ST 6, 颊车), transverse to *shuǐ gōu* (DU 26, 水沟), circle around the lips, and end at *chéng jiāng* (RN 24). The procedure is the same on both sides.

⑤ Push *bǎi huì* (DU 20, 百会): Use the lateral side or the pad of the thumb to perform thumb pushing on *bǎi huì* (DU 20). The thumb needs to focus firmly on the acupoint to avoid slipping and deviation.

(2) *Grasping the five meridians:* Place the five fingers on points along the frontal hairline of the *du mai* (Governing Vessel) and both sides of bladder and gallbladder meridians, that is, a total of five meridians. Push towards the back of the head until the occipital region, and ends on both sides, level with the left and right *fēng chí* (GB 20, 风池).

(3) *Sweep scattering:* Ask the patient to sit. Use the tip of the thumb and other four fingers to push from *tài yáng* (EX-HN 5), move to *tóu wéi* (ST 8) and the mastoid process, and end at *fēng chí* (GB 20). Perform the procedure three to five times.

(4) *Palmar smearing:* Ask the patient to be seated. Use the lateral margin of both the thenar eminences to press firmly on the forehead, then push from the center to the side, move to *yáng bái* (GB 14, 阳白), *tài yáng* (EX-

HN 5), above the ears, go up and end at *fēng chí* (GB 20).

2. Neck and Back

(1) *Thumb Pushing* (in a sitting position)

① Push up and down three to five times from the area under the occipital bone, move to *fēng chí* (GB 20) of both sides, and end at *dà zhuī* (DU 14).

② Place the lateral edges of both thumbs firmly on both *fēng chí* (GB 20) respectively. Use what is called "paired butterfly flying" thumb pushing with both hands working at the same time. Push up and down three to five times from *fēng chí* (GB 20), move to *tiān zhù* (BL 10, 天柱), and reach *dà zhù* (BL 11, 大杼).

(2) *Straight Thumb Pushing on Qiáo Gōng* (in a sitting position)

While working on left *qiáo gōng* (bridge arch, 桥弓), one must use the right hand. With the four fingers press firmly on the neck, and the lateral edge of the thumb to push one way from *yì fēng* (SJ 17, 翳风) to *quē pén* (ST 12, 缺盆) 10 to 20 times.

(3) Rolling: Ask the patient to sit. Apply the rolling maneuver from the region under the occipital bone, move to *fēng fǔ* (DU 16, 风府), *dà zhuī* (DU 14), *jiān zhōng shù* (SI 15, 肩中俞), and end at *jiān wài shù* (SI 14, 肩外俞). At the same time, combine with the passive movements of flexion, extension, left and right rotation, and lateral flexion of the neck.

(4) *Grasping* (in a sitting position)

① Grasping both sides of *fēng chí* (GB 20) with one hand five to 10 times.

② Grasping both sides of *jiān jǐng* (GB 21, 肩井) eight to 10 times.

(5) *Pressing* (in a sitting position): Use the pulp of the thumb to press *fēng chí* (GB 20), *jiān zhōng shù* (SI 15), *jiān wài shù* (SI 14) and *tiān zōng* (SI 11, 天宗).

(6) *Rotation* (in a sitting position): Hold the occiput with one hand, and hold under the chin with the other. First have the cervical vertebra in neutral position, then perform passive rotation to the left and right, each for three times.

(7) *Spontaneous Torquing* (in a sitting position): Press one thumb against the spinous process of the cervical vertebra, use the other

hand to hold the patient's head and perform spontaneous rotation torquing. Note this reduction method is only applicable when one cervical spinous process is deviated.

3. Chest and Abdomen

(1) *Thumb Pushing* (in the supine position): Perform thumb pushing on *dàn zhōng* (RN 17, 膻中), *rǔ gēn* (ST 18, 乳根), *shàng wǎn* (RN 13, 上脘), *zhōng wǎn* (RN 12, 中脘), *tiān shū* (ST 25, 天枢) and *qì hǎi* (RN 6, 气海) using the lateral tip or pad of the thumb.

(2) *Bilateral Outward-pushing*: (in a supine position). Use the lateral tips of both thumbs to perform bilateral outward-pushing from *dàn zhōng* (RN 17) to the edge of the two nipples.

(3) *Scrubbing* (in a sitting position): Use the whole palm to perform scrubbing three to five times from the region right under the clavicles horizontally, and gradually move down to *dàn zhōng* (RN 17), both *rǔ gēn* (ST 18), and *jiū wěi* (RN 15, 鸠尾).

(4) *Foulage* (in a sitting position): Clamp the hypochondriac regions with the four fingers and palms and perform foulage top to bottom three to five times.

(5) *Rubbing* (in the supine position)

① Rubbing *dàn zhōng* (RN 17) with the index, middle and ring fingers.

② Rubbing *zhōng wǎn* (RN 12), *tiān shū* (ST 25), *qì hǎi* (RN 6) and the abdomen with the index, middle and ring fingers, or the whole palm in circular motion, both clockwise or counterclockwise.

(6) *Pushing Rubbing* (compound maneuver, take a supine position): Use the lateral tip of the thumb to perform thumb pushing on *zhōng wǎn* (RN 12), *tiān shū* (ST 25) and *qì hǎi* (RN 6), and the index, middle and ring fingers to perform rubbing on these acupoints. Alternatively, perform the three-finger rubbing first and thumb pushing second to the same acupoints.

(7) *Kneading* (in the supine position): Use the pad of the middle finger to perform kneading on *tiān tū* (RN 22, 天突), *dàn zhōng* (RN 17), *zhōng wǎn* (RN 12), and *shén què* (RN 8, 神阙), 50 to 300 times for each acupoint.

(8) *Pressing* (in the supine position): Press *zhōng wǎn* (RN 12), *qì hǎi* (RN 6) and *zú sān lǐ* (ST 36, 足三里) with the tip or pad of the thumb. It is better to obtain the *de-qi* sensation during the maneuver.

4. Shoulder and Upper Limbs

(1) *Thumb Pushing* (in a sitting position)

① Perform thumb pushing in the order of *jiān yú* (LI 15, 肩髃), *jiān nèi líng* (EX-UE 12, 肩内陵), *bì nào* (LI 14, 臂臑), *qū chí* (LI 11, 曲池), and *shǒu sān lǐ* (LI 10, 手三里).

② Perform thumb pushing in the order of *jiān jǐng* (GB 21, 肩井), *jiān liáo* (SJ 14, 肩髎), *jiān zhēn* (SI 9, 肩贞), and *tiān zōng* (SI 11).

(2) *Rolling* (in a sitting or lying position)

① The performance of rolling at the anterior margin of the shoulder can be combined with passive movements of the shoulder including internal rotation, external rotation, and abduction.

② The performance of rolling at the lateral margin of the shoulder, can be combined with passive movements of the shoulder including internal rotation, and posterior extension.

③ The performance of rolling at the posterior margin of the shoulder, can be combined with passive shoulder movements including adduction and upward rotation.

④ The performance of rolling on elbow, forearm, wrist and metacarpophalangeal joints can be combined with corresponding passive movements of the joints.

(3) *Pressing* (in a sitting position): Perform pressing on *jiān nèi líng* (EX-UE 12), *jiān yú* (LI 15), *jiān zhēn* (SI 9), *tiān zōng* (SI 11), *bì nào* (LI 14), and *qū chí* (LI 11) with the pad of the thumb and obtain a sense of *de-qi*.

(4) *Grasping* (in a sitting position): Perform grasping to the shoulder and on *qū chí* (LI 11), *hé gǔ* (LI 4, 合谷), *jí quán* (HT 1, 极泉), and *shào hǎi* (HT 3, 少海).

(5) *Twirling* (in a sitting position): Twirling is performed to the interphalangeal joints.

(6) *Rotation* (in a sitting position)

① Hold the shoulder with one hand, support the elbow with the other, and perform rotation to the shoulder clockwise and counterclockwise, three to five times in each direction.

② Perform rotation to the shoulder with a wide range of motion, clockwise and counterclockwise, three to five times in each direction.

(7) *Foulage* (in a sitting position): Hold the shoulder with both palms, perform foulage in circular motion, gradually move down to the arm without pause, change to up and down foulage to the wrist.

(8) *Shaking* (in a sitting position): Hold the wrist with both hands, perform slow shaking from wrist up to elbow and shoulder.

(9) *Scrubbing* (in a sitting position): Ask the patient to expose the affected shoulder, elbow, arm, wrist, palm and fingers, and perform the thenar eminence scrubbing method until each area being treated feels the heat.

5. Lumbar Area and Lower Limbs

(1) *Rolling* (in the prone position)

① Perform rolling on the back, lumbar and sacral regions along both sides of the spine, in combination with passive lumbar and hip extension

② Perform rolling from the hip, posterior aspect of the thigh, popliteal fossa, gastrocnemius, and the Achilles tendon back and forth for three times, same for the left and right side.

③ Ask the patient to change to a supine position. Perform rolling on the inguinal region, adductor muscle of the thigh, quadriceps, knee, anterolateral aspect of the shin, ankle, and dorsal aspect of the foot.

(2) *Pressing* (in the prone and supine position): Perform pressing to the acupoints on the back and lumbar region, including *pí shù*

(BL 20, 脾俞), *wèi shù* (BL 21, 胃俞), *shèn shù* (BL 23, 肾俞), *dà cháng shù* (BL 25, 大肠俞), *shàng liáo* (BL 31, 上髎), *cì liáo* (BL 32, 次髎), *huán tiào* (GB 30, 环跳), *yīn mén* (BL 37, 殷门), *wěi zhōng* (BL 40, 委中), *chéng shān* (BL 57, 承山), *kūn lún* (BL 60, 昆仑), *tài xī* (KI 3, 太溪), *qiū xū* (GB 40, 丘墟), *shāng qiū* (SP 5, 商丘), and *zú sān lǐ* (ST 36).

(3) *Scrubbing* (in a sitting position)

① Use horizontal scrubbing to work from the shoulder and back, and gradually travel down to the lumbosacral areas for three to five times.

② Perform straight scrubbing along the spine and sacrospinalis on both sides until a heat sensation is thoroughly felt in the region.

③ In the supine position, perform scrubbing on the medial and lateral aspects of the knee.

④ Also in the supine position, perform scrubbing on the medial and lateral aspects of the ankle.

(4) *Rotation* (in the supine position): Perform rotation to the hip joint, the knee and ankle.

(5) *Spontaneous Torquing*

① Perform the spontaneous oblique lumbar torquing method in lateral position; first left, then right.

② Perform the lumbar rotation and spontaneous torquing in a sitting position.

③ Perform the straight leg raise test in the supine position.

Chapter **Nine**

Application of *Tuina* in Common Adult Diseases

Section One　Locomotor Diseases

I. Neck Pain

(I) Cervical Spondylosis

Cervical spondylosis is due to degenerative changes of the cervical spine, joints, joint capsules, ligaments, and discs, causing cervical instability, bone hyperplasia, hypertrophy of the ligaments and joint capsules, or calcification. Such pathological changes stimulate or oppress the nerve root, vertebral artery, spinal cord, or sympathetic nerve, resulting in a series of symptoms that are also known as cervical degenerative disease and cervical syndrome. Depending on what tissue is damaged, types of cervical spondylopathy include nerve root type, vertebral artery type, cervical spondylotic myelopathy, sympathetic type and mixed type.

> *Note:*
>
> Previous to studying the chapter, it is recommended that you review the knowledge of local anatomy, physiology, pathology of the cervical vertebrae and maneuvers of joint movements.

▶ Diagnosis

1. Clinical Symptoms

(1) *Nerve Root Type of Cervical Spondylosis*

A. Neck and shoulder discomfort accompanied by pain or numbness in the upper limbs, often spreading to the fingers. The pain manifests as dull pain, soreness, distended pain, ambiguous pain, or radiating pain. The symptoms become worse in case of exhaustion or stiff neck.

B. Symptoms of dizziness, heaviness of the head, neck soreness, and feeling of oppression on the back may also occur.

C. Neck activity is limited, muscle spasm of the neck, and tilted head can be seen. Muscle atrophy may appear in patients with a long-term chronic condition .

D. There may be disorders of autonomic vascular nutrition and dysfunction with manifestations such as upper extremities feeling cold or hot, blushing, pale complexion, cyanosis or swelling. The nails can be deformed, brittle and lacking luster.

(2) *Vertebral Artery Type of Cervical Spondylosis*

A. Cervical dizziness: Dizziness that happens when the head is at a particular angle, is known as positional vertigo. The occurrence is episodic, and intermittent. The patient can experience feelings of spinning, floating, or rocking, and the lower limbs can be weak and unstable, with feelings of ground movement, often accompanied by symptoms such as diplopia, nystagmus, tinnitus, deafness, nausea , and vomiting.

B. Cataplexy: Cataplexy can occur while doing neck activities, or when the dizziness is severe, with symptoms such as sudden numbness of the four limbs, weakness and falling. At the same time, the patient is conscious, and normally able to get up.

C. Headache: Headaches are mostly paroxysmal and can last several minutes, hours, and even days. The pain, usually throbbing or distending, is often located in the occipital, occipitoparietal, and temporal areas. Pain may radiate to the posterior aspect of the ear, face, teeth, occipitoparietal and even the eye area. The headache may also be the result of insufficient blood supply of the vertebrobasilar artery and collateral vessel dilatation.

D. Ocular symptoms: Blurred vision, diplopia, visual hallucinations, blindness and other visual impairment is possible with cervical spondylosis. Visual symptoms are related to the symptoms of the neck, especially when there is neck movement and eye discomfort occurs.

E. There may be paralysis and other symptoms associated with the cranial nerves such as unclear language, difficult swallowing, disappearance of pharyngeal reflex, choking while drinking water, soft palate paralysis, and hoarseness. Facial paralysis, limb paralysis, and balance disorders may also manifest.

F. Paresthesia: There may be facial, circumoral, and glossal numbness, and numbness of the four limbs or one side of the body. Some parastetic pain can have pricking pain, formication (sensation of insects crawling on the skin), and deep sensory disturbances.

G. Neck muscle spasm, tenderness, restricted neck movement, and spinous process deviation.

(3) *Spinal Cord Type of Cervical Spondylosis*
A. Initially, symptoms such as unilateral or bilateral numbness, and drowsiness, appear on the lower extremities, followed by walking difficulties, and instability.

B. Later, symptoms of the torso emerge, including sensory dysfunction below the second to fourth rib, and tightness of the chest, abdomen and pelvis.

C. Finally, upper extremity symptoms occur, including unilateral or bilateral numbness, pain, weakness. Failure to do fine movements of the upper limbs can occur, and even to the point that patients are unable to feed themselves.

D. Limitation in neck extension or flexion, spinous process tenderness, and paraspinal muscle tenderness.

(4) *Sympathetic Cervical Spondylosis*
A. *Sympathetic Excitement Type*: Headache, dizziness, increased eye fissure, blurred vision, mydriasis, increased heart rate and blood pressure, arrhythmia, precordial pain, vasospasm of the limbs, coldness of the limbs, decreased local temperature, profuse sweating, and tinnitus.

B. *Vagus Excitement Type*: Headache, dizziness, tearing, stuffy nose, decreased heart rate and blood pressure, increased gastrointestinal motility or belching. Horner's syndrome, marked by ipsilateral ptosis, miosis and anhidrosis, would appear.

(5) Mixed Type of Cervical Spondylosis: Cervical spondylosis mixed clinical signs and symptoms of two or more types.

2. Clinical Signs
(1) *Nerve Root Type of Cervical Spondylosis*
A. Decreased biceps tendon reflex.
B. Positive foraminal compression test.
C. Positive brachial plexus traction test.
(2) *Vertebral Artery Type of Cervical Spondylosis*: Cervical torsion test is positive.
(3) *Spinal Cord Type of Cervical Spondylosis*
A. Positive Hoffmann's sign.
B. Positive Babinski's sign.

Note:

Orthopedic disorders and physical traumas require not only diagnostic imaging of the affected skeletal structures and intervertebral discs and surrounding tissues but also functional performance testing must be evaluated. This includes testing the impairment of the spinal column and the joints of the four limbs. Damage to soft tissue often results in decreased stability of skeletal structures and joints. Functional performance assessment of joint integrity includes mobility, gait, locomotion and balance, axial tilt and trunk rotation, to name a few. Clinically, many problems are not caused by osteoproliferation but by soft tissue conditions and unstableness of bone structures and joints; therefore, an orthopedic diagnosis cannot be made with medical imaging alone.

3. Examinations

(1) X-ray examination shows joint hyperplasia on the posterior aspect of the vertebral body or the lateral aspect of the uncovertebral joint that correspond to the clinical manifestations and examination;

(2) CT or MRI are showing deformity of spinal cord due to the compression;

(3) Vertebral Artery Angiography or MRA shows visible vertebral artery distortion, and deformity.

▶ Treatment

1. Treatment Principles Soothing tendons, invigorating blood, dissolving spasm, relieving pain, and dislocation reduction.

2. Maneuvers Rolling, press-kneading, grasping, traction, plucking, traction-shaking, et cetera.

3. Operation

(1) Ask the patient to sit, and stand behind him/her. And performs press-kneading on both sides of *fēng chí* (GB 20) with the pads of the thumb and index fingers respectively.

(2) Use the pads of the thumb, forefinger and middle finger to perform grasping to the soft tissue of the neck symmetrically, starting from *fēng chí* (GB 20) and working down to the bottom of the neck.

(3) Apply rolling to relax the patient's muscles of the neck, shoulder, upper back and upper limbs.

(4) Hold the patient on both sides of *jiān jǐng* (GB 21) and kneading the affected limbs, mainly biceps and triceps.

(5) Plucking the subaxillary branches of the brachial plexus with several fingers horizontally.

> *Note:*
> It is an appropriate manipulation to make the patient experience a radiating numbness in his/her fingers.

(6) The physician places both forearms on top of the patient's shoulders, presses downward with appropriate power, and uses the thumb to press the region above *fēng chí* (GB 20) on both sides. Next, use the other four fingers and palms to support the mandible, instruct the patient to sink, and apply the power upwards. At the same time, the forearms and hands should use power towards opposite directions, so that traction is applied to the neck. Simultaneously, perform passive flexion, extension and rotation to the neck.

(7) Apply traction-shaking to the upper limbs to end the procedure.

▶ Prognosis

Relapse of the disease is common, herefore, instruct the patient to rest well, keep warm, and avoid prolonged office work and neck trauma. Moreover, make functional exercises of the neck a daily routine, pay attention to sleeping position, avoid pillows that are too full or too thin. Patients with vertebral artery type of cervical spondylosis should not seek employment as such as drivers, electricians, high altitude workers, or underwater workers.

▶ Exercise Methods

Neck Rotation: ① The patient stands upright, legs straight and apart at shoulder width, hands at the side, and eyes looking straight; ② Turn the head to the left side to its maximum extent, pause for five seconds, and return to the neutral position; ③ Turn the head to the right side to its maximum extent, pause for five seconds, and return to the neutral position. Perform the procedure six times daily.

(II) Stiff Neck (*lào zhěn*)

Stiff neck, also known as "fall off from the pillow", is one of the common neck soft tissue injuries, often seen in young adults, with a higher incidence rate in winter and spring. Clinically, the main symptoms include acute neck muscle spasm, rigidity, soreness, and pain, so that the neck is unable to rotate. In mild cases, the symptoms may disappear in four to five days. Patients with severe pain that radiating to the head, back and upper extremities, however, may get no relief from pain for a few weeks. The use of *tuina* is normally very effective and produces rapid results

▶ Diagnosis

1. Clinical Symptoms
(1) Neck pain that increases with physical activity.
(2) Neck movements, such as left and right rotation, left and right lateral flexion, forward flexion and backward extension, are significantly limited.
(3) The neck is relatively restricted in certain positions. Some patients have to support the neck with one hand to reduce neck activity, and relieve symptoms.
2. Clinical Signs   Increased muscle tension and tenderness can be palpated at the sternocleidomastoid, trapezius, levator scapula or lateral ⅓ of the clavicular region, *jiān jǐng* (GB 21), or the medial edge or the medial upper corner of the scapula.
3. Examination   Before treating this condition, rule out diseases such as cervical spondylosis, and cervical subluxation. If necessary, refer out for a cervical X-ray.

▶ Treatment

1. Treatment Principles   Soothing tendons, invigorating blood, warming meridians, unblocking collaterals, rectifying muscles and tendons.
2. Maneuvers   Rolling, pressing, kneading, grasping, traction, and scrubbing.
3. Operation
(1) Ask the patient to sit, and stand behind him/her. Apply soft rolling on the affected side of the neck and shoulder for three to five minutes.
(2) Perform lift-grasping in the soft tissue 1.5 cun lateral from the cervical spine, focus especially on the affected region, and perform plucking on tight muscles to gradually loosen them up.
(3) Ask the patient to naturally relax the neck muscles. The physician holds the patient's mandible with the left hand, and supports the occiput with the right hand, so that the patient's neck is in slight forward flexion position with mandible in adduction position. Lift both hands up at the same time, and

slowly rotate the patient's head left and right for about 10 to 15 times to move the cervical facet joints.
(4) Perform press-kneading *fēng chí* (GB 20), *fēng fǔ* (DU 16, 风府), *fēng mén* (BL 12, 风门), *jiān jǐng* (GB 21), *tiān zōng* (SI 11, 天宗), and *jiān wài shù* (SI 14), each point for 30 seconds with the power gradually increasing from gentle to heavy.
(5) Apply scrubbing on the affected area as the ending maneuver.

▶ Prognosis

To prevent relapse, it is necessary to do functional exercise strengthening the back, and actively participate in sports such as light gymnastics, and *tai chi* to enhance the strength of the neck and the overall physique. Moreover, avoid catching cold.

II. Shoulder Pain

(I) Frozen Shoulder

Shoulder periarthritis is due to extensive adhesions on the shoulder, characterized by wide range of pain and dysfunction. The disease has a few alternative names in Chinese. Since it occurs more often among people over the age of 50, one of the names literally means "50's Shoulder". Due to limited shoulder movements, as if it is frozen or solidified, it is also known as "frozen shoulder" or "shoulder solidifying disease". Moverover, because patients often feel that cold air is entering the shoulder, it is also known as "leaking wind shoulder". It affects more women than men, and is more common on the left side.

▶ Diagnosis

1. Clinical Symptoms
(1) *Shoulder pain*: The pain is characterized by extensive pain in the shoulder that is aggravated at night, and with traction or impact. In patients with severe pain, it may radiate to the upper limbs and ears.
(2) *Restricted motor function of the shoulder*: Frozen shoulder normally involves extensive range of movement limitations, and both active and passive movement limitation of the shoulder joint.

2. Clinical Signs

(1) Widespread tenderness around the shoulder joint that is often located at coracoid process, greater tubercle, lesser tubercle, intertubercular groove, acromion, deltoid insertions, supraspinatus, infraspinatus, teres minor, and scapula levator.

(2) Muscle atrophy: Due to long-term adhesions in the shoulder, resulting in limited function, it is not unusual to see muscle atrophy in chronic cases. Muscle atrophy is especially obvious in the deltoid and supraspinatus.

3. Examination

(1) X-ray examination: osteoporosis, supraspinatus tendon calcification, widened or narrowed joint, and shadow indicating increased density of the greater tubercle may appear at late stage.

(2) MRI or CT examination is valuable for evaluating lesions of rotator cuff and other soft tissue.

▶ Treatment

1. Treatment Principles   Unblocking the meridians and collaterals, invigorating blood, and relieving pain. In later stage, loosening the adhesion, smoothing the joints and promoting the recovery of joint function.

2. Maneuvers   Rolling, precision pressing, rotation, shaking, and kneading method.

3. Operation

(1) Ask the patient to be seated. The doctor stands at the posterolateral aspects of the patient's ipsilateral side. Clamp the affected upper limb with the forearm and body side, and perform deep and wide-range rolling on the anterior, superior and posterior regions of the shoulder.

(2) Apply precision pressing on the coronoid process, acromion, greater tubercle, lesser tubercle, intertubercular groove, deltoid ending, *bǐng fēng* (SI 12, 秉风), *tiān zōng* (SI 11), *jiān zhēn* (SI 9, 肩贞), *hé gǔ* (LI 4, 合谷), *hòu xī* (SI 3, 后溪), and *zhōng zhǔ* (SJ 3, 中渚) with the thumb, forefinger or middle fingers.

(3) The patient remains seated. Stand at the affected side of the patient, apply rotation to the shoulder.

(4) Stand on the affected side of the patient, and hold the patient's fingers with both hands. First, perform passive abduction to the upper limb of the affected side. Then, apply traction and combine with even and fast shaking up and down with small range.

(5) Place both hands to the anterior and posterior aspects of the affected shoulder, and apply kneading in circular motion.

▶ Prognosis

To some extent, the disease is self-healing, although recovery can take anywhere from eight months to two years. Patients should keep the shoulder warm, avoid direct blowing of cold-wind, and reduce bearing weight. In addition to active treatment, patients need to keep doing functional exercises, which is beneficial to speed up the recovery of the shoulder area from inflammation and reduce the incidence of sequelae.

▶ Exercise Method

(1) Bend forward and shake the shoulders: Start in standing position, bend forward, and stretch the arms. Perform shoulder rotations, and gradually increase the range from small to large, and slow to fast.

(2) Wall stretching: In standing position, face the wall. Use both hands or the affected shoulder to reach up and stretch the arm to the highest point on the wall that the patient can reach. Recover and repeat. Gradually increase the daily limit.

(3) Stretch from the back: In a standing position, have both hands placed on the back of the body. Use the contralateral hand to grab the wrist of the ipsilateral limb, pull it gradually upward and toward the contralateral side to its maximum. Slowly relax and repeat.

(4) Hand swing: In standing position, relax shoulder, and swing the upper limb vigorously to make the shoulder joint do passive flexion, extension, adduction, and abduction, with the movement range from small to large until its maximum.

(5) Exercise using pulley: Fix a pulley to the ceiling and feed a rope through the pulley. Standing immediately below the pulley, the patient should grab each end of the rope with both hands alternately. The contralateral side of the hand should pull harder in order

to passively pull the affected shoulder up.

(II) Subacromial Bursitis

Subacromial bursa, also known as the sub-deltoid bursa, is one of the largest bursae in the body and is located below the acromion, the coracoacromial ligament, and the deep fascia of the deltoid, above the rotator cuff and greater humeral tuberosity. Subacromial bursitis is the condition with main symptoms include pain and limited mobility of the shoulder caused by irritation and inflammation of the subacromial sac as the result of acute and chronic shoulder injury.

▶ Diagnosis

1. Clinical Symptoms
(1) Shoulder pain: The pain increases gradually, and is generally worse at night. The pain also intensifies in abduction and external rotation position, so the patient often holds the shoulder in adduction and internal rotation position. The pain is located deep in the shoulder joint involving the ending of the deltoid point, which may also radiate to the scapula, neck, and hands.
(2) Limited shoulder function: In the early stage, shoulder pain can make the patient avoid active shoulder movement. Passive movement, however, is not limited. As the disease progresses with thickening of the bursa wall and tissue adhesion, the range of motion of the shoulder gradually reduces. In the later stage, it can complicate with shoulder periarthritis.
(3) Muscle atrophy may occur over time.
2. Clinical Signs   Tenderness can be found in the area below the deltoid, acromion, and the greater tubercle, which moves around along with the rotation of the humerus. When there is synovial swelling and effusion, tenderness is found around the shoulder joint and in the deltoid area.
3. Examination   X-ray examination can detect calcareous infarct of the supraspinatus.

▶ Treatment

1. Treatment Principles   Invigorating blood, dissolving stasis, resolving swelling, relieving pain, and smoothening and benefit-ing the joints.
2. Maneuvers   Rolling, precision pressing, kneading, plucking, grasping, and rotation.
3. Operation
(1) Ask the patient to be seated. The physician stands at the posterolateral aspect of the patient's ipsilateral side. Use the forearm and lateral side of the body to clamp the patient's ipsilateral limb, and perform a wide range of deep rolling with the other hand on the affected shoulder.
(2) Perform precision pressing with the index finger, middle finger or thumb on the coracoid process, acromion, the greater and lesser tubercles, intertubercular groove, deltoid ending, *bǐng fēng* (SI 12, 秉风), *tiān zōng* (SI 11), and *jiān zhēn* (SI 9).
(3) Apply plucking on the acromion, the greater and lesser tubercles, the intertubercular groove, and the deltoid ending.
(4) Ask the patient to be seated. The doctor should stand lateral to the affected side of the patient, and perform shoulder rotation.
(5) Perform five-finger grasping on the lateral side and superior aspect of the shoulder, and the supraspinatus.

▶ Prognosis

In general, the prognosis is good after the treatment. Ask patients in acute stage to reduce shoulder movements in order to have the damaged tissue repaired. Encourage the patients to do functional exercise after the pain and swelling relieved.

(III) Biceps Tenosynovitis

Biceps tenosynovitis is an inflammation of the biceps tendon sheath. Long-term friction between the biceps long head and its tendon sheath, or excessive shoulder activity causes congestion, edema, and thickening of the tendon sheath, further resulting in adhesion and tendon degeneration. Thus, the disease occurs more commonly among athletes involved in sports such as throwing, gymnastic rings, horizontal bars, weightlifting, and volleyball. For middle-aged people suffering the disease, if it is not treated in time, it often triggers frozen shoulder.

▶ Diagnosis

1. Clinical Symptoms

(1) *Anterior shoulder pain*: Severe pain in acute stage, which gets worse at night. The pain can radiate to underneath the deltoid muscle. In the chronic phase, the shoulder experiences soreness.

(2) Limited shoulder flexion, and abduction.

2. Clinical Signs

(1) Tenderness on the intertubercular groove, sometimes its posterior region as well.

(2) Biceps long head tension test is positive.

3. Examination   Anterior posterior X-ray usually does not show obvious abnormalities. If one suspects biceps tenosynovitis, the routine X-ray should be the tangential projection of the bicipital groove. Some patients can have narrowing and shallowing of the bicipital groove, or formation of spur at the edge or bottom of the groove.

▶ Treatment

1. Treatment Principles   In the acute stage, the treatment principles should be dissolving blood stasis and swelling, while in the chronic phase, it is appropriate to invigorate blood, dissolve swelling, promote the movement, and warm and unblock the channels.

2. Maneuvers   Rolling, kneading, plucking, rotating, and scrubbing.

3. Operation

(1) The patient takes a sitting position, while the physician stands on the affected side with one hand supporting the affected limb to move it into an abduction position. The other hand should perform kneading at the anterior aspect of the shoulder.

(2) Perform pressing with one thumb at the bicipital groove and plucking left and right to separate the adhesions.

(3) Hold the patient's shoulder with one hand, and the elbow with the other hand, and apply the shoulder rotation maneuver. Focus more while performing rotation in the abduction and external rotation position.

(4) Perform scrubbing around the shoulder until the area feels thoroughly warm.

▶ Prognosis

Tuina is very effective in treating this disease. The maneuvers should be gentle, while the selection of the treatment area should be accurate. In the acute stage, reduce activities involving the affected shoulder. For athletes, it is a good idea to stop training. Among middle-aged and elderly patients, ensure shoulder movement in all directions a few times a day to prevent adhesions.

III. Elbow Pain

(I) Lateral Humeral Epicondylitis

Lateral humeral epicondylitis refers acute or chronic strain with localized pain at the lateral side of the elbow and the supracondylar humerus that affects wrist extension and forearm rotation. It is also known as tennis elbow and blacksmith's elbow. The disease tends to affect people doing labor-intensive work involving excessive use of forearm, such as barber, carpenter, blacksmith and chef. Also, it is commonly seen in tennis, badminton, and table tennis players. In Chinese medicine, it is called "elbow exhaustion", which pertains to the category of tendon damage.

▶ Diagnosis

1. Clinical Symptoms   The pain in the lateral side of the elbow is persistent and gradually increases in severity. The nature of the pain is soreness or tingling. Some patients may have pain that radiates to the forearm, wrist or the upper arm. The pain increases while lifting, pulling, and holding heavy items, or rotating with power (such as twisting a towel). The forearm is often weak due to pain, with weakened grasping power. Rest reduces the pain significantly or can make it disappear. Patients often state that they cannot twist a towel, sweep the floor, or hold an item firmly.

2. Clinical Signs

(1) Lateral elbow tenderness on the humer-

al supracondylar, annular ligaments, or bra-chioradial joint space.

(2) The forearm extensor tendon traction test is positive.

3. Examination   X-ray examination is mostly negative. Sometimes increased bone density is visible at the humeral lateral epicondyle, or there is light calcified plaque around the epicondyle.

▶ Treatment

1. Treatment Principles   Soothing sinews, dispelling stasis, and stretching tendons.

2. Maneuvers   Precision kneading, plucking, rotation, traction, and pushing et cetera.

3. Operation

(1) The physician holds the patient's elbow with one hand, and performs finger kneading on the lateral aspect of the elbow with the thumb of the other hand.

(2) Use the tip of the thumb to apply plucking left and right on tender points.

(3) Press a thumb on the tender point and apply kneading, hold the affected wrist with the other hand, and perform passive forearm pronation and supination.

(4) The physician holds the medial side of the affected elbow with one hand, and the radial side of the wrist with the other hand . Use opposing force to apply traction to the lateral side of the elbow.

(5) With the pad of the thumb, push the lateral side of the elbow up and down.

▶ Prognosis

Tuina is very effective in treating tennis elbow. In the acute phase, avoid violent activities as much as possible, especially the extensor carpius. If it is necessary, splint the elbow properly until the pain is relieved. Then, gradually start function activities of the elbow, but avoid obvious tractions of the wrist extensor muscles.

▶ Exercises

(1) *Forearm extensor extension training*: ① Stand facing the wall with the five fingers of the affected limb naturally hanging; ② Press the dorsal side of the hand against the wall, and then slowly slide the hand and

forearm upward. The stretch tension of the forearm extensor should be more and more obvious; ③ When the tension peaked, maintain this position for about 30 seconds. Then slowly return to the original position. Perform the complete procedure for six to eight times each time, three times a day.

(2) *Muscle strength training*:   ① In a sitting or standing position, lift up the affected limb, keep it level with the shoulder, and straighten the forearm with the wrist naturally hanging; ② Slowly perform wrist flexion and dorsiflexion. As long as the pain is tolerable, keep the palm in flexion or dorsiflexion position for five to eight seconds. Then slowly relax to complete the exercise. Do it six to eight times per session, and three sessions per day.

(II) Olecranon Bursitis

Olecranon bursitis refers to an aseptic inflammation of the olecranon bursa due to acute trauma or chronic strain, characterized by increased bursa swelling and hypertrophic cystic mass at the posterior side of the elbow. Generally, there is no pain or dysfunction. In the past, since the disease was more common in miners, it is also known as "miner's elbow".

▶ Diagnosis

1. Clinical Symptoms

(1) The patient has a clear history of acute trauma or frequent and excessive use of the posterior side of the elbow.

(2) Local swelling, cystic mass can be seen on the olecranon. If the patient suffers acute injury with infection, there will be local swelling and skin redness.

(3) There maybe varying degrees of pain and tenderness on the olecranon.

(4) Elbow movements may be slightly limited. In acute injury, the elbow is often held in semi-extension position.

2. Clinical Signs

(1) Visible hemispherical bulging on the back of the elbow which is more obvious when the elbow is in flexion position.

(2) The cystic mass, mostly between two to four centimeters in size, is soft in texture with smooth surface and clear edge. When it

is pressed, slight fluctuations can be felt with significant tenderness.

3. Examinations   X-ray examination does not detect any abnormal lesions of the elbow, although some may have calcification shadow.

▶ Treatment

1. Treatment Principles   Soothing the tendons, unblocking the collaterals, nvigorating blood, and dispelling stasis.

2. Maneuvers   Press-kneading, grasping, scrubbing, pressing, and passive joint movements.

3. Operations

(1) Hold the elbow in one hand, and apply finger kneading using the thumb of the other hand from the elbow to the wrist on the lateral aspect of the affected limb.

(2) Perform grasping to the whole triceps tendon from top to bottom.

(3) Use the thumb to perform press-kneading on the olecranon, *qū chí* (LI 11), *zhǒu liáo* (LI 12, 肘髎), *tiān jǐng* (SJ 10, 天井), *shǒu sān lǐ* (LI 10, 手三里), and *shào hǎi* (HT 3, 少海).

(4) Use the thumb of one hand to press on the tenderness point and apply kneading, and the other hand to hold the wrist of the patient and perform passive forearm pronation and supination.

(5) Use scrubbing around the elbow and focus more at the triceps, olecranon and ulnar margin of the forearm until these area feels thoroughly warm.

▶ Prognosis

Tuina is very effective in treating olecranon bursitis. During the treatment, once the bursa is broken because of squeezing, apply pressure to the area and dress it. Avoid excessive physical activities involving elbow support that stimulates the elbow. Keep the elbow warm, in order to promote absorption of local inflammation.

IV. Wrist Pain

(I) Carpal Tunnel Syndrome

Carpal tunnel syndrome, also known as delayed median nerve paralysis, is due to compression of the median nerve in the carpal tunnel, causing a series of symptoms, mostly associated with overuse, infection, dislocation, or fracture. Especially with the advancement and popularization of computers, more and more people are prone to the disease due to the long-term improper position or the use of the mouse with excessive involvement of the wrist.

▶ Diagnosis

1. Clinical Symptoms

(1) Persistent numbness and pain, more often of the thumb, the index finger, and the middle finger, that progressively increases at night or after overuse;

(2) Muscle atrophy and weakness of the thenar eminence. In severe cases, the patients are not able to perform movements such as holding, grasping, and twisting.

(3) Disappearance of sensation in index finger, middle finger and the radial side of the thumb.

2. Clinical Signs

(1) The Finkeisten's sign is tested positive.

(2) The wrist flexion test is positive.

(3) The Tinel's sign is positive.

3. Examinations

(1) *X-ray*: To provide a basis for diagnosis of fractures of the wrist and trauma of the surrounding area.

(2) *Angiography*: The positive rate is high. The test is not popular since it is invasive.

(3) *MRI*: It can be used to confirm the degree of compression and degeneration of the median nerve. MRI's examination has a higher accuracy with respect to diagnosis of the condition.

(4) *Ultrasound*: The test result offers a high degree of accuracy, comparable to that of the MRI, and it is easy to operate, affordable, and valuable in early diagnosis.

(5) *Electrophysiological testing*: As the most commonly used examination method, the test is important in diagnosis, differential diagnosis, efficacy evaluation, and identification of surgical indications.

▶ Treatment

1. Treatment Principles   Invigorating

blood, dissolving stasis, soothing tendons, and unblocking the collaterals.

2. Maneuvers   Pressing, kneading, pushing, scrubbing, and traction.

3. Operation

(1) Ask the patient to take a sitting position and place the affected wrist on a cushion with the palmar side up. Sit opposite from the patient, use the thumb to press *wài guān* (SJ 5, 外关), *yáng xī* (LI 5, 阳溪), *yú jì* (LU 10, 鱼际), *hé gǔ* (LI 4) and *ashi* points, each point for one minute.

(2) Use the thumb pad to gently apply press-kneading along the forearm flexor tendon for one minute.

(3) Use both thenar eminences to perform split pushing on the wrist, palm and forearm repeatedly for one minute. Then, with a light and quick scrubbing maneuver applied on the affected side of the wrist until the area feels thoroughly warm.

(4) Hold the affected wrist with both hands and slowly perform stretching to the joint. When the wrist is loosened, continue with passive flexion, dorsiflexion, radial deviation, ulnar deviation, for one minute with the wrist stretched.

▶ Prognosis

Due to the popularity of the computer and other electronic devices, the disease is susceptible to relapse.

▶ Exercise

1. Finger Pulling   Sit down and use the contralateral hand to hold and stretch every finger of the ipsilateral side for a total of two minutes. The traction should be gently and violent action should be avoided.

2. Circling Movement of the Fingers   While sitting, whirl the thumb and other four fingers 360° in turn with each finger doing it for 50 times. The movement should not be too fast to ensure a complete a 360° circle each time.

(II) Wrist Sprain

Wrist sprain, characterized by symptoms such as wrist pain, swelling and wrist movement disorders, refers wrist ligament damage due to external force beyond the normal range.

▶ Diagnosis

1. Clinical Symptoms

(1) Wrist swelling and pain;

(2) Localized blood stasis;

(3) Weakened gripping strength;

(4) Wrist movement disorders, or snapping sound while moving the wrist;

(5) Sometimes the wrist may have fluid.

2. Clinical Signs   Diffuse tenderness of the wrist.

3. Examination

X-ray: A simple wrist X-ray examination cannot be used alone as the standard diagnosis of wrist sprain. X-rays, however, can be an important differential diagnostic method to rule out wrist dislocation or fracture.

▶ Treatment

1. Treatment Principles   Invigorating blood, dissipating stasis, dissolving swelling and relieving pain.

2. Maneuvers   Press-kneading, pushing, and scrubbing.

3. Operation

(1) Ask the patient to be seated and place the wrist on a cushion with the palm facing down. The physician sits opposite the patient, applies press-kneading with the thumb to *wài guān* (SJ 5), *yú jì* (LU 10) and *hé gǔ* (LI 4), at each acupoint for one minute.

(2) Use both the thenar eminences to perform split pushing to the wrist, palm and forearm repeatedly for one minute. Then, with a light and quick scrubbing maneuver applied on the affected side of the wrist until the area feels thoroughly warm.

▶ Prognosis

With timely treatment, the prognosis of wrist sprain is fairly good. At the same time, pay attention to protecting the wrist, exercise to enhance its strength, and avoid recurring damage to the wrist after recovery.

▶ Exercise Methods

(1) *Making and Relaxing a Fist:* In a sitting position, make a fist with the affected hand,

and relax. Repeat 10 to 20 times, and the action should not be too fast to ensure a full fist is made and the relaxation is complete each time.

(2) *Wrist Rotation with Fingers Crossed*: In a sitting position, have the hands clenched, perform rotation for 20 times, and change to the opposite direction for 20 times as well. The movement of the affected wrist should be gentle with calm and even speed.

V. Finger Pain

(I) Finger Tenosynovitis

Finger tenosynovitis is a disease caused by stenosis of the tendon sheath of the finger flexor tendon or a thickening of the finger flexor tendon. Patients suffer from the sense of bounce while performing finger flexion and extension. Therefore, it is also called snapping finger or trigger finger. The disease has a slow onset, and is more commonly seen among craftsmen, with more occurrence in the thumb, middle finger, and ring finger. Moreover, there are more women than men suffering the disease.

▶ Diagnosis

1. Clinical Symptoms
(1)There is a sense of bouncing and limited range while doing finger flexion and extension. In some cases, the finger may even locked in position.

(2) The affected finger is stiff and painful in the morning. The pain disappears after physical activities. When the finger encounters cold, such as washing hands with cold water, symptoms become more obvious.

2. Clinical Signs Tenderness in palmar side of the affected finger, sometimes there are palpable nodules. When the finger is doing finger flexion or dorsiflexion, there is a sense of bouncing or locking.

3. Examination Although X-ray is not the standard diagnostic method of the disease, it can help to rule out joint dislocation or fracture.

▶ Treatment

1. Treatment Principles Invigorating

blood, dissolving stasis, soothing tendons, and unblocking the collaterals.

2. Maneuvers Kneading, pushing, and traction.

3. Operation
(1) Ask the patient to remain seated. Sit across from the patient, and use one hand to support the affected wrist. At the same time, use the thumb of the other hand to apply press-kneading to the metacarpophalangeal, proximal interphalangeal and distal interphalangeal joints of the affected hand, for one minute at each joint until the patient feels soreness and distended feeling on the area.

(2) Smear a small amount of *tuina* butter to the palmar side of the metacarpophalangeal joint, use the thumb to apply power and push the metacarpophalangeal joint of the affected finger along the direction of the flexor tendon. If there are palpable knots at the metacarpophalangeal joint, use more effort while doing pushing, and add pressing with more power.

(3) Hold the ipsilateral wrist in one hand, use the thumb of the other hand to apply physical power on the treatment site, and place the other four fingers on the corresponding positions to help with the stretching to the opposite direction. The stretch should last for five seconds and be repeated for five times.

▶ Prognosis

With timely treatment, the prognosis of this disease is generally fairly good. Pay attention to balancing work and rest, and avoid the use of cold water.

▶ Exercise Methods

Raise both arms, palms up to level with the shoulder and at shoulder width, fingers naturally bent. Stretch fingers and make a loose fist repeatedly. Keep both hands palms up at all time.

(II) Sprain of Interphalangeal Joint

Interphalangeal joint sprain is due to violent lateral force to the joint sprain, leading to laceration of the collateral ligament. In severe cases, it can lead to complete destruction of the interphalangeal collateral ligament, resulting in lateral dislocation of the interphalangeal joint. It is common in volleyball and basketball players, while the sprain often occurs in the first and second interphalangeal joints.

▶ Diagnosis

1. Clinical Symptoms
(1) Interphalangeal joint pain and swelling.
(2) Pain is aggravated when the injured interphalangeal joint is in the semi-flexion, flexion and extension position, or lateral movement.
(3) Limited interphalangeal joint movement.
2. Clinical Signs   Obvious tenderness of the interphalangeal joint.
3. Examination   Although X-ray is not the standard diagnostic method of the disease, it can help to rule out joint dislocation or fracture.

▶ Treatment

1. Treatment Principles   Invigorating blood, dissolving stasis, resolving swelling and relieving pain.
2. Maneuvers   Pressing, scrubbing, pushing, and traction.
3. Operations
(1) Ask the patient to take the sitting position, place the affected wrist on a cushion, with the palm facing down. Sit across from the patient, and press *hé gǔ* (LI 4), *yáng xī* (LI 5), *yú jì* (LU 10), and *ashi* with the thumb, for one minute at each acupoint.
(2) Use the thenar or hypothenar eminence to apply scrubbing the interphalangeal joints along the fingers until the area feels thoroughly warm.
(3) Use both the thenar eminences to perform split pushing to wrist, palm, and fingers of the affected side repeatedly for one minute.
(4) Hold the injured wrist in one hand, while placing the thumb of the other hand on the patient's joint to be treated. The other four fingers should help the thumb in applying the stretching as the opposite force. Stretch the joint continuously for five sec-

onds, and repeat the operation for five times.

▶ Prognosis

The disease is acute injury, the prognosis is fairly good if it is a appropriate treatment.

▶ Exercise method

Fist relaxation exercises: in a sitting position, make a fist with the affected hand, and relex. Repeat 10 to 20 times, the action should not be too fast to ensure a full fist and complete relaxation.

VI. Lumbar Pain

(I) Acute Lumbar Sprain

Acute lumbar sprain is the acute damage to the waist muscles, ligaments, and fascia due to uncoordinated contraction of the waist muscles in daily life and work. The condition is more common in adults, mostly young and middle-aged people. It is not common among elderlies, and generally affects men more than women. Laborers and people who do not do physical exercise are often susceptible to the problem.

▶ Diagnosis

1. Clinical Symptoms
(1) Severe stabbing or tearing pain in the lumbar area that is usually unilateral, and sometimes bilateral. The pain is often located in the lumbosacral region, while some may also experiencing referred pain in hips and lower extremities that is obscure and hard to locate. In order to relieve waist pain, patients often have their hands place on the waist;
(2) Limited lumbar motor function and weight-bearing ability;
(3) Decreased or absent lumbar curvature and scoliosis may appear;
(4) Spasm and stiffness of the lumbar muscle.
2. Clinical Signs   Tenderness of the lumbar that often located between L4 and L5, L5 and S1, the transverse process of L3, and the starting point of the erector muscle of spine. The points are in fixed locations, and the pain can be unbearable while pressing these points.

3. Examination X-ray often detects lumbar scoliosis at the posterior lateral view, while the lateral view shows reduced or even absent physiological curvature. X-ray examination helps to illustrate whether there is any problems such as congenital anomalies, fracture of the transverse process, facet joint, spinous process, or bone spurs. The lateral flexion view is helpful to diagnose whether there is any rupture of the supraspinal or interspinous ligaments.

▶ Treatment

1. Treatment Principles Soothing tendons, invigorating blood, dispersing swelling, and relieving pain.

2. Maneuvers Precision pressing, rolling, kneading, and scrubbing.

3. Operation

(1) Ask the patient to lie in the prone position. Apply precision pressing with more force on both sides of *shèn shù* (BL 23, 肾俞), *qì hǎi shù* (BL 24, 气海俞), *wěi zhōng* (BL 40, 委中), and *xuán zhōng* (GB 39, 悬钟), at each acupoint for one minute.

(2) Perform kneading top-down on the muscles of the lumbar region with the force perpendicular to the muscle bellies, and put more focus on both sides of the sacrospinalis of the lumbar region. Repeat the step three to five times.

(3) Apply rolling on both sides of the sacrospinalis of the lumbar region back and forth for three to five times.

(4) Perform straight scrubbing on both bladder meridians with the hypothenar eminence until the area feels thoroughly warm.

▶ Prognosis

Acute lumbar sprain has a good prognosis, if it is treated in a timely manner. After it is cured, keep doing exercises strengthening the lumbar area to prevent the disease from recurring.

▶ Exercise Method

Lie in a supine position and use both hands to hold the knee close to the chest. Remain in this position for three to five seconds, then slowly return to the original position.

Three to five times is considered a set, and perform it three sets a day.

(II) Chronic Lumbar muscle Strain

Chronic lumbar muscle strain refers to long-term, chronic and damaging stimulation of the soft tissue in the lumbar region, resulting in chronic injuries of the lumbar muscles, ligaments, and fascia, such as ischemia, degeneration, exudation, adhesions and other pathological changes, which causes localized pain. The disease occurs more often in adults, especially those who do not engage in physical exercise.

▶ Diagnosis

1. Clinical Symptoms

(1) Wide-spread and recurrent soreness on one or both sides of the lumbar area that increases after work and at night. The pain is reduced after rest and upon waking up.

(2) Lumbar functions are mostly normal. However, physical activity may cause discomfort of the lumbar area. In acute attacks, the spine may seem to have scoliosis and referred pain on the lower extremities may occur.

2. Clinical Signs

(1) The straight leg raise test and accelerated straight leg raise test are negative.

(2) The neck flexion test is negative.

(3) The lower limb extension test is negative.

3. Examination Mostly, the X-ray examination of the lumbar spine in posterior lateral view does no reveal any positive manifestation.

▶ Treatment

1. Treatment Principles Relaxing tendons, unblocking the collaterals, resolving spasm and relieving pain.

2. Maneuvers Pushing, pressing, rolling, rotating, and scrubbing.

3. Operation

(1) Ask the patient to lie in a prone position. Stand to the side of the patient. Use both the thenar and hypothenar eminences to perform pushing along the *du mai* from *dà zhuī* (DU 14) to *cháng qiáng* (DU 1, 长强),

both sides of the *hua tuo jia ji*, and both bladder meridians from *dà zhù* (BL 11, 大 杼) to *kūn lún* (BL 60, 昆仑), and *fù fēn* (BL 41, 附分) to *kūn lún* (BL 60). Push along each meridian three to five times.

(2) Apply kneading along the both bladder meridians bottom-up three to five times, the power from light to forceful. Then, perform rolling following the same direction on the same area three to five times.

(3) Use the thumbs to perform precision pressing on *shèn shù* (BL 23, 肾俞), *yāo yáng guān* (DU 3, 腰阳关), and *dà cháng shù* (BL 25, 大 肠 俞) of both sides, each acupoints for a minute until it feels thoroughly warm.

(4) Ask the patient to change a supine position with the hips and knees in a flexion position. The physician holds the patient's knees to perform lumbosacral rotation clockwise and anticlockwise, eight to ten times each direction. Next, let the patient hold his/her knees with both hands and rolls forward and backward on the treatment table for 10 to 20 times.

(5) Ask the patient to lie in the prone position. The physician uses his/her palms to perform straight scrubbing on the lumbosacral area with a penetrating force. Treatment should last for about five minutes till the area is thoroughly warm.

▶ Prognosis

The disease is caused by long-term and cumulative strain, and is therefore prone to recur. The patient needs to maintain a balance between work and rest.

▶ Exercise Method

"Double Bridge" exercise: Take a supine position with knees and hips flexed, hands at the sides of the body, feet forced downward, at the same time waist, abdomen and hips slowly leave to arch the lower back. Maintain this position 10 seconds, then slowly down, this is a complete action. Repeat the action 10 times / group, 3 groups / day

(III) Lumbar Disc Herniation

Lumbar disc herniation, also known as lumbar slipped disc, is one of the more common diseases involving low back and leg pain. The disease is due to degenerative changes in the lumbar intervertebral disc, resulting in mechanical imbalance within and outside the spine. Due to external force, the annulus fibrosus bursts, so that the herniated nucleus pulposus stimulates or oppresses a nerve root, blood vessels or spinal cord, causing a series of clinical symptoms including lumbar pain, and pain and numbness of both lower limbs. Herniation often occurs in the intervertebral disc between L4 and L5, or L5 and S1 disc and accounts for nearly 95% of the cases.

▶ Diagnosis

1. Clinical Symptoms

(1) Lower back pain with radiating pain on the lower limb even reaching the calf or the foot;

(2) Stiffness and physical activity dysfunction of the lower back;

(3) For patients with chronic symptomology, subjective numbness are often seen in posterolateral aspect of the calf, dorsal aspect of the foot, the heel or the sole.

2. Clinical Signs

(1) The straight leg raise test and the accelerated straight leg raise test are positive.

(2) The neck flexion test is positive. In severe cases, the patient cannot even complete the test.

(3) Lower limb extensor test is positive.

(4) When there is increased abdominal pressure, lower back pain aggravates, which is accompanied by radiation pain of the lower extremity.

(5) There are tender points lateral to the interspinal ligament between L4 and L5 or L5 and S1, which can cause radiating pain in the lower leg or foot with pressure.

(6) Reduced skin sensory on the anterolateral or posterolateral aspect of the calf, muscle weakness of the toes, decreased or disappeared reflexes of the knee and Achilles tendon of the affected side.

3. Examination

(1) *X-ray*: Plain radiography alone cannot be used as the only evidence for the diagnosis of lumbar disc herniation. The degenerative

changes such as narrowing of intervertebral space and hyperplasia of vertebrae, however, can sometimes be seen on X-ray film, which is an indirect indication. In addition, X-ray can detect if there are diseases such as tuberculosis or tumor of the bone. Therefore, it is an important differential diagnostic method.

(2) *CT scan*: Computer Tomography can clearly show the location, size, and shape of the disc herniation, as well as shifting of the nerve root or the dural sac due to the pressure of herniated disc. Moreover, it reveals hypertrophy of the lamina, ligamentum flavum and facet, and stenosis of the vertebral canal and lateral recess. Therefore, it is widely used now for its greater diagnostic value of the disease.

(3) *MRI*: An MRI can be of great significance in diagnosing lumbar disc herniation and provides a comprehensive view observing the lumbar disc lesion. Furthermore, it clearly shows the shape of the disc herniation, its relationship with surrounding tissues such as the dural sac, and the nerve root through sagittal images of different levels and transverse cross-sectional images of the affected disc. In addition, an MRI can identify whether there are other space-occupying lesions in the spinal canal. MRI's are however, not as effective as the CT scan in reflecting calcification of the disc.

▶ Treatment

1. Treatment Principles Relaxing the sinews, unblocking the collaterals, reducing the injured tendons and bones, invigorating blood, and dissolving stasis.

2. Maneuvers Rolling, pressing, grasping, and passive joint movements.

3. Operation

(1) Ask the patient to lie in a prone position. Apply rolling along the first lateral line of the bladder meridian top-down to the sacroiliac joint on the affected side first, and then the contralateral side for three to five minutes.

(2) Use the thumb or have the index and middle fingers overlapped to perform pressing along the bladder meridian from *dà zhù* (BL 11) to *bái huán shù* (BL 30, 白环俞). It is necessary to control the amount of force being applied and requires the physician to stand to the side of the patient with the elbow in extension position and the shoulder stabilized. Control the power of pressing by shifting the body forward and backward. Press each acupoint three times.

(3) The patient needs to hold the front edge of the treatment table or ask an assistant to hold the patient's shoulders. The physician stands to the side of the patient's foot. Hold and separate both ankles of the patient with each hand respectively. Have the body tilt backwards and gradually stretch to the direction of the toes, and retain the position for about a minute.

(4) The patient brings his/her legs close together. The physician presses the patient's waist with one hand, holds the region just above both of the patient's knee from underneath, and slowly raises them to move the patient's back into an extension position. When the stretch reaches the maximum, coordinate the force of both hands and use the "dexterous force and agile strength" to perform a quick spontaneous torquing by pressing the waist down and lifting the lower limbs up with substantial range.

(5) Ask the patient to lie on their side, with the hip and knees of the leg on the top in flexion position while the leg on the bottom in extension position. The physician should use one hand or elbow to push and press firmly on the anterior or posterior aspect of the patient's shoulder, and the other hand or elbow to press against the patient's anterior superior iliac spine. Both hands need to coordinate the force to perform slight twisting to the patient's waist until it is completely relaxed. Then, rotate the patient's waist to its maximum while obvious resistance is sensed. Pause for a while, use "dexterous force and agile strength" to perform a sudden spontaneous torquing; a snapping sound may be heard.

(6) Ask the patient to lie in a prone position. Press *huán tiào* (GB 30, 环跳) using the elbow for 30 seconds.

(7) Have the patient lie on his/her side with hip and knees in flexion position, and apply

pressing with the elbow on *jū liáo* (GB 29, 居髎) for 30 seconds.

(8) Ask the patient to take a prone position. Stand close to the patient's lumbosacral region. Perform perpendicular pressing on *yāo yǎn* (EX-B7, 腰眼), continue to press the third lumbar transverse process, slowly increase the pressure, and relax. Repeat three to five times.

(9) Ask the patient to lie in a prone position. Stand on the left side of the patient, use the palm to cover the anterior aspect of the thigh root with the thumb separated from the other four fingers. Perform a combined maneuver of pinching, grasping, pressing and rubbing from top-down and all the way to the ankle with a good amount of force. Repeat the action three to five times.

▶ Prognosis

Although relapse is common, the effect of *tuina* is obvious, especially combined with functional exercise that increases the strength of the waist muscles.

▶ Exercise Method

(1) *Backwards bending*: Begin in the prone position, both lower extremities straight, hands on the sides of the body, and legs still. Look up and have the upper body bend backwards. Each set is 20 to 50 times, and perform it three sets a day. When the body adjusts to the exercise over time, change to have both legs in the extension position while looking up and the waist bending backwards as far as possible. Each set is 50 to 100 times, and perform this five to ten sets daily to strengthen the muscles of the back.

(2) *Backwards walking*: Practice backwards walking on a flat and open space. While walking backwards, swing both arms to keep the body balanced. Be careful and avoid falls initially, while the length of the practice should be about 10 minutes. After getting skilled on this, extend the exercise time accordingly. The method can adjust the function of the back muscle, and perseverance is the key.

(IV) Degenerative Lumbar Osteoarthritis

Degenerative lumbar osteoarthritis refers to bone hyperplasia due to spine degeneration, so that bone spurs can often stimulate the surrounding tissue directly or indirectly, causing inflammation. The disease often occurs among middle-aged or elderly people, more commonly in men than women, especially in long-term laborers.

▶ Diagnosis

1. Clinical Symptoms

(1) Soreness, pain and discomfort of the lower back, which prevents the patient from sitting or standing for a long time. The symptoms are more severe in the morning just after getting up, and often reduce after physical activity. Excessive activity or hard work, however, also aggravates the symptoms.

(2) Lumbar dysfunction.

(3) The lumbar physiological curvature is decreased or disappeared.

(4) Local muscle spasms and mild tenderness, generally without radiating pain.

2. Clinical Signs　Generally, the result of the special examinations can be close to normal.

3. Examination　X-ray shows visible various degree of hyperplasia, intervertebral space narrowing, or physiological curvature changes.

▶ Treatment

1. Treatment Principles　Moving qi, invigorating blood, dissolving spasm, and relieving pain.

2. Maneuvers　Precision pressing, rolling, kneading, spontaneous torquing and scrubbing.

3. Operation

(1) Ask the patient to lie in a prone position, while the physician performs precision pressing with the thumb on *shèn shù* (BL 23), *dà cháng shù* (BL 25, 大肠俞), *yāo yáng guān* (DU 3, 腰阳关) and *jū liáo* (GB 29), one minute each point.

(2) Apply rolling on both sides of the sacrospinalis top-down three to five times, and then use the palm root rub to perform press-kneading three to five times.

(3) The patient lies on their side. The physician performs lumbar oblique spontaneous torquing once for each side.

(4) Ask the patient to lie in a supine position. Apply scrubbing along both sides of the bladder meridian, and then the lumbosacral region until these areas are thoroughly warm.

▶ Prognosis

The disease is degenerative, and the symptoms recur easily. Although the effect of *tuina* is obvious, relapse is common, if the patient does not take self-care seriously.

▶ Exercise Method

(1) *Supine pedaling*: Lie in a supine position with hands on the side, legs lifted, knee in the flexion status, and pedal in the air as if riding a bicycle. Left and right count as a complete action, and 20 to 30 times as a set. Three sets per day. The movements should be slow and powerful, and neither the waist nor the buttocks should leave the treatment table while pedaling.

(2) *Waist swinging*: Lie in a supine position with the hip and knees in the flexion position, and hands at the sides. Make both knees lean to the left towards the table. Swing back to the starting position, repeat the tilt to the right, and swing back to the starting position. Perform both sides six times as a set, and perform three sets a day. Keeping the hands close to the sides, helps to stabilize the waist, and not to move along with the swing of the knees. The angle formed by the knee swing should not be too great, and within the controllable range for the feet.

VII. Hip Pain

(I) Hip Bursitis

Hip bursitis is a disease due to long-term friction and oppression, causing effusion of synovial fluid and swelling around the hip joint, further leading to a chronic aseptic inflammation. Hip bursitis can be classified as ischial bursitis, trochanteric bursitis, iliopectineal bursitis and so forth. The disease is more common in the elderly.

▶ Diagnosis

1. Clinical Symptoms
(1) *Ischial bursitis*: The patient's ischial tuberosity region suffers from pain, swelling. The patient is unable to sit down for an extended period of time, and pain is worse when sitting on a hard surface. Gluteal muscle contraction can produce pain that radiates to the buttock. When sciatic nerve is irritated, there may be sciatic nerve pain.

(2) *Trochanteric bursitis*: The patient cannot lie on the affected side, and internal rotation of the hip can aggravate the pain. In order to reduce the pain, patients often have the affected limb in abduction or in external rotation to relax the muscles.

(3) *Iliopectineal bursitis*: Pain in the lateral aspect of the femoral triangle that exacerbates during iliopsoas contraction, flexion of the hip, gluteus maximus contraction, and extension of the hip. As a result hip activity is limited, and the pain can radiate along the anterior aspect of the thigh to the medial side of the calf.

2. Clinical Signs
(1) *Ischial bursitis*: Swelling and tenderness can be found in the ischial tuberosity region. During the physical examination, an oval-shaped mass with clear edge that connected with the ischial tuberosity can be palpated in the deeper part of the ischial tuberosity.

(2) *Trochanteric bursitis*: Swelling and tenderness can be found posteriorly and superiorly to the greater trochanter, while the hip rotation is limited. When the swelling of the bursa is obvious, a palpable mass can be detected in the region, and sometimes with a sense of fluctuation.

(3) *Iliopectineal bursitis*: Tenderness is apparent in the lateral aspect of the femoral triangle. When there is excessive swelling of the bursa, the normal groove of the groin disappears and the area can bulge outward. In addition, hip activity is limited.

3. Examinations
(1) *X-ray*: When there is a large amount of joint effusion, the anterior and lateral views of the hip show increased joint space.

(2) The total number of leukocytes and erythrocyte sedimentation rate are generally normal with occasional increase. The bacterial culture is negative.

▶ Treatment

1. Treatment Principles   Relaxing tendons, assisting the movement, invigorating blood, and resolving swelling.

2. Maneuvers   Pressing-kneading, plucking, pushing, scrubbing, and rolling.

3. Operations

(1) *Ischial bursitis*:

① Ask the patient to be in the prone position. Use press-kneading method on the ischial tuberosity and its surrounding areas for about six minutes.

② Apply plucking on the same area for about three minutes.

③ Perform press-kneading and pushing on the same area for about three minutes.

④ Ask the patient lie on their side, with the affected side away from the table, hip and knees in a flexion position, apply scrubbing to the ischial tuberosity area until the area is thoroughly warm.

(2) *Trochanteric bursitis*:

① Ask the patient lie on their side, with the affected side away from the table. Perform rolling to relax the lateral hip muscles for about six minutes.

② Apply plucking on the bursa for about three minutes.

③ Use the thumb for kneading on the affected region for about three minutes.

④ Perform scrubbing to the area until it feels thoroughly warm.

(3) *Iliopectineal bursitis*:

① Ask the patient to lie in a supine position, with knees and hip slightly flexed. Use the thumb to perform kneading in the groin area, and combine with passive hip flexion and extension at the same time for about six minutes;

② Apply plucking on the lateral side of the femoral triangle for about three minutes.

③ Perform scrubbing on the region till it feels thoroughly warm.

▶ Prognosis

(1) Reduce hip activities during the treatment period.

(2) Avoid sitting on cold or hard surfaces.

(3) For patients with ischial bursitis, the use of a soft cushion while sitting can prevent the ischial tuberosity being oppressed for a long time.

▶ Exercise method

Squatting and backward extension of the lower limbs while standing.

(II) Hip Sprain

Hip sprain is defined as the injury occurs when the hip moves out of its normal range or position, so that the abnormal wrenching causes the muscles, ligaments and articular capsule surrounding the hip to tear, bleed and swell with a series of other symptoms.

▶ Diagnosis

1. Clinical Symptoms

(1) Ipsilateral hip pain, swelling, dysfunction after injury.

(2) Pain that increases with physical activities, and reduces with rest.

(3) Limited mobility of the affected limb while walking and weight-bearing, appearing to have protective gait, such as halting step, dragging, or with pelvic tilt.

2. Clinical Signs

(1) During physical examination, tender points can be found on the ipsilateral groin, posterior aspect of the greater trochanter, and specific muscles in the buttock. The pain aggravates in all directions of passive hip movement.

(2) Occasionally, the affected limb appears to be longer.

(3) The Thomas sign is positive.

3. Examinations

(1) X-ray does not show any abnormality.

(2) MRI may show joint effusion, intermuscular effusion, or discontinuous signals of the muscles, ligaments, and joint capsule.

▶ Treatment

1. Treatment Principles   Relaxing sinews, unblocking collaterals, reducing injured tendons and bones, invigorating blood, and dissolving stasis.

2. Maneuvers   Precision pressing, pressing, kneading, rubbing, grasping, passive joint movements.

3. Operation

(1) Ask the patient to lie in the prone position. The physician applies precision pressing, kneading, and rubbing on tenderness points of the hip.

(2) Change to the supine position. Use tendon rectifying and collateral quickening maneuvers such as pressing, kneading, and grasping on the tender points of the hip area.

(3) Lastly, the physician holds the pelvis with one hand and the knees with the other hand. Perform passive rotation, with the hip and knees in the flexion position, pressing the hip down, and passive abduction, external rotation and stretching to the lower extremity simultaneously several times. In this way, it is possible to release the trapped round ligament or the joint capsule, eliminate muscle cramps caused by pain, and restore hip mobility.

▶ Prognosis

During the treatment period it is necessary to limit activities or weight-bearing of the affected limb. Keep the limb and joint warm and avoid cold.

▶ Exercise Method

(1) Lie in a supine position with the hip and knee of the affected side in a flexed position. Clamp and hold the proximal tibia on the affected side with both hands. Put the elbow up and actively flex the hip to increase the strength and range of hip flexion. Repeat the action and continue with the exercise for three to five minutes. Gradually increase the frequency and range every day.

(2) Lie in a supine position with the feet flat to the bed, hip and knees in maximum flexion position. Use both feet as the axis, have the knees perform adduction, abduction, internal rotation, and external rotation for five to ten minutes. Gradually increase the range of the exercise, especially the abduction.

VIII. Knee Pain

(I) Traumatic Knee Synovitis

Traumatic knee synovitis is caused by traumatic injury of the knee, resulting in a variety of intra-articular injuries, damage to the synovial membrane of the joint capsule, and congestion, exudation, and massive effusion or in the joint cavity. Consequently, the situation will lead to a clinical syndrome with symptoms of inflammation of synovial membrane, and hematocele and effusion of the knee joint.

▶ Diagnosis

1. Clinical Symptoms

(1) *Joint swelling*: Mostly diffuse swelling that gradually aggravates. Acute trauma may cause a joint hematoma immediately or within one to two hours after the injury, while extensive bleeding spots can be seen on the knee and calf.

(2) *Joint pain*: Pain can occur right after the injury and can gradually exacerbate. The pain also becomes worse during physical activity, especially squatting.

(3) *Restricted physical activities*: Limited knee movement, limping, difficulty in squatting can all occur after the injury. Reactive synovial effusion appears usually six to eight hours after the incident with obvious knee swelling, heat sensation and limited flexion and extension ability.

2. Clinical Signs

(1) Widespread knee tenderness.

(2) Obvious and mostly diffuse swelling of the knee. Increased local skin temperature.

(3) Knee movement difficulty, and unable to hyperextend and hyperflex. Knee pain aggravates especially extension while encountering resistance.

(4) Patella tap test is positive.

3. Examinations

(1) Yellowish or light red liquid can be extracted during knee puncture, but fluid culture is negative for bacteria.

(2) X-ray does not found any abnormalities of the bone, loose body in the joint, or bone spurs at the edge.

▶ Treatment

1. Treatment Principles   Relaxing tendons, unblocking the collaterals, invigorating blood, relieving pain, and lubricating joints.

2. Maneuvers   Rolling, pressing, kneading, precision pressing, pushing, plucking, rotation, and stretching.

3. Operation

(1) Ask the patient to lie in a supine position. Stand to one side of the patient, apply rolling repeatedly along the medial, lateral and anterior aspects of the thigh top-down for three minutes.

(2) Use both hands to perform push-pressing slowly from the root of the thigh to the knees until the upper edge of the patella repeatedly for three minutes, and gradually increase the intensity.

(3) Apply kneading along the lateral aspect of the calf from top to bottom repeatedly for three minutes.

(4) Perform precision pressing on points including *bì guān* (ST 31, 髀关), *fú tù* (ST 32, 伏兔), *wěi zhōng* (BL 40), *nèi xī yǎn* (EX-LE 4, 内膝眼), *xī yǎn* (EX-LE 5, 膝眼), *zú sān lǐ* (ST 36), *yáng líng quán* (GB 34, 阳陵泉), and *sān yīn jiāo* (SP 6, 三阴交) for 30 seconds each point with just enough force to make them feel sore.

(5) Next, use gentle force to perform circular plucking around the patella for about two minutes.

(6) Lastly, apply press-kneading around the knee for about two minutes.

(7) Ask the patient to lie in a supine position. Stand on the lateral side of the patient, flex the affected hip and knee to a 90°. Support from under the patient's popliteal fossa with one hand while the other holding his/her ankle, and perform gentle rotation to the knee combining with a slight traction, six to seven times.

(8) Gently use passive action to move the knee into a maximum flexion position and a complete extension position. Repeat five times.

▶ Prognosis

During the treatment period avoid excessive use of the knee. At the same time, moderate functional exercise is necessary to prevent muscle atrophy and tissue adhesion. Keep the knee warm and avoid the invasion of cold and dampness.

▶ Exercise Method

(1) In early stage of the trauma, intentionally contract the quadriceps to prevent muscle atrophy.

(2) In the later stage, have the knee involved in movements including flexion and extension to prevent or resolvie adhesions.

(3) Avoid violent movements while doing functional exercise of the knee, and excessive activity is not recommended.

(II) Chondromalacia Patellae

Chondromalacia patellae, also known as "runner's knee", is softening of the cartilage under the patella caused by trauma or chronic strain of the knee joint. It occurs mainly in people 15 to 40 years old while women are more likely to than men. Generally, it happens on both knees, or one knee first then the other one, especially among athletes, and people that stand a lot or involve in repeated knee flexion and extension.

▶ Diagnosis

1. Clinical Symptoms

(1) *Knee pain*: The onset of the disease is slow. Initially, the patient has frequent and vague knee pain while going downstairs. Gradually, the pain would occur both going upstairs and downstairs. When the patient stands up after squatting, the knee feels weak and pain. Usually, it happens on one knee, then the other one.

(2) False locking phenomenon can happen to the knees.

2. Clinical Signs

(1) *Tenderness*: Tenderness on the particular surface of the patella or around the patella, especially at the medial edge, sometimes both *nèi xī yǎn* (EX-LE 4) and *xī yǎn* (EX LE 5).

(2) The patellar grind test is positive.

(3) The single leg squat test is positive.

(4) A negative patellar inhibition test (a.k.a. the Zohlen's sign) helps to exclude patellar chondromalacia.

(5) *Patellar mobility*: Compare the movement range of the patellas of both sides. If the ipsilateral side has a reduced range of movement, it suggests osteoarthritis of the

knee, quadriceps tension, knee stiffness, or intra-articular adhesions. Increased mobility is seen in the unstable patella and loosening of joint ligaments.

(6) There might be slight quadriceps atrophy, but the joint activity is not limited.

3. Examinations

(1) *X-ray*: The axial view of the patellar is mostly normal in the early stage of the disease. In the late stage though, visible abnormalities may include narrowing of the space between the femoral joint and the patella, eburnation and roughness of the cartilage of the underside patella articular surface, sometimes cystic degeneration, and bone hyperplasia on the edge.

(2) Arthroscopy can confirm the diagnosis.

▶ Treatment

1. Treatment Principles Relaxing tendons, dispersing stasis, unblocking collaterals, and assisting movements.

2. Maneuvers Precision pressing, kneading, rolling, scrubbing, and rotating.

3. Operation

(1) Ask the patient to lie in a supine position. Stand laterally to the patient, and perform kneading around the knee for about one minute until the area feels sore.

(2) Apply rolling on the knee joint and its surrounding area, especially the superior and inferior edges of the patella and the quadriceps for about five minutes.

(3) Apply knead-grasping to the quadriceps and calf muscles for about five minutes.

(4) Ask the patient to lie in a supine position. Stand to the side of the patient and use precision kneading on points such as *xuè hǎi* (SP 10, 血海), *yīn líng quán* (SP 9, 阴陵泉), *yáng líng quán* (GB 34, 阳陵泉), *xī yǎn* (EX-LE 5), *hè dǐng* (EX-LE 2, 鹤顶), and *xī yáng guān* (GB 33, 膝阳关) for about three minutes. Contiue until the points to feel sore.

(5) Ask the patient to lie in a prone position. The physician should stand on to the side, and perform palm-scrubbing to both sides of the patient's knees and the popliteal fossa until there is a thorough warm sensation.

(6) Ask the patient to change to a supine position. Stand on one side of the patient to apply knee rotation for three to five times, and then perform passive traction for half a minute.

▶ Prognosis

While the knee is in a flexed position, the patella bears more weight and is prone to damage of the articular surface. Therefore, the patient should avoid continuous squatting to reduce the pressure on the patellar articular surface.

▶ Exercise Method

Start non-weight-bearing exercises as soon as possible, especially the exercise to strengthen the quadriceps, such as active knee extension and flexion in a sitting position.

(III) Osteoarthritis of the Knee

Osteoarthritis refers to the hyperplasia of bone around the joints that irritates the surrounding tissue, and often affects more elderly patients. Since most cases of knee osteoarthritis are caused by hyperplasia, it is also known as proliferative osteoarthritis. Joint deformity often occurs, so that it is also called deformability arthritis. Moreover, the disease is degenerative; therefore, it is also known as degenerative arthritis. Knee osteoarthritis has the highest incidence among all types of osteoarthritis. Osteoarthritis of the knee is closely related to factors including age, occupation, trauma, obesity, knee deformity, cold and humidity. It affects more women than men, especially post-menopausal women.

Note:

It is recommended that you review the knowledge of local anatomy, physiology and pathology of knee joint before studying this chapter.

▶ Diagnosis

1. Clinical Symptoms

(1) Knee pain: The severity of the pain var-

ies. In mild cases, there may be slight pain or even no pain; and in severe cases, the pain can be unbearable. The following are the characteristics of the pain:

① *Initial pain*: Pain often occurs when the patient starts activities involving the affected knee or after it stays in a certain position for an extended period of time. Pain can occur after the beginning of exercise , after a brief moment of activity, or prolonged activity .

② *Weight-bearing pain*: Knee pain occurs in weight-bearing activities, such as going up and down the stairs, or climbing a hill;

③ *Active movement pain*: The knee pain is more intense while doing active movement involving the knee due to muscle contraction comparing with passive movement;

④ *Rest pain*: Knee pain occurs after the knee remains in a static position for a long time. The pain is related to increased marrow cavity and intra-articular pressure due to poor venous return, and can be alleviated with the change of body position;

⑤ The pain is related to weather changes.

(2) *Restricted knee function*: The extent of restriction of knee function varies. Both the weight-bearing and motor function can be limited to varying degrees, according to the severiry of the condition.

2. Clinical Signs

(1) *Knee deformities*: Some patients may develop deformity of the knee with varying severity. Deformity can lead to osteoarthritis, and in turn, osteoarthritis can make the deformity worse. Clinically, bowlegs (O-shaped), and knock-knee (X-shaped or K-shaped) deformities are commonly seen. Sometimes, knee flexion contracture and hyperextension deformity can also be seen.

(2) *Tenderness*: Tender points are commonly located in the regions of the medial femoral condyle, lateral femoral condyle, medial tibial condyle, lateral tibia condyle, upper and lower edge of the patella, and *xī yǎn* (EX-LE 5).

(3) *Articular crepitus*: During knee movement, the joint may have a frictional sound, known as crepitus. Depending on cause and duration of the disease and the severity of hyperplasia, the existence or level of the crepitus may vary. Soft crepitus often suggests

lighter degeneration and hyperplasia, while louder crepitus usually indicates more severe degeneration and hyperplasia.

(4) *Swelling*: Some patients may have mild swelling. Swelling can also be aggravated when hyperplastic bone stimulates the synovial membrane.

3. Examinations　The frontal view of X-ray may show problems including sharpened intercondylar spine of tibia, narrowed or unequal joint space, hyperplasia of the medial femoral condyle and tibia lateral condyle, bone spurs due to pressure or traction, and blurred joint surface. The lateral view may show hyperplasia of the upper or lower edge of patella bone, and patellar ligament calcification. Lastly, the axial view of the patella film can indicate problems such as narrowing of the patellofemoral joint surface, rough articular surface, and hyperplasia at the edge of the patella.

▶ Treatment

1. Treatment Principles　Relaxing tendons, dispersing stasis, loosing up the tissues, and benefiting the movements.

2. Maneuvers　Rolling, kneading, grasping, plucking, scrubbing, and rotating.

3. Operation

(1) Ask the patient to lie in the supine position. Stand to one side of the patient, and apply rolling on the quadriceps with more focus on the upper part of the patella for about five minutes.

(2) Perform precision kneading on points such as *hè dǐng* (EX-LE 2), *nèi xī yǎn* (EX-LE 4), *xī yǎn* (EX-LE 5), *yáng líng quán* (GB 34), *xuè hǎi* (SP 10), *liáng qiū* (ST 34, 梁丘), *fú tù* (ST 32, 伏兔) and *fēng shì* (GB 31, 风市) for about three minutes.

(3) Ask the patient to change to the prone position. Stand to one side and use rolling to the posterior aspect of the thigh and calf, and the popliteal fossa for about three minutes.

(4) Apply grasping on *wěi zhōng* (BL 40) and *chéng shān* (BL 57, 承山) several times.

(5) Ask the patient to lie in a supine position. Stand to one side of the patient and perform press-kneading and plucking alternately to the patellar ligament, and medial

and lateral collateral ligament, focusing on *hè dǐng* (EX-LE 2), *nèi xī yǎn* (EX-LE 4), *xī yǎn* (EX-LE 5), *yáng líng quán* (GB 34), *xuè hǎi* (SP 10), *liáng qiū* (ST 34) for about three minutes.

(6) Use the lift-grasping maneuver to the patella several times.

(7) Apply scrubbing to the ipsilateral knee and its surrounding area with the palm until the frictional heat penetrating the area.

(8) Ask the patient to lie in a supine position with hip and knees flexed. Stand to one side of the patient, use one hand to support the patella of the affected knee and the other hand to hold the distal aspect of the calf, and perform rotation with the knee in the flexion position. Afterwards, extend and flex the knee several times. Repeat this step several times

▶ Prognosis

For patient with severe knee pain and swelling, instruct the patient to rest in bed. When the symptoms are alleviated, get involved in appropriate physical exercises.

Note:

Advise the patients that are obese to perform more physical exercises, curb their appetite, and reduce their body mass index (BMI) to less than 25 in order to reduce the burden of their knees.

▶ Exercise Method

1. Do more functional exercise of the knee joint, for example, knee flexion and rotation to restore the motor function of the knee.

2. The quadriceps contraction exercises can help to reduce swelling, restore the strength of the quadriceps, and prevent and treat quadriceps atrophy.

IX. Ankle and Heel Pain

（Ⅰ）Soft Tissue Injury of the Ankle
Ankle joint soft tissue injuries refer to the damage to the ligaments and joint capsule around the ankle, and are commonly known as ankle sprain. The disease can occur in people of any age, and often happens when the ankle is in the plantar flexion varus position.

Note:

It is recommended that you review the knowledge about the anatomy and physiology of the ankle before you study this chapter.

▶ Diagnosis

1. Clinical Symptoms
(1) *Pain*: The pain can happen immediately after the ankle is injured. The severity of the pain is proportional to the severity of the injury. If the pain is on the medial side then the medial collateral ligament has been injured, when it is on the lateral side, the lateral collateral ligament has been injured. Since more cases of the injury happen while the ankle is in plantar flexion varus position, the damage is often in the anterior talofibular ligament and the calcaneal ligament. Therefore, anterolateral and lateral pain of the ankle are more common. At the time the lateral collateral ligament is stretched due to the injury, the medial malleolus may have pain due to the compression of the talus.

(2) *Limited function*: After the ankle is injured, active movement in any direction is restricted and there will be difficulty in walking.

(3) *Swelling and ecchymosis*: After the injury, there will be various degrees of swelling and ecchymosis that may occur three to four hours later and gradually increase in intensity. Medial swelling reveals medial injury, while lateral swelling suggests lateral injury. Ecchymosis often appears below or distal to the site of injury, which is often cyan in color. If severe swelling and ecchymosis emerges immediately after the injury, suspect the presence of a fracture.

2. Clinical Signs There is obvious tenderness on the site of injury. The tenderness is often inferior to the lateral malleolous in anterior talofibular ligament injury. Pay attention to the presence of any tenderness on the medial and lateral malleolus, the process of the medial and lateral malleolus, and the region of the fifth metatarsal base during the examination to rule out any fractures.

3. Examination X-ray helps to rule out fractures. The film for the ankle is usually taken laterally. If a complete rupture of the ligament is suspected, a varus or valgus stress film should be taken for the ankle. If the joint gap of the injury side is significantly widened or there is talus dislocation, it suggests complete fracture of the ligament.

▶ Treatment

1. Treatment Principles Dispelling stasis, dispersing swelling, relieving pain, and improving movements.

2. Maneuvers Pressing-kneading, rubbing, pushing, and rotating.

Note:

The treatment scope of *tuina* in treating soft tissue injury of the ankle does not include bone fracture or third degree sprain. First degree sprain has mild ligament tearing, second degree has moderate tearing, and the third degree has complete tearing.

3. Operations

(1) *Tuina* manual treatment should not be used in the acute phase of this injury. If there is tarsometatarsal joint dislocation, traction of the toe can be used to reduce it. Then according to the specific circumstances, refer out to fix the joint and advise the patient to limit physical activities involving the injured joint. Wait for 72 hours prior to perform *tuina*.

(2) The specific treatment in the period of convalescence is as follows: ① Ask the patient to sit on the treatment table with the affected limb extended. Use the thumb and the thenar eminence to press-knead the injured foot. The force should be gentle to invigorate

blood and dispel blood stasis. ② Smear a small amount of *tuina* butter on the injured area, perform finger rubbing, and perform pushing from the distal to the proximal side to speed up swelling elimination. ③ Support the heel with one hand, hold the dorsal aspect of the foot, and perform circular rotation without causing pain.

Note:

This method should not be used too early, generally used for two to three weeks after injury when there is still pain and limited function. When shaking, do not use strong shaking so as to avoid repeated damage of the repaired ligament. Be especially mindful when using the shaking technique in patients with the most pain.

▶ Prognosis

1. During the acute phase, if the injury is mild, use gentle *tuina* maneuvers for treatment. Then, fix the area by wrapping it with bandage to limit the movement of the injured foot to ensure the complete repair of damaged tissue and prevent repeated injury in the future. Ask the patient to keep the affected limb elevated above the heart to promote swelling elimination. If the damage is serious, be cautious while using *tuina* maneuvers, especially passive joint movements to avoid aggravating the injury.

2. In the early acute stage, apply cold pack to the area. As soon as the area is no longer swollen, use heat pack instead to invigorate blood and dispel stasis.

3. In the recovery period, instruct the patient to do functional exercise to promote the elimination of swelling.

▶ Exercise Method

In the recovery period, the patient can perform varus, valgus, plantar flexion, and dorsiflexion without causing pain in order to prevent the formation of adhesions. After adapting to the exercise, start walking slowly.

(II) Calcaneodynia

Calcaneodynia, or heel pain, refers to the pain in the plantar side of the heel. According to the different causes, it can be name as calcaneal periostitis, calcaneus spur, and attachment ending region ailment of the plantar fascia. It is common among people 40 to 60 years old. Among sports injuries, it is generally seen in athletes such as long-distance runners, jumpers, gymnasts, and basketball players.

Note:

Review knowledge related to the heel such as topographic anatomy, physiology, and pathology.

▶ Diagnosis

1. Clinical Symptoms

(1) *Pain*: The pain is generally localized to the plantar side of the heel. The pain is most severe when the patient stands up in the morning, or starts to move after resting for a while. After a short walk, the pain is alleviated; however, it increases after a long walk. Lastly, the pain can be aggravated while the patient rests, and it frequently disappears after a while.

(2) *Swelling and numbness*: Localized swelling of the sole accompanied by sense of distension and numbness.

2. Clinical Signs   Tenderness posteromedial to the calcaneal tuberosity often indicates calcaneus spur or plantar fasciitis, while tenderness inferior to, or at posterior inferior margin of the calcaneal tuberosity, is mostly due to calcaneal fat pad degeneration. If the tenderness is posterior superior to the heel, it is commonly Achilles tendonitis or subcutaneous calcaneal bursitis.

3. Examination   Among elderly patients, the lateral view of the X-ray can detect calcaneal spur. In acute injury, X-ray is helpful to rule out fractures.

▶ Treatment

1. Treatment Principles   Dispelling stasis and unblocking collaterals.

2. Maneuvers   Precision pressing, pressing, kneading, grasping, plucking, rotating, and scrubbing.

3. Operation

(1) Ask the patient to lie in the supine position. Stand to the patient's affected side, and perform precision pressing on acupoints including *sān yīn jiāo* (SP 6), *jīn mén* (BL 63, 金门), *rán gǔ* (KI 2, 然谷), *tài chōng* (LR 3, 太冲), *zhào hǎi* (KI 6, 照海), *kūn lún* (BL 60, 昆仑), *shēn mài* (BL 62, 申脉), *yǒng quán* (KI 1, 涌泉) and the heel area, each point for half a minute.

(2) Use the palm heel or fist to perform tapping on the tenderness point continuous for a few dozen times.

(3) Ask the patient to lie in a prone position. Stand beside the affected limb and apply grasping and press-kneading starting from the gastrocnemius to the base of the calcaneus up and down repeatedly for five minutes.

(4) Perform plucking to the plantar fascia transversely to foot toe direction for a minute.

(5) Ask the patient to lie in the supine position. Stand to the side of the patient, gently perform passive rotation, flexion and extension to the ankles for a few dozen times.

(6) Apply scrubbing using the hypothenar along the direction of plantar fascia on the heel and *yǒng quán* (KI 1) until the area feels thoroughly warm.

Note:

The method is suitable for calcaneal bone spur, calcaneus bursitis, and fat pad inflammation of the heel. *Tuina* manual treatment is forbidden for calcaneodynia due to calcaneal osteomyelitis, and calcaneal tuberculosis.

▶ Prognosis

A patient in the acute stage of the disease should rest well, while an athlete should refrain from training. Shoe-pads helps to reduce irritation in the area.

▶ Exercise Method

Persist in plantar metatarsophalangeal plantar flexion movement, dorsiflexion and foot muscle contraction exercise.

Section 2   Internal Diseases

I. Common Cold

Common cold refers to acute upper respiratory tract infection. The incidence shows no differences among age, gender, occupation and region. People with a weak constitution are, however, more vulnerable to the disease. The disease can occur at any time of the year, but especially in spring and winter. In general, the condition is mild, with shorter duration, and self-healing, but can sometimes be accompanied by serious complications. The disease is somewhat contagious. In Chinese medicine, common cold pertains to the disease category of "wind damage" and "cold damage". If the disease is widespread at a particular time of year and the symptoms are similar among all people, and can be bio-medically defined as influenza, then it is known as seasonal cold in Chinese medicine rather than common cold.

Note:

Chinese medicine believes that the main cause of cold is wind pathogen or epidemic virus entering from the mouth, nose or pores and invading the body. At the same time, since the function of the lung-*wei* fails to defend the human body, a series of lung system symptoms emerge.

▶ Diagnosis

1. Clinical Symptoms   Nasal congestion, runny nose, sneezing, cough, headache, aversion to cold, fever, general malaise and so on.

2. Chinese Medicine Pattern Differentiation

(1) *Common cold of wind-cold pattern*: An aversion to cold is more severe than fever, there is no sweating, headache, body aches, nasal congestion, hoarse voice, running nose, scratchy throat, or cough. There may be a thin white sputum, and the patient may not be thirsty or thirsty with a preference for warm water. The tongue coating is thin, white and moist while the pulse is floating, or floating and tight.

(2) *Common cold of wind-heat pattern*: Symptoms may include fever, slight aversion to cold, sweating, headache, stuffy nose, yellow drainage, cough, dry mouth and thirst. The throat may be swollen, inflamed and painful and the sputum is yellow and sticky. The tongue coating is thin and yellow with floating pulse.

(3) *Common cold of summer-dampness pattern*: As the name suggests, this variant of the common cold is seen in the summer. Symptoms include fever, aversion to cold, headache, dizziness, drowsiness and distention of the head, nasal congestion, turbid nasal discharge, vexation, thirst, no sweat or a little sweat, chest tightness, nausea, and scanty dark urine. The tongue body is red with yellow and greasy coating, while the pulse is soggy and rapid.

(4) *Common cold of deficient pattern*: In patients with qi deficiency, symptoms include aversion to cold, fever, headache, nasal congestion, sleepiness, fatigue, weakness, shortness of breath, no desire to talk, and a propensity to sweat easily. Often the patient may be elderly with multiple chronic conditions. The tongue body is pale with thin white coating and the pulse is floating and powerless. On the other hand, in patients with yin deficiency, symptoms can include headache, fever, dizziness, palpitation, dry mouth, heat sensation in the center of the palms and feet, dry cough with little sputum, night sweats,

and insomnia. The tongue is red with peeled coating or no coating, while the pulse is thready and rapid.

3. Clinical Signs   Generally, auscultation of the lungs is normal, although coarse breathing sounds can be found among a small number of patients.

4. Examinations   Laboratory tests normally indicate a viral infection with normal or slightly low white blood cell count, and increased proportion of lymphocytes. Among those that have bacterial infection, the white blood cell and neutrophil are increased while the nuclei shift to the left.

> *Note:*
>
> Common cold needs to be differentiated from as allergic rhinitis, acute tracheitis, acute bronchitis, and some acute infectious diseases.

▶ Treatment

1. Purpose   Opening the surface to release the pathogens.

2. Treatment Principle   Disperse the lung to release the surface.

3. Acupoints   *Yìn táng* (EX-HN 3), *tài yáng* (EX-HN 5), *shàng xīng* (DU 23, 上星), *bǎi huì* (DU 20), *fēng chí* (GB 20), *fēng mén* (BL 12), *fēng fǔ* (DU 16), *tiān zhù* (BL 10), *dà zhù* (BL 11), *fèi shù* (BL 13, 肺俞), *xīn shù* (BL 15, 心俞), *pí shù* (BL 20), *wèi shù* (BL 21), *shèn shù* (BL 23, 命门), *jiān jǐng* (GB 21), *qū chí* (LI 11), *zú sān lǐ* (ST 36), and *fēng lóng* (ST 40).

4. Maneuvers   Thumb pushing, palmer pushing, press-kneading, grasp-pinching, scrubbing, and patting.

5. Basic Operation

(1) Ask the patient to be seated. Stand to the side of the patient, apply thumb pushing to the neck top-down repeatedly for five to ten times, and perform the thenar eminence kneading method on the forehead with more focus on *yìn táng* (EX-HN 3) and *tài yáng* (EX-HN 5) for about five minutes.

(2) Pinch-grasping the five meridians of the head repeatedly for five to eight times.

(3) Stand in front of the patient and apply the sweep-scattering maneuver to both side of the head for about five minutes.

(4) Ask the patient to lie in a prone position. Use the heel of the palm to perform straight scrubbing the *du mai* and the both bladder meridians on the back till the area feels warm.

(5) Perform press-kneading the acupoints on the back such as *fēng mén* (BL 12), *fēng fǔ* (DU 16), *tiān zhù* (BL 10), *dà zhù* (BL 11), and *fèi shù* (BL 13), each point for a minute.

(6) Ask the patient to be seated. Stand behind the patient and apply grasping *jiān jǐng* (GB 21) for one to two minutes.

6. Modification Based on Pattern Differentiation

(1) *Wind-cold pattern*: Apply press-kneading with the focus on *fēng mén* (BL 12), *fēng chí* (GB 20) and *fēng fǔ* (DU 16), until the neck and upper back are relaxed. Perform pushing and scrubbing along the first and second lateral lines of both sides of the bladder meridians until the area feels thoroughly warm.

(2) *Wind-heat pattern*: Perform thumb pushing along the *du mai* from *yìn táng* (EX-HN 3) to *shàng xīng* (DU 23) repeatedly for five minutes. Then apply press-kneading on *bǎi huì* (DU 20) and *qū chí* (LI 11) for one to two minutes.

(3) *Summer-heat pattern*: Perform press-kneading on *pí shù* (BL 20) and *wèi shù* (BL 21) for two minutes, rub-kneading on the abdomen for five minutes, and press-kneading on *fēng lóng* (BL 40) for two minutes.

(4) *Deficient pattern*: Apply press-kneading on *shèn shù* (BL 23), *mìng mén* (DU 4) and *zú sān lǐ* (ST 36), each point for two minutes. Then use thumb pushing on *qì hǎi* (RN 6) and *guān yuán* (RN 4, 关元), each point for two minutes.

> *Note:*
>
> During the *tuina* treatment, if there are symptoms such as persistent high fever, aggravated cough, and cough up with bloody phlegm, take immediate comprehensive treatment measures.

▶ Precautions

1. During the disease period of a common cold, the patient needs to rest, drink plenty of warm water, eat healthy, and diet should be light, and maintain indoor air circulation.

2. Participate more in physical exercise, such as jogging, and swimming to enhance physical fitness.

Note:

Not only does *tuina* treat common cold, but also it can prevent the disease by press-kneading acupoints such as *yíng xiāng* (LI 20) and *fēng chí* (GB 20).

II. Chronic Bronchitis

Chronic bronchitis refers to any nonspecific chronic inflammation of the mucosa and the surrounding tissue of the trachea and bronchia. Bronchitis can be caused by a variety of factors. Clinical symptoms include cough, phlegm or asthma, which can last for more than three months per year and more than two consecutive years. In the early stage, the symptoms are mild, mostly occur in the winter, and are relieved after the spring while it is warm. In the advanced stage, the inflammation is aggravated, and the symptoms exist year round, regardless of the season. Along with the progression of the disease, it can be complicated by chronic obstructive pulmonary emphysema that seriously affect life and work. The disease pertains to the scope of "cough" and "panting pattern" defined in Chinese medicine.

▶ Diagnosis

1. Clinical Symptoms   The disease has a slow onset, and prolonged course, while recurrent acute attacks often lead to exacerbation of the disease. The main symptoms are cough, expectoration, sometimes accompanied by wheezing. Coughing generally happens in morning. During sleep, there is intermittent cough, sometimes with expectoration

that is generally sticky, white, serous, and foamy, occasionally with a tinge of blood. Shortness of breath after labor or activity may occur if the disease is accompanied by emphysema. Morning is the time of expectoration of a large amount of sputum, because getting up and standing stimulate the process. In asthmatic bronchitis, wheezing is significant, while some cases may be complicated by bronchial asthma. If the bronchitis is complicated with emphysema, shortness of breath can be manifested after participating in work or physical activities.

2. Chinese Medicine Pattern Differentiation

(1) *Wind-cold attacking the lung*: Clear or white and sticky sputum, chest distension, cough with hoarse sound, and body aches. The tongue body is normal or pale and swollen with thin white or white greasy coating, while the pulse is floating or floating tight.

(2) *Wind-heat invading the lung*: Yellow or green phlegm that may be sticky, purulent or bloody, chest fullness or shortness of breath, dry stool, and dark urine. The tongue is red with yellow and dry coating, while the pulse is slippery or rapid.

(3) *Phlegm-damp Accumulation in the lung*: The disease course of this pattern is a longer than other ones. Symptoms include cough with rough sound, profuse and sticky sputum which is white or gray, chest tightness, sensation of blockage of the middle abdomen, poor appetite, thin stool, and fatigue. The tongue coating is white and greasy while the pulse is soggy and slippery.

3. Signs   There is no abnormal signs in the early stage. In the acute stage, rhonchi or wet rales can be heard on the back or at the base of both lungs. The sound reduces or disappears after coughing. If bronchitis complicates with asthma, a wide range of wheezing and prolonged exhalation can be heard.

4. Examinations

(1) X-ray examination for the early stage of the disease may not show any abnormality. Recurrent attacks, however, would cause thickening of the bronchial wall, and inflammatory cell infiltration or fibrosis of the bronchioles or alveolar stroma. Under X-ray, these would be manifested as increased lung markings and the

texture is abnormal, which can be reticular or chord-like with speckled shadows, especially the lower part of the lungs.

(2) A pulmonary function test in the early stage does not produce abnormal findings. In the case of small airway obstruction, the flow volume is significantly reduced while the maximum expiratory flow volume curve is between 75% and 50% of the lung volume.

(3) If bacterial infection exists, the blood test findings may show the increase of the total leukocytes and/or neutrophils.

(4) Sputum culture can have positive result for certain pathogenic bacteria. The smear can detect Gram-positive or Gram-negative bacteria, or many damaged white blood cells and ruptured goblet cells.

Note:

During the diagnosis of chronic bronchitis, it is necessary to rule out other diseases such as cough-variant asthma, lung cancer, tuberculosis, bronchiectasis, pneumoconiosis, cardiac insufficiency, and bronchial asthma with manifestations of cough, expectoration and wheezing.

▶ Treatment

1. Purpose   Disperse phlegm, stop coughing and panting.

2. Treatment Principles   Scattering wind, diffusing the lung, drying dampness, dissolving phlegm, relieving cough, and calming panting.

3. Acupoints and Areas   Use acupoints such as *tiān tū* (RN 22), *dàn zhōng* (RN 17), *zhōng fǔ* (LU 1, 中府), *yún mén* (LU 2, 云门), *shēn zhù* (DU 12, 身柱), *dà zhù* (BL 11), *fēng mén* (BL 12), *fèi shù* (BL 13), *dìng chuǎn* (EX-B 1, 定喘), *chǐ zé* (LU 5, 尺泽), *wài guān* (SJ 5), *liè quē* (LU 7, 列缺), *tài yuān* (LU 9, 太渊), *yú jì* (LU 10), and *hé gǔ* (LI 4). The treatment areas can include the pathways of the lung meridian on the upper limbs, the hypochondriac region, the chest and the back.

4. Maneuvers   Thumb pushing, split pushing, pressing, kneading, multi-finger grasp-pinching, scrubbing and patting.

5. Basic Operations

(1) Ask the patient to be seated. Use thumb pushing on *tiān tū* (RN 22), *dàn zhōng* (RN 17), *zhōng fǔ* (LU 1), and *yún mén* (LU 2), each acupoint for one to two minutes. Then use the middle-finger kneading on these acupoints for a minute each.

(2) Use the thumbs to perform split pushing from the sternum xiphoid along the arc of the ribs to the hypochondriac areas on both side, and repeat five to eight times.

(3) Apply press-kneading on *dà zhuī* (DU 14), *dìng chuǎn* (EX-B 1), *shēn zhù* (DU 12), *dà zhù* (BL 11), *fēng mén* (BL 12), *fèi shù* (BL 13), *liè quē* (LU 7), and *yú jì* (LU 10) , each point for a minute.

(4) Use palmar scrubbing on the back horizontally until the region feels warm.

(5) Perform thumb pushing on *chǐ zé* (LU 5), *wài guān* (SJ 5), and *tài yuān* (LU 9), each point for two minutes.

(6) Perform grasp-kneading on *hé gǔ* (LI 4) for one to two minutes.

6. Modification Based on Pattern Differentiation

(1) *Wind-cold attacking the lung*: Perform press-kneading on *fēng chí* (GB 20) and *fēng fǔ* (DU 16), each point for one to two minutes. Then apply scrubbing along both the inner lines of the bladder meridians on the back using the hypothenar eminence until the area feels thoroughly warm. Next, perform grasping on *jiān jǐng* (GB 21) for one to two minutes.

(2) *Wind-heat invading the lung*: Press-kneading *qū chí* (LI 11) and *fēng lóng* (ST 40), each point for one to two minutes. Next, apply hypothenar scrubbing on *dà zhuī* (DU 14) until the region is thoroughly warm. Then, perform grasping to *jiān jǐng* (GB 21) for one minute.

(3) *Phlegm-damp Accumulation of the lung*: Press-kneading *shǒu sān lǐ* (LI 10), *fēng lóng* (ST 40), *zhāng mén* (LR 13, 章门), *tài chōng* (LR 3), and *xíng jiān* (LR 2), each point for one minute. Then, apply thumb-pushing to *tiān zhù* (BL 10), *zhōng wǎn* (RN 12), *pí shù* (BL 20) and *sān yīn jiāo* (SP 6), each point for one to two minutes. Next, use palmar scrubbing on the chest horizontally, and the hypochondriac regions obliquely until each area is warm.

Note:

Tuina is effective in treating this disease, especially increasing the patient's vital capacity, and alleviating symptoms after the treatment. When symptoms are severe, however, comprehensive treatment is necessary.

▶ Precautions

1. The patient should quit smoking, and keep the air in the living and workplace fresh. In the winter, take extra measures to keep warm and avoid cold, and actively prevent respiratory diseases such as the common cold.
2. Participate in physical exercise such as jogging, brisk walking, and *tai chi* to enhance physical fitness and improve cold tolerance.

Note:

Patients with chronic bronchitis should usually choose strengthening acupoints for self *tuina*, such as *zú sān lǐ* (ST 36), *shèn shù* (BL 23), *mìng* mén (DU 4), *qì hǎi* (RN 6), and *guān yuán* (RN 4) to enhance physical fitness, and prevent chronic bronchitis attack.

III. Stomachache

Stomachache refers to the pain of the stomach, and is a disorder of the spleen and stomach system, also known as the "heartburn" and "pain below the heart" in ancient China. Clinically, it is a common gastrointestinal symptom, often seen in problems such as acute and chronic gastritis, stomach ulcer and functional gastrointestinal disorder. The disease frequently recurs, and the condition often lingers.

Note:

Chinese Medicine believes that the disease is a disorder pertaining to the spleen and stomach system. Stomachache of cold pattern is caused by externally contracted cold pathogen attacking the stomach or eating too much cold food and drink, while that of the heat or food accumulation patterns are the final results of endogenous dampness owing to overeating too much oily and greasy food. The pain of the abnormal liver qi flow pattern can also cause stomach qi rebellion. Furthermore, if the spleen yang is weak, or the patient is often overworked, overeating or hungry, it may lead to deficient cold in the center, resulting in stomach pain. Lastly, the accumulation of parasites can cause stomach pain as well.

▶ Diagnosis

1. Clinical Symptoms   Pain in the upper abdomen right under the heart with noisy stomach, belching, acid reflux or spitting clear fluid, poor appetite, constipation or thin stool, and even vomiting blood or blood in the stool. If the course of the disease is long, the patient can be physically frail and lack luster.

2. Chinese Medicine Pattern Differentiation

(1) *Cold pathogen invading the stomach*: Sudden onset of the stomachache, aversion to cold, fond of warmth, reduced pain with heat pack on the stomach, and no thirst or desire for warm drinks. The tongue coating is white while the pulse is tight.

(2) *Food stagnation damaging the stomach*: Stomachache with distension and even pain, rotten acid regurgitation, vomiting of undigested food, and reduced pain after vomiting. The tongue coating is thick and greasy, while the pulse is slippery.

(3) *Liver qi attacking the stomach*: Pain due to distension and bloating of the stomach, and even radiating to both hypochondria, belch-

ing, and inhibited bowel movement. The tongue coating is usually thin white, while the pulse is wiry.

(4) *Deficient cold of the spleen and stomach*: Dull stomach pain, acid reflux with clear fluid, preference for warmth and pressing on the stomach area, cold limbs, and thin or watery stool. The tongue is pale with white coating, while the pulse is soft and weak or deep and thready.

3. Clinical Signs   Tenderness in gastric area.

4. Examinations   Gastroscopy can detect chronic superficial gastritis, gastric ulcer or gastric hemorrhage.

Note:

Stomachache is a symptom that can be caused by a variety of diseases. Therefore, it is important to confirm the diagnosis. In case of a severe situation, such as bleeding or gastric perforation, the patient needs to be sent to an emergency room.

▶ Treatment

1. Purpose   Rectifying qi, harmonizing the stomach, and relieving pain.

2. Treatment Principles   Warming the stomach, dissipating cold, promoting digestion, guiding out food stagnation, soothing the liver, resolving constraint, warming the center, and fortifying the spleen.

3. Acupoints and Areas   The acupoints may include *zhōng wǎn* (RN 12), *tiān shū* (ST 25), *qì hǎi* (RN 6), *gān shù* (BL 18, 肝俞), *pí shù* (BL 20), *wèi shù* (BL 21), *sān jiāo shù* (BL 22), *jiān jǐng* (GB 21), *shǒu sān lǐ* (LI 10), *nèi guān* (PC 6), and *hé gǔ* (LI 4). The areas may include the upper epigastric region, left and hypochondriac regions, and the regions lateral to the hypochondria.

4. Maneuvers   Thumb pushing, rubbing, kneading, pressing, scrubbing, grasping, and foulage.

5. Basic Operation

(1) Ask the patient to lie in a prone posi-

tion. Apply thumb pushing top-down along both sides of the bladder meridians until reaching the *sān jiāo shù* (BL 22) for five times.

(2) Use moderate force to perform press-kneading on *gān shù* (BL 18), *pí shù* (BL 20), *wèi shù* (BL 21), and *sān jiāo shù* (BL 22) for about five minutes.

(3) Apply scrubbing on the back from top to bottom along both sides of the bladder meridians until the area feels thoroughly warm.

(4) Ask the patient to lie in a supine position. Perform thumb pushing and rubbing on the epigastric region briskly so as to make the frictional heat penetrate the stomach.

(5) Perform press-kneading on *zhōng wǎn* (RN 12), *qì hǎi* (RN 6) and *zú sān lǐ* (ST 36) for about 20 minutes.

(6) Ask the patient to be seated. Apply grasping to *jiān jǐng* (GB 21) and along the upper arm top to the wrist to stimulate strongly with press-kneading to *shǒu sān lǐ* (LI 10), *nèi guān* (PC 6) and *hé gǔ* (LI 4). Then, perform foulage to the shoulder and arms to unblock the meridian. Next, apply foulage and smearing on the lateral hypochondria from top to bottom, five times.

6. Modification Based on Pattern Differentiation

(1) *Cold pathogen invading the stomach*: Use precision pressing or pressing to operate on *pí shù* (BL 20), and *wèi shù* (BL 21) for about two minutes. Perform scrubbing on the back until the area feels warm.

(2) *Food stagnation*: Apply the rubbing abdomen maneuver clockwise, precision-pressing method on *zhōng wǎn* (RN 12) and *tiān shū* (ST 25). Perform the press-kneading *pí shù* (BL 20), *wèi shù* (BL 21) and *zú sān lǐ* (ST 36).

(3) *Liver qi attacking the stomach*: Apply gentle thumb pushing or kneading to operate in the top-down direction from *tiān tū* (RN 22) to *zhōng wǎn* (RN 12) with more focus on *dàn zhōng* (RN 17). Then, perform gentle press-kneading to both sides of *zhāng mén* (LR 13) and *qī mén* (LR 14, 期门). Both steps take about 10 minutes. Next, work on the *gān shù* (BL 18) and *dǎn shù* (BL 19) with press-kneading maneuver.

(4) *Deficiency cold of the spleen and stomach*: Apply press-kneading on *qì hǎi* (RN 6), *guān*

yuán (RN 4), and *zú sān lǐ* (ST 36) for about two minutes at each point, however, the press-kneading time on *qì hǎi* (RN 6) may be extended. Then, perform straight scrubbing on *du mai*, and transverse scrubbing on the left side of the back and *shèn shù* (BL 23) and *mìng mén* (DU 4) until the area is thoroughly warm.

Note:

Patients with ulcerous bleeding should not have *tuina* treatment. The operation on the epigastric area should be one hour before or after meals. If the stomachache is severe, it should be treated with comprehensive method including herbal prescriptions or drugs.

▶ Precautions

1. Patients with stomach pain need to maintain a good mood, and exercise proper. Avoid overeating, or irregular eating habit. Generally, it is a good idea to have multiple meals in small proportion with food easy to digest. Avoid hard liquor and spicy food.
2. For patients with bleeding due to stomach or duodenal ulcer, *tuina* in general is not applicable.

Note:

If the attack of stomach pain is mild, the patient can press-knead *zhōng wǎn* (RN 12), *liáng qiū* (ST 34, 梁丘) and *zú sān lǐ* (ST 36), at each acupoint for one minute to relieve symptoms.

IV. Gastroptosis

Gastroptosis is caused by decreased tension of the stomach muscle layer and weakness of the surrounding tissue, and affects the lowest point of the lesser curvature below the iliac crest line when the patient is standing, or left deviation of the duodenal bulb.

The disease pertains to the scope of "stomach loose" and "stomach drop" defined in Chinese medicine.

Note:

Chinese medicine believes that the disease is closely related to the function of the spleen and stomach. The spleen and stomach system is the postnatal foundation and the source of qi and blood production. The spleen governs ascent of the clear qi, keeping organs in their normal position. Only when the spleen is not deficient, causing qi to sink, or food accumulation drags the stomach, the gastroptosis would happen. Moreover, it can happen after illness or postpartum weakness due to deficiencies of qi and blood, and spleen and stomach.

▶ Diagnosis

1. Clinical Symptoms   Patients have symptoms including chronic abdominal pain, a sense of bulging after eating, a conscious sense of sagging stomach and bowel sounds. Occasionally, there are constipation and diarrhea. In severe cases, there may be multiple visceral ptosis.

2. Chinese Medicine Pattern Differentiation

(1) *Liver qi stagnation*: Depression, poor mood, distension and pain in the hypochondriac area, or chest tightness, sensation of a foreign body in the throat, belching, nausea, and decreased food intake. The tongue coating is thin and white, while the pulse is thready and wiry.

(2) *Qi and blood deficiency*: Shortness of breath, reluctance to talk, lassitude of the four limbs, spontaneous sweating, insomnia, palpitation, pale or sallow facial complexion, and poor appetite. The tongue is light or swollen with teeth marks on the edge, and the tongue coating is thin and white fur. The pulse is thready, weak and powerless.

3. Clinical Signs   Patients often have

slender physique and the stomach area is concave with prominent lower abdomen. Strong beat of the abdominal aorta of the upper abdomen is palpable, while there is often vibration sound in the lower abdomen.

4. Examination   X-ray barium meal examination can detect that the stomach is visibly lowered in a standing position with the lowest point of the lesser curvature below line connecting the two iliac crests. Due to the traction of the sagging stomach, the upper corner of the duodenal ball seems sharper.

Note:

Gastroptosis should be differentiated from peptic ulcer, chronic gastritis, chronic hepatitis, neurosis, chronic cholecystitis, gastric cancer, gastric distension and pyloric obstruction.

▶ Treatment

1. Purpose   Raising yang and lifting the sunken.

2. Treatment Principles   Fortifying the spleen, harmonizing the stomach, supplementing the center, boosting and lifting qi.

3. Acupoints and Treatment Areas   *Zhōng wǎn* (RN 12), *qì hǎi* (RN 6), *guān yuán* (RN 4), *pí shù* (BL 20), *wèi shù* (BL 21), *qì hǎi shù* (BL 24), and *guān yuán shù* (BL 26).

4. Main Maneuvers   Kneading, thumb pushing, lifting, vibrating, and rubbing.

5. Operating Method

(1) Ask the patient to lie in a supine position. Use gentle thumb-pushing and kneading to operation with the focus on *zhōng wǎn* (RN 12).

(2) Start from *zhōng wǎn* (RN 12) and work down sequentially to the abdomen and lower abdomen. Focus more on the area around the umbilicus, *qì hǎi* (RN 6), and *guān yuán* (RN 4) for about 10 minutes.

(3) Apply lifting bottom-up from the lower edge of the stomach depending on the degree of gastroptosis.

(4) Use vibration on *zhōng wǎn* (RN 12) and the upper abdomen for about two minutes. Then, apply rubbing on the abdomen counterclockwise operation for about 10 minutes.

(5) Ask the patient to lie in a prone position, and perform press-kneading on *pí shù* (BL 20), *wèi shù* (BL 21), *qì hǎi shù* (BL 24), and *guān yuán shù* (BL 26) for about three minutes at each point.

6. Modification Based on Pattern Differentiation

(1) *Liver qi stagnation*: Apply press-kneading on *zhāng mén* (LR 13), *qī mén* (LR 14), *gān shù* (BL 18) and *tài chōng* (LR 3), at each point for two minutes. Next, perform scrubbing on both hypochondria until the warmth is thoroughly felt.

(2) *Qi and blood deficiency*: Perform straight scrubbing on the back portion of *du mai* and transverse scrubbing to the back until the area is thoroughly warm. Next, use gentle precision kneading on *wèi shù* (BL 21) and *zú sān lǐ* (ST 36).

Note:

while using *tuina* to treat gastroptosis, the maneuver should be gentle and even. At the same time, pay attention to anatomical location to ensure accurate treatment. Gastroptosis takes a long time to treat using *tuina* with 10 times as a treatment course, once every other day. If the symptoms get worse, comprehensive treatment should be sought as soon as possible.

▶ Precautions

1. Patients with gastroptosis should do exercises to strengthen the chest and abdomen muscles and ligaments. For patient with severe ptosis, use an abdominal binder to support the stomach.

2. Pay attention to the diet by eating easy to digest food and have a regular for meals. Do not overeat or skip meals. Avoid spicy food. Keep the mind relaxed, and maintain a positive attitude.

Note:

Gastroptosis patients can perform *tuina* to themselves by pressing on *qì hǎi* (RN 6), *zú sān lǐ* (ST 36) and foot relaxation zones such as the kidney, stomach, duodenum, small intestine, large intestine, and diaphragm on the sole for 10 minutes every time and once a day.

V. Diarrhea

Diarrhea is a condition characterized by an increase in the number of defecations (> 3 times per day), an increase in the amount of stools (> 200 g/d) and a thin fecal matter (water content > 85%), which can often be seen in diseases including acute enteritis, chronic enteritis, and intestinal disorders. The disease can occur at any time of the year, but is more common in summer and autumn.

Note:

Chinese medicine believes that the main pathologic changes of diarrhea happens in the system of spleen, stomach and intestines. One cause is invasion of external pathogens, commonly damp-cold, summer-damp, and damp heat. The other causes are food damage, emotional disorders and spleen and kidney yang deficiency.

▶ Diagnosis

1. Clinical Symptoms Main clinical symptoms include significantly increased frequency of bowel movements, fluffy stool, and even watery feces.

2. Chinese Medicine Pattern Differentiation

(1) *Acute diarrhea*: ① *Invasion of dampness*: Sudden onset, thin stool or mixed with mucus, several to a dozen times a day, abdominal pain, borborygmus, and body aches. The tongue coating can be white and greasy or yellow and greasy, while the pulse is soggy or slippery and rapid. ② *Food damage*: A history of overeating or unclean diet, sudden onset, abdominal pain and distension, the fecal odor resembling rotten eggs, reduced abdominal pain after the diarrhea, eructation with fetid odor, and acid reflux. The tongue coating is thick and greasy, while the pulse is soggy or slippery and rapid.

(2) *Chronic diarrhea*: ① *Spleen and stomach weakness*: The stool is loose sometimes and watery at other times with recurrent onset. Even a little bit of greasy food would increase the frequency of bowel movement with loss of appetite. The color of the tongue is pale with white coating, while the pulse is weak and moderate. ② *Spleen and kidney yang deficiency*: Multiple attacks before dawn with pain around the umbilicus. Diarrhea follows borborygmus with a reduction of pain after diarrhea. The patient's abdominal area is averse to cold with backache and cold limbs. The tongue is pale with white coating, while the pulse is deep and thready. ③ *Liver qi over-controlling the spleen*: Diarrhea is often induced by mental stimulation, and mood swings. Usually there may be abdominal pain, borborygmus, chest and hypochondriac fullness, belching, and poor appetite. The tongue coating is thin, while the pulse is wiry and thready.

3. Clinical Signs Abdominal palpation may have tenderness, severe diarrhea will be associated with signs of dehydration.

4. Examination

(1) *Blood and biochemical tests*: Help to understand the presence of anemia, increased white blood cell count, electrolyte and acid-base balance situation.

(2) *Stool examination*: Fresh stool examination is the most important method for the diagnosis of etiology of acute and chronic diarrhea. It can detect red and white blood cells, phagocytes, protozoa, parasite eggs, fat droplets and undigested food. The occult blood test can detect bleeding. Fecal culture can discover pathogenic microorganisms.

(3) *X-ray barium examination and abdominal plain film*: Both tests can reveal gastrointesti-

nal lesions, and intestinal motility status.

> **Note:**
>
> Diarrhea is a symptom that can be associated with various diseases. Therefore, the exact diagnosis needs to be confirmed. If the disease is severe or contagious, seek immediate emergency care.

▶ Treatment

1. Purpose Arresting diarrhea, and rescuing yang from desertion.

2. Treatment Principles Strengthening the spleen, harmonizing the stomach, warming the kidney, boosting yang, soothing liver qi, rectifying qi. Treat acute diarrhea with comprehensive methods including arresting and regulating, while chronic diarrhea needs to be treated by warming, tonifying, and supporting the healthy qi, so that the transporting function of the intestines can be restored.

3. Acupoints and Areas *Zhōng wǎn* (RN 12), *tiān shū* (ST 25), *qì hǎi* (RN 6), *guān yuán* (RN 4), middle abdomen; *pí shù* (BL 20), *wèi shù* (BL 21), *shèn shù* (BL 23), *dà cháng shù* (BL 25), *cháng qiáng* (DU 1), and lumbar area and sacral area.

4. Maneuvers One-finger pushing, rubbing, rolling, pressing-kneading, and scrubbing.

5. Basic Operations

(1) Ask the patient to lie in a supine position. Use thumb pushing, work slowly, start from *zhōng wǎn* (RN 12), and move down to operate on *qì hǎi* (RN 6) and *guān yuán* (RN 4) in turn. Repeat the procedure five to six times.

(2) Use a palm to perform counterclockwise abdomen rubbing for about eight minutes.

(3) Ask the patient to lie in a prone position. Apply rolling along both sides of the spine from *pí shù* (BL 20) to *dà cháng shù* (BL 25) for three to four times.

(4) Perform press-kneading on *pí shù* (BL 20), *wèi shù* (BL 21), *dà cháng shù* (BL 25), and *cháng qiáng* (DU 1), at each point for one to two minutes. Then, perform scrubbing on the left side of the back until the area feels thoroughly warm.

6. Modification Based on Pattern Differentiation

(1) *Spleen and stomach weakness*: Apply press-kneading *qì hǎi* (RN 6), *guān yuán* (RN 4) and *zú sān lǐ* (ST 36) for about two minutes at each point. The length of time working on *qì hǎi* (RN 6) can be extended. Apply counterclockwise abdominal rubbing for about three minutes with focus on the epigastric area. When working in the middle and lower abdomen, apply rubbing clockwise.

(2) *Spleen and kidney yang deficiency*: Perform press-kneading on *qì hǎi* (RN 6) and *guān yuán* (RN 4) for about three minutes at each acupoint. Then, apply straight forward scrubbing on the back portion of *du mai* and horizontal scrubbing on *mìng mén* (DU 4), *shèn shù* (BL 23), and the eight *liáo* (BL 31 to BL 34) points until the area is warm thoroughly.

(3) *Liver qi over-restricting spleen*: Apply press-kneading on both sides of *zhāng mén* (LR 13) and *qī mén* (LR 14), at each point for about two minutes. Then, perform oblique scrubbing on both hypochondria until the areas are thoroughly warm. Next, apply press-kneading on acupoints such as *gān shù* (BL 18), *dǎn shù* (BL 19), *gé shù* (BL 17), *tài chōng* (LR 3) and *xíng jiān* (LV 2), at each point for a minute.

> **Note:**
>
> *Tuina* is fairly effective in treating both acute and chronic diarrhea.For patients with serious diarrhea,however, it is necessary to take a comprehensive approach involving Chinese medicine and other measures.

▶ Precautions

1. *Tuina* is very effective for chronic diarrhea. On the other hand, severe acute diarrhea with fulminant vomiting in the summer should be treated using a comprehensive approach.

2. Maintain a lifestyle with a regular schedule.

Do not overeat food with high fat, cold food or food that is not easy to digest. Pay attention to keep warm, and avoid being too tired.

> **Note:**
>
> Patients can perform press-kneading to themselves on *bǎi huì* (DU 20) and *zú sān lǐ* (ST 36) at each acupoint for a minute. Then, apply scrubbing on *yǒng quán* (KI 1) until it feels warm. Using these self care techniques would improve the symptoms of diarrhea.

VI. Constipation

Constipation is the condition of dry and hard stool with prolonged defecation, or having the urge to defecate yet difficulty in producing a bowel movement. Constipation can appear alone or as a symptom in a variety of diseases. There is no obvious seasonal pattern of onset and no gender and age differences but it can be related to eating habits and a lack of physical activities. It is similar to biomedically defined illnesses such as "habitual constipation".

> **Note:**
>
> Chinese medicine believes that food and drinks enter into the stomach, which kicks off the transportation and transformation function of the spleen and stomach system, so that first, the essence from the food can be absorbed. Then, the large intestine would purge the remaining waste in the form of feces. If the transportation and transformation of the spleen and stomach, and the conducting and transmitting functions of the large intestine are normal, the patency of the defecation is ensured. On the other hand, if there is damage to the gastrointestinal functions, constipation may occur.

► Diagnosis

1. Clinical Symptoms Dry stools with defecation difficulty once every three days or even once every week. Alternatively, the frequency of the bowel movement may be normal, but the stool is dry and hard, making it difficult to defecate. In some cases, patients they often have the desire for a bowel movement, and the stool is not dry, but there is hardship in emptying their bowel. Other symptoms may include abdominal distension, hemorrhoids or anal fissure.

2. Chinese Medicine Pattern Differentiation

(1) *Dryness-heat of the stomach and intestines*: Dry stool, dark urine, red face, hot sensation of the body, dry mouth, and vexation. The tongue is red with yellow coating, while the pulse is slippery and rapid.

(2) *Qi stagnation*: Constipation with dry stool and difficult defecation, frequent belching, and fullness of the hypochondria and the abdomen. The tongue coating is thin and greasy, while the pulse is wiry.

(3) *Qi and blood deficiency*: ① *Constipation of qi deficiency* - Defecation difficulty, sweating and shortness of breath after bowel movement, but the stool is not dry. The tongue is pale with thin coating, while pulse is weak and deficient. ② *Constipation of blood deficiency* - Dry stool, pale facial complexion, dizziness, and palpitation. The lips and tongue are pale, while the pulse is thready.

(4) *Yin-cold coagulation*: Difficult defecation, clear urine with larger amount, cold limbs, aversion to cold, and backache with cold feeling. The tongue is pale with white coating, while the pulse is deep and slow.

3. Signs Fullness of the abdomen, abdominal muscle tension, and palpable shape of the intestine.

4. Examination

(1) *Stool examination*: May not find any abnormalities among patients with functional constipation.

(2) *Rectal examination*: Rectum dilatation and fecal matter can be detected. At the same time, examination can also reveal rectal cancer, hemorrhoids, anal fissure, inflammation,

stenosis and foreign pressure.

(3) *Barium enema X-ray exam and abdominal plain film*: Barium X-rays can provide a comprehensive understanding of the function of colon movement (peristalsis), which is beneficial to the diagnosis of lesions such as colon tumor, rectal tumor, colon stenosis or spasm, megacolon, and intestinal obstruction.

(4) *Colonoscopy*: Endoscopic examination is of great help in diagnosing a variety of colorectal lesions causing constipation, such as colon cancer, rectal cancer, intestine polyps and so on which cause organic intestinal stenosis. While combining with biopsy, it can be used to confirm a diagnosis.

> **Note:**
>
> Functional constipation needs to be differentiated from constipation caused by diseases such as rectal cancer, intestinal obstruction, intestinal polyps, and hemorrhoids.

▶ Treatment

1. Purpose   Harmonizing the intestines, and promoting defecation.

2. Treatment Principles   Unblocking the bowels, directing qi downwards, and rectifying qi movements.

3. Acupoints and Areas to be Used   *zhōng wǎn* (RN 12), *tiān shū* (ST 25), *dà héng* (SP 15, 大横), *gān shù* (BL 18), *pí shù* (BL 20), *wèi shù* (BL 21), *shèn shù* (BL 23) and *dà cháng shù* (BL 25).

4. Maneuvers   Thumb pushing, rubbing, pressing, and kneading.

5. Basic Operations

(1) Ask the patient to lie in a supine position. Use the thumb pushing method to gently work on *zhōng wǎn* (RN 12), *tiān shū* (ST 25), and *dà héng* (SP 15), each point for about a minute.

(2) Use the palmar rubbing method on the abdomen clockwise for about five minutes.

(3) Ask the patient to lie in a prone position. Use gentle thumb pushing maneuver along both sides of the spine back and forth between *gān shù* (BL 18) and *pí shù* (BL 20) for

about five minutes.

(4) Apply the press kneading method gently on *shèn shù* (BL 23) and *dà cháng shù* (BL 25), each point for about two minutes.

6. Modification Based on Pattern Differentiation

(1) *Dryness-heat in the stomach and intestines*: Perform the press-kneading method on *dà cháng shù* (BL 25), *zhī gōu* (SJ 6, 支沟) and *qū chí* (LI 11) until each point feels sore. Then, apply the pushing method from *zú sān lǐ* (ST 36) down to *xià jù xū* (ST 39) for five minutes.

(2) *Qi stagnation*: Apply the press-kneading maneuver to *dàn zhōng* (RN 17), *gé shù* (BL 17), *zhōng wǎn* (RN 12), *zhāng mén* (LR 13), *qī mén* (LR 14), *fèi shù* (BL 13), and *gān shù* (BL 18) until each point feels sore. Next, use the scrubbing method to the upper chest horizontally until the region feels thoroughly warm. Lastly, apply the oblique scrubbing maneuver on both the hypochondria until the areas are slightly warm.

(3) *Qi and blood deficiency*: Perform the horizontal scrubbing maneuver to the upper chest until it is thoroughly warm. Then, apply the press-kneading method on *zú sān lǐ* (ST) and *pí shù* (BL 20) for two minutes at each point. Press-kneading can also be combined with the pinching *jǐ* (spine) method for three times.

(4) *Yin-cold coagulation*: Perform the horizontal scrubbing method to the shoulders, back, *shèn shù* (BL 23), *mìng mén* (DU 4) and the sacral area, and vertical scrubbing method on *du mai* until these areas are thoroughly warm.

> **Note:**
>
> *Tuina* maneuvers that unblock the bowels to purge feces is applicable once a day for treating constipation of excess patterns. When using *tuina* for constipation of deficient patterns, the maneuvers should be gentle, while the treatment time and treatment course should be longer.

▶ Precautions

1. Patients suffering from constipation should intentionally develop the habit of a

regular schedule for bowel movement and drink plenty of water. When getting up in the morning, light salt boiled water is recommended. Add more fruits and vegetables to the diet and avoid spicy food.

2. Participate in more outdoor activities, avoid being sedentary, do more squatting, standing up and movement with a supine position. At the same time, maintain a positive attitude.

Note:

Patients having constipation can perform clockwise pushing and rubbing by placing their overlapped hands on top of the navel. Clockwise rubbing is a great purging method.

VII. Hypertension

Hypertension, also known as essential hypertension, is a syndrome with the main clinical manifestation as vascular hypertension of systemic circulation with or without a variety of cardiovascular risk factors. The diagnostic criteria for hypertension are based on clinical and epidemiological data. Currently, the international standard for the diagnosis of hypertension is a systolic blood pressure ≥ 140mmHg and (or) diastolic blood pressure ≥ 90mmHg. Hypertension can affect the structure and function of heart, brain, kidney and other vital organs, and eventually lead to functional failure of these organs. Therefore, it is one of the major causes of cardiovascular death. In Chinese medicine, the disease is in the scope of "headache" or "dizziness".

Note:

Chinese medicine believes that hypertension is closely related to factors including diet, fatigue from excessive strain, emotional disorders, age, and daily life routines.

▶ Diagnosis

1. Clinical Symptoms   Symptoms may include dizziness, headache, neck stiffness, fatigue, palpitations, tinnitus, forgetfulness, and insomnia that are mild and persistent. Many of the symptoms may ease on their own, yet will be aggravated after being stressed or after a period of hard-working. In the late stage, there may be symptoms of organ damage to the heart, brain, and kidney.

2. Chinese Medicine Pattern Differentiation

(1) *Ascendant hyperactive liver yang*: Symptoms can include dizziness, headache, red face and eyes, impatience, irritability, dry and bitter mouth, insomnia, stiff neck, and limb numbness. Mood swings can induce or aggravate the symptoms. The tongue is red, while the pulse is wiry and rapid.

(2) *Turbid phlegm obstructing the center*: Symptoms may include dizziness, vertigo, heavy-headedness, sticky feeling in the mouth, nausea, vomiting, excessive sputum, poor appetite, fatigue, and abdominal fullness. The tongue body is red with greasy coating, while the pulse is wiry and slippery.

(3) *Kidney essence deficiency*: Headache with physical feeling of emptiness, dizziness, tinnitus, heat in the five centers, soreness and weakness of the lumbar and knees, palpitation, fatigue, forgetfulness, and nocturnal emission. The tongue is red with less coating, while the pulse is thready and rapid.

3. Clinical Signs   Systolic blood pressure ≥ 140mmHg, and (or) diastolic blood pressure ≥ 90mmHg. Auscultation can detect a loud second heart sound, systolic murmur or clicks in the early contraction period. In patients with second or third stage hypertension, signs such as left ventricular hypertrophy, retinal artery spasm and stenosis can be seen.

4. Examination

(1) Urinalysis, blood glucose, blood cholesterol, triglycerides, renal function, serum uric acid and electrocardiogram may help to detect related risk factors and target organ damage.

(2) Some patients can further take fundus

examination, echocardiography, blood electrolytes, LDL-C, HDL-C, plasma renin activity (PRA), and 24-hour ambulatory blood pressure monitoring (ABP monitoring) to understand the process of hypertension.

Note:

Hypertension should be differentiated from conditions such as transient hypertension and secondary hypertension.

▶ Treatment

1. Purpose   Clearing the liver, and lowering the blood pressure.

2. Treatment Principles   Calming the liver and mind, dissolving the phlegm, and directing turbidity downwards. For patients with ascendant liver yang hyperactivity pattern, supplement with clearing fire and extinguishing wind. For those with phlegm-dampness obstructing the center, add spleen fortifying and damp dispelling techniques. Lastly, supplement the treatment by adding kidney tonifying and essence boosting for patients that are showing kidney essence deficiency pattern.

3. Acupoints and Areas   *Qiáo gōng* (bridge arch), *yìn táng* (EX-HN 3), the hairline, *tài yáng* (EX-HN 5), *bǎi huì* (DU 20), *fēng chí* (GB 20), *fēng fǔ* (DU 16), *tóu wéi* (ST 8), *gōng sūn* (SP 4, 公 孙), *cuán zhú* (BL 2), *dà zhuī* (DU 14), *guān yuán* (RN 4), *qì hǎi* (RN 6), *zhōng wǎn* (RN 12), *dà héng* (SP 15), *shèn shù* (BL 23), *mìng mén* (DU 4), *yǒng quán* (KI 1), the forehead and so on.

4. Maneuvers   Straight pushing, thumb pushing, kneading, split pushing, sweep scattering, smearing, grasping, rubbing, pressing, and scrubbing.

5. Basic Operations

(1) Ask the patient to be seated. Use the straight pushing method top down on *qiáo gōng* (bridge arch), first on the left, then on the right, each side for a minute.

(2) Apply the thumb pushing on both sides from *yìn táng* (EX-HN 3) up to the front hairline, and from *yìn táng* (EX-HN 3) to *tài yáng* (EX-HN 5) along the eyebrows for three to

five times. Next, push from *yìn táng* (EX-HN 3) to one side of *jīng míng* (BL 1) around the orbit, each side for three to five times, and perform this for four minutes. Then, perform the kneading maneuver on the forehead with the thenar eminence from one side of the *tài yáng* (EX-HN 5) to the other for three to five times, and continue for about four minutes. Lastly, use the split pushing from the forehead to *yíng xiāng* (LI 20) for three to five times and repeat for two to three times.

(3) Perform the sweep scattering along the head portion of gallbladder meridian starting from the anterior-superior to the posteroinferior aspect for 20 to 30 times each side. Then apply the smearing method on the forehead and face combined with press kneading *jiǎo sūn* (SJ 20, 角 孙), *jīng míng* (BL 1) and *tài yáng* (EX-HN 5) for about three minutes.

(4) Apply the five-finger grasping to the top of the head, and change it to three-finger grasping when reaching neck, continue to work along the cervical vertebra on both sides until the level of *dà zhuī* (DU 14), and repeat three to four times. Then, perform the press grasping method on *bǎi huì* (DU 20) and *fēng chí* (GB 20) for about three minutes.

(5) Use the thumb pushing maneuver, start from *fēng fǔ* (DU 16) and go down along both sides of the cervical vertebra until *dà zhuī* (DU 14) back and forth for about four minutes.

(6) Ask the patient to lie in a supine position. Use the palmar rubbing clockwise on the abdomen for about five minutes.

(7) Apply the press kneading method on points such as *guān yuán* (RN 4), *qì hǎi* (RN 6), *zhōng wǎn* (RN 12) and *dà héng* (SP 15), one minute at each point.

(8) Have the patient be in a prone position. Apply horizontal scrubbing with the palm on the region crossing *shèn shù* (BL 23) and *mìng mén* (DU 4), and oblique scrubbing with the hypothenar eminence on *yǒng quán* (KI 1) until the areas are thoroughly warm.

6. Modification Based on Pattern Differentiation

(1) *Ascendant hyperactive liver yang*: Use the precision pressing method on *tài chōng* (LR 3) and *xíng jiān* (LR 2), a minute or two each

point. Then, apply the press kneading maneuver on *gān shù* (BL 18), *shèn shù* (BL 23) and *yǒng quán* (KI 1), for a minute at each point.

(2) *Phlegm-dampness obstructing the center*: Apply the thumb pushing method on *zhōng wǎn* (RN 12) and *tiān shū* (ST 25) for one to two minutes at each point. Then, apply the press kneading method on *fēng lóng* (ST 40), *jiě xī* (ST 41, 解溪) and *zú sān lǐ* (ST 36), for a minute at each point.

(3) *Kidney essence deficiency*: Perform the precision pressing on *gān shù* (BL 18) and *shèn shù* (BL 23), every point for one to two minutes. Next, apply the press kneading method on *tài xī* (KI 3), *sān yīn jiāo* (SP 6) and *yǒng quán* (KI 1), for a minute at each point.

> **Note:**
>
> Avoid using violent and brute force while treating hypertensive patients with *tuina*. Especially when applying the pushing method on *qiáo gōng* (bridge arch), the stroke must be gentle, unilateral, and alternating between the left and right sides.

▶ Precautions

1. *Tuina* is applicable to hypertensive patients with mild and moderate hypertension that is slowly progressing. *Tuina* can produce moderate and satisfactory effects in lowering the blood pressure. Unlike antihypertensive drugs, however, *tuina* does not have side effects.

> **Note:**
>
> Hypertensive patients can perform self *tuina* by using the press kneading method on *nèi guān* (PC 6), *fēng chí* (GB 20), *tiān zhù* (BL 10), *shuài gǔ* (GB 8, 率谷), *qū chí* (LI 11) and *tài yáng* (EX-HN 5), for one minute at each point. Also, the split-smearing manuever can be used on *qiáo gōng* (bridge arch), alternating between the left and right sides, 30 times each side, once in the morning and once in the evening.

2. Hypertensive patients should maintain a cheerful and optimistic attitude. Avoid stress and fatigue, ensure adequate sleep time, engage in appropriate physical exercise under the guidance of a doctor, avoid being overweight and obesity, quit smoking and alcohol, and maintain a low fat, low sodium and light diet.

VIII. Headache

Headache is usually associated with pain confined to the upper part of the head, including the eyebrows, the upper edge of the ear and the area above the line of the external occipital protuberance. It can appear alone, or also be found in a variety of acute and chronic diseases. Headache can be divided into two types, primary and secondary. The former can also be called idiopathic headache, and includes common form of headaches such as migraine and tension headache, while the latter includes headaches caused by a variety of intracranial lesions such as cerebrovascular diseases, intracranial infections, craniocerebral trauma, systemic diseases and psychoactive drug abuse. Headache can occur at any time, and in any age groups. In Chinese medicine, it is often referred as the "head wind" or "brain wind". In this section, only primary headache will be discussed.

> **Note:**
>
> Chinese medicine believes that the head is the convergence of all yang meridians, where all external pathogens and internal damages can cause situations such as qi and blood blockages, meridian disorders, and failure of the clear yang to rise, resulting in various types of pain in different parts of the head.

▶ Diagnosis

1. Clinical Symptoms The primary symptom is the headache that may occur in the forehead, or frontotemporal, parietal, and parieto-occipital areas, and even the whole head. The types of the headache can be throbbing, stabbing, distending, fainting and dull. In some cases, a headache can have a sudden onset with stabbing and persistent pain, while in other cases, it is recurrent, intermittent and refractory. The length of the headache episode can last for several minutes, hours, days or even weeks.

2. Chinese Medicine Pattern Differentiation

(1) *Headache due to wind-cold*: Commonly occur after being contacted with cold wind, and the pain can radiate to the neck, shoulders and even the back. Other symptoms include aversion to cold wind, associated with a preference to wrap the head with a scarf. Patients usually do not feel thirsty. The tongue coating is thin and white, while the pulse is floating or tight.

(2) *Headache due to wind-heat*: Wind-heat headaches exhibit distending pain, some patients may even describe the pain as "splitting headache". Other symptoms may include aversion to wind, low grade to medium fever, red eyes, flushing, and thirst with desire for water. The throat can be inflamed, sore, and swollen, and the urine is dark. The patient may be constipated. The tip of the tongue may be red and the tongue coating thin and yellowish, the pulse is floating and rapid.

(3) *Headache due to summer-damp*: Headache, heavy-headedness, abdominal fullness, poor appetite, general fatigue, fever, sweating, vexation, and thirst. The tongue coating is greasy, while the pulse is rapid.

(4) *Headache due to hyperactive liver yang*: Headache, dizziness, irritability, restless sleep, flushing, and dry mouth. The tongue coating is thin and yellow, or the tongue is red with very little coating, while the pulse is wiry or wiry, thready and rapid.

(5) *Headache due to phlegm turbidity*: Headache with distended feeling, obstruction in the chest and diaphragm region, poor appetite, fatigue, spitting of frothy saliva, and nausea. The tongue coating is white and greasy, while the pulse is slippery.

(6) *Headache due to blood deficiency*: Headache, dizziness, mental and physical fatigue, lack of skin luster, palpitations, and shortness of breath. The tongue is pale, while the pulse is thready and weak.

(7) *Headache due to kidney deficiency*: Headache, empty headedness feeling, tinnitus, dizziness, backache, weak legs, and nocturnal emission or abnormal vaginal discharge. Patients with yang deficiency have cold limbs, and pale and swollen tongue, while the pulse is deep, thready and weak. Patients with yin deficiency will have dry mouth, lack of fluid, while the tongue is red and the pulse is thready and rapid.

(8) *Headache due to blood stasis*: Refractory headache with stabbing pain in fixed areas that comes and goes. Stasis macules can be seen on the tongue, and the pulse is choppy.

3. Clinical Signs   There is no specific positive signs.

4. Examinations   The examinations that helps to rule out organic diseases include routine blood test, transcranial Doppler, electroencephalogram, cerebrospinal fluid, brain CT, MRI, and the relevant ENT examination.

Note:

Primary headache should be differentiated with headaches caused by intracranial lesions, craniocerebral trauma, various encephalopathies, cerebrovascular accident, and ENT diseases.

▶ Treatment

1. Purpose   Regulating and unblocking the meridians, and raising and lifting clear yang.

2. Treatment Principles   Relaxing sinews, unblocking the collaterals, invigorating blood, dissolving stasis, resolving spasm, and relieving pain. Additions:

(1) *Wind-cold pattern*: Dissipating wind and dispelling cold;

(2) *Wind-heat pattern*: Dissipating wind and clearing heat;

(3) *Summer-damp pattern*: Removing summer-heat and conquering dampness;

(4) *Liver-yang rising*: Calming the liver and extinguishing wind;

(5) *Turbid phlegm*: Fortifying the spleen to

resolve the phlegm;

(6) *Blood deficiency*: Enriching yin and nourishing blood;

(7) *Kidney deficiency*: Supplementing the kidney to generate bone marrow;

(8) *Blood stasis*: Invigorating blood and dissolving stasis

3. Acupoints and Areas *fēng chí* (GB 20), *fēng fǔ* (DU 16), *tiān zhù* (BL 10), *yìn táng* (EX-HN 3), *tóu wéi* (BL 8), *tài yáng* (EX-HN 5), *yú yāo* (EX-HN 4), *bǎi huì* (DU 20), neck and forehead.

4. Maneuvers Thumb pushing, grasping, pressing, and kneading.

5. Basic Operations

(1) Ask the patient to be seated. Apply the thumb pushing method along both sides of the nape from top to bottom for three to five minutes.

(2) Use the press-kneading method on acupoints such as *fēng chí* (GB 20), *fēng fǔ* (DU 16) and *tiān zhù* (BL 10) for two to three minutes.

(3) Perform the grasping maneuver on both sides of *fēng chí* (GB 20) and along the neck from top to bottom four to five times.

(4) Apply the thumb pushing method from *yìn táng* (EX-HN 3), push up and continue along the front hairline to *tóu wéi* (ST 8), then go down to *tài yáng* (EX-HN 5). Repeat three to five times.

(5) Use the press kneading maneuver to work on *yìn táng* (EX-HN 3), *yú yāo* (EX-HN 4), *tài yáng* (EX-HN 5), and *bǎi huì* (DU 20) for two to three minutes.

(6) Apply the five-finger grasping method to start from the top of the head to both the *fēng chí* (GB 20) points. Then, change to the three-finger grasping method to work along the bladder meridians along both sides until level with *dà zhuī* (DU 14). Repeat three to five times.

6. Modification Based on Pattern Differentiation

(1) *Wind-cold headache*: Apply the press kneading method on the nape of the neck and the upper back for two to three minutes, focusing on *fēng mén* (BL 12) and *fèi shù* (BL 13). Next, perform the grasping method on *jiān jǐng* (GB 21) for 30 times. Then, use straight scrubbing method with hypothenar eminence on both sides of the bladder meridians on the back until the area is thoroughly warm.

(2) *Wind-heat headache*: Use the press kneading method on *dà zhuī* (DU 14), *fèi shù* (BL 13), and *fēng mén* (BL 12), for a minute at each acupoint. Then, apply the grasping method *jiān jǐng* (GB 21) for 30 times. Next, perform the press grasping on *qū chí* (LI 11) and *hé gǔ* (LI 4) until the points feel sore. Then, use the patting-striking maneuver on both sides of the bladder meridian of the back until the skin of the area is reddish.

(3) *Summer-damp headache*: Apply the press kneading method on *dà zhuī* (DU 14) and *qū chí* (LI 11), for one minute at each point. Then, use the grasping method on *jiān jǐng* (GB 21) and *hé gǔ* (LI 4) until there is the feeling of soreness and distention. Next, perform the patting-striking method on both sides of the bladder meridian of the back until the skin of the area is reddish. Lastly, apply the lift-pinching maneuver to the skin of *yìn táng* (EX-HN 3) and the nape of the neck until the skin is red.

(4) *Headache due to liver-yang rising*: Push *qiáo gōng* (bridge arch) from top to bottom, about 20 times on each side. Then, use the sweep-scattering maneuver along the gallbladder meridians from the anterosuperior to the posterior-inferior aspect of the head, on both sides for a few dozen times each side. At the same time, apply the pressing method on *jiǎo sūn* (SJ 20). Next, perform the press-kneading maneuver on *tài chōng* (LR 3) and *xíng jiān* (LR 2) until there is soreness sensation. Lastly, apply oblique palmar scrubbing method on *yǒng quán* (KI 1) until the acupoint feels thoroughly warm.

(5) *Phlegm-turbidity headache*: Apply the thumb-pushing method on *zhōng wǎn* (RN 12) and *tiān shū* (ST 25), for one to two minutes at each point, then abdomen rubbing method for three minutes, and the press-kneading maneuver on *pí shù* (BL 20), *wèi shù* (BL 21), *dà cháng shù* (BL 25), *zú sān lǐ* (ST 36), *fēng lóng* (ST 40) and *nèi guān* (PC 6) for one minute at each point. Lastly, perform horizontal palmar scrubbing along the left side of the back until the area is thoroughly warm.

(6) *Blood deficiency headache*: Perform abdominal rubbing for five minutes with the focus on *zhōng wǎn* (RN 12), *qì hǎi* (RN 6) and *guān yuán* (RN 4). Next, use palmar scrub-

bing straightly on *du mai* of the back until the area feels thoroughly warm. Then, apply the press-kneading maneuver on *xīn shù* (BL 15), *gé shù* (BL 17), *zú sān lǐ* (ST 36) and *sān yīn jiāo* (SP 6) to make these points slightly sore.

(7) *Kidney deficiency headache*: Apply abdominal rubbing for five minutes with the focus on *qì hǎi* (RN 6) and *guān yuán* (RN 4). Use straight palmar scrubbing to *du mai* on the back and horizontal scrubbing over *shèn shù* (BL 23), *mìng mén* (DU 4) and the lumbosacral area until each area is thoroughly warm.

(8) *Blood stasis headache*: Apply press-rubbing on *tài yáng* (EX-HN 5) and *cuán zhú* (BL 2) for one minute each. Next, perform split-smearing to the forehead and both sides of the gallbladder meridians on the head for three to five times. Lastly, apply palmar scrubbing to the forehead and *tài yáng* (EX-HN 5) of both sides until they feel thoroughly warm.

Note:

The *tuina* maneuvers used to treat headache should be gentle; particularly while operating on the head and face, avoid the use of violent force to prevent iatrogenic injury.

▶ Precautions

1. *Tuina* should be avoided for organic intracranial diseases such as acute cerebrovascular diseases, intracranial space-occupying lesions, cerebral contusion, or traumatic intracranial hematoma.

Note:

Suggest that patients with headache perform the daily press-kneading maneuver on their own on *fēng chí* (GB 20), *tiān zhù* (BL 10), *shuài gǔ* (GB 8) and *tài yáng* (EX-HN 5) for one minute at each point. Also, apply the split-smearing method to the forehead and temporal areas for one minute each area, once in the morning and once in the evening.

2. Patients suffering from headaches should avoid excessive stress and fatigue owing to hard-work, maintain emotional stability and adequate sleep, and eat light meals. In addition, it is important to keep warm, especially pay attention to the warmth of the head while being outside in the winter. Moreover, get involved in physical exercises to enhance physical strength, and actively seek treatment.

IX. Insomnia

Insomnia is a subjective experience that affects social functioning during daytime due to the difficulty of falling asleep and/or maintaining a normal sleep. During bouts of insomnia, the hours or quality of sleep fail to meet normal physiological needs. Insomnia is the most common sleep disorder. In mild cases, a patient may have difficulties in fallig asleep, may not enter deep sleep, may wake up often, or not be able to fall back sleep after waking up. In serious cases, a patient can be sleepless the whole night. Patients with a long history of insomnia may complicate with other conditions such as anxiety, obsessive-compulsive disorder or depression. In addition, insomnia can stand alone, or exist with co-morbidities, commonly neurosis, and perimenopause. Insomnia pertains to the scope of sleeplessness in Chinese medicine.

Note:

Chinese medicine believes that many factors can cause insomnia, such as intemperate diet, thinking too much, fatigue from overstrain, genetic factors, emotional factors, being chronically ill, and aging. Any of factors can lead to situations including internal damages of heart-spleen, failure of yin-yang interaction, failure of the heart-kidney interaction, excessive fire owing to yin deficiency, qi deficiency of the heart and the gallbladder, and disharmony of the stomach, so that it affects the heart spirit, causing insomnia.

▶ Diagnosis

1. Clinical Symptoms In mild cases, patients have difficulty in falling asleep, wake up easily, or have difficulty in falling back to sleep after waking up. In severe cases, a patient is sleepless all night long. Insomnia is often accompanied by headache, dizziness, palpitation, forgetfulness, mental and physical fatigue, restlessness, dreaminess, attention deficit and so on. The onset time can be short or long, some can gradually improve, while other patients can suffer for years.

2. Chinese Medicine Pattern Differentiation

(1) *Heart-spleen deficiency*: Dreaminess, waking easily, palpitations, forgetfulness, mental and physical fatigue, tastelessness, and pale or sallow facial complexion. The tongue is pale with thin coating, while the pulse is thready and weak.

(2) *Yin-deficient fire*: Vexation, insomnia, dizziness, tinnitus, dry mouth, lack of saliva, and vexing heat in five centers. The tongue is red, while the pulse is thready and rapid. Or dreaminess, forgetfulness, palpitations, and backache.

(3) *Phlegm-heat disturbing the interior*: Insomnia, chest tightness, heavy headedness, vexation, bitter mouth, and dizziness. The tongue coating is greasy and yellow, while the pulse is slippery and rapid.

(4) *Liver constraint transforming into fire*: Insomnia, irritability, poor appetite, thirst with desire for drinking water, red eyes, bitter mouth, dark urine, and constipation. The tongue coating is yellow, while the pulse is wiry and rapid.

3. Clinical Signs Generally speaking, there is no particular positive sign of organic lesion interfering with sleep.

Note:

Insomnia should be differentiated from temporary insomnia, reduced sleep time, and menopausal insomnia.

4. Examination Polysomnography examination is useful in demonstrating that the sleep onset latency exceeds 30 minutes, the actual sleep time is less than six hours every night, and waking time during the night is more than 30 minutes.

▶ Treatment

1. Purpose Regulating and harmonizing yin and yang.

2. Treatment Principles Nourishing the heart and calming mind.

3. Acupoints and Areas *Yìn táng* (EX-HN 3), *shén tíng* (DU 24), *jīng míng* (BL 1), *cuán zhú* (BL 2), *tài yáng* (EX-HN 5), *jiǎo sūn* (SJ 20), *fēng chí* (GB 20), *xīn shù* (BL 15), *gān shù* (BL 18), *pí shù* (BL 20), *wèi shù* (BL 21), *shèn shù* (BL 23) and *mìng mén* (DU 4).

4. Maneuvers Thumb-pushing, kneading, smearing, pressing, sweep-scattering, grasping, and rolling.

5. Basic Operation

(1) Ask the patient to be seated. Apply the thumb-pushing method or kneading with the thenar eminence to operate from *yìn táng* (EX-HN 3) up to *shén tíng* (DU 24) for five to six times, from *yìn táng* (EX-HN 3) to *tài yáng* (EX-HN 5) of both sides along the eyebrows five to six times, and around the orbits three to four times. Then, use the same method to operate from *yìn táng* (EX-HN 3) down to *yíng xiāng* (LI 20), continue to the cheekbones, and reach the anterior sides of the ears two to three times. Focus more on *yìn táng* (EX-HN 3), *shén tíng* (DU 24), *jīng míng* (BL 1), *cuán zhú* (BL 2) and *tài yáng* (EX-HN 5).

(2) Perform the split-smearing maneuver on the forehead three to five times, combining with pressing *jīng míng* (BL 1) and *yú yāo* (EX-HN 4).

(3) Apply the sweep-scattering to both sides of the gallbladder meridians on the head, combining with pressing *jiǎo sūn* (SJ 20).

(4) Use the five-finger grasping to work from the top of the head, switch to three-finger grasping when reaching the region below the occipital bone, and combine with grasping on *fēng chí* (GB 20) for two to three minutes.

(5) Ask the patient to lie in a prone position. Apply rolling on the back and lumbar areas of the patient, with more focus on *xīn shù* (BL 15), *gān shù* (BL 18), *pí shù* (BL 20), *wèi shù* (BL 21), *shèn shù* (BL 23) and *mìng mén*

(DU 4) for three to five minutes.

(6) Perform the thumb-pushing or press-kneading method on *xīn shù* (BL 15), *gān shù* (BL 18), *pí shù* (BL 20), *wèi shù* (BL 21), *shèn shù* (BL 23) and *mìng mén* (DU 4), at each point for one to two minutes.

6. Modification Based on Pattern Differentiation

(1) *Heart-spleen deficiency*: Use the press-kneading method on *xīn shù* (BL 15), *gān shù* (BL 18), *wèi shù* (BL 21), *xiǎo cháng shù* (BL 27) and *zú sān lǐ* (ST 36), at each point for a minute. Then, apply horizontal scrubbing on the left side of the back and straight scrubbing *du mai* of the back area until each is thoroughly warm.

(2) *Yin-deficient fire*: Apply pushing on *qiáo gōng* (bridge arch) one side then the other, each side for 20 to 30 times. Next, perform horizontal scrubbing on *shèn shù* (BL 23), *mìng mén* (DU 4) and *yǒng quán* (KI 1) until each area is thoroughly warm.

(3) *Phlegm-heat disturbing the interior*: Apply the press-kneading method on *zhōng wǎn* (RN 12), *qì hǎi* (RN 6), *tiān shū* (ST 25), *shén mén* (HT 7), *zú sān lǐ* (ST 36) and *fēng lóng* (ST 40), for a minute at each point. Then, use horizontal scrubbing on the left side of the back and the eight *liáo* points (BL 31~34) with the palm until the area is thoroughly warm.

(4) *Liver constraint transforming to fire*: Apply the press-kneading method on *gān shù* (BL 18), *dǎn shù* (BL 19), *qī mén* (LR 14), *zhāng mén* (LR 13) and *tài chōng* (LR 3), for one to two minutes at each point. Next, perform foulage of both the hypochondria top down for one to two minutes.

> **Note:**
>
> The force should not be too strong while using *tuina* to treat insomnia. On the head and face, *tuina* should be especially gentle. If the treatment is performed in the evening, the effect is even better.

▶ Precautions

1. Patients with insomnia should develop the habit of going to sleep early and getting up early, they should also balance work and rest, participate in appropriate amount of physical work and exercise to enhance physical fitness.

2. Maintain an optimistic mood, eliminate mental burden, and avoid mood swing and and worries. Do not smoke, drink tea and coffee before bedtime.

> **Note:**
>
> Patients with insomnia can apply press-kneading on *tài yáng* (EX-HN 5), *yì fēng* (SJ 17), *ān mián* (Extra point, midpoint between SJ 17 and GB 20), *fēng chí* (GB 20), *nèi guān* (PC 6), and *zú sān lǐ* (ST 36), for one minute at each point, once every night before sleep.

X. Sequelae of Apoplexy

Sequelae of apoplexy is characterized by a series of serious symptoms including unilateral paralysis and numbness, deviated facial expression, and difficulty of speaking or even aphasia after cerebral vascular accident, also known as hemiplegia. The sequelae of apoplexy is more common in elderly patients, and many of the patients have a history of hypertension or heart disease. The disease can occur at any time of the year but has a higher occurrence in the winter and spring seasons. The earlier the treatment, the better the effect. The disease is in the scope of "wind stroke" in Chinese medicine.

> **Note:**
>
> Chinese medicine believes that stroke can be caused by conditions such as organ dysfunction, weakness of healthy qi, emotional stress, fatigue from overstrain, interior damage, intemperate diet, and sudden climate change can result in blood stasis, formation of phlegm-heat, excess of heart fire, ascendant hyperactivity of liver yang, stirring of liver wind, and colliding of wind and fire, finally leading to the rising of qi and blood counter-flow rushing to the brain.

▶ Diagnosis

1. Clinical Symptoms   Some main clinical manifestation of sequalae of apoplexy are unilateral paralysis and weakness of an upper and lower limb, facial distortion, and speech difficulty. Some patients can also have pain, numbness, movement difficulty of the limb, while others may have local edema that is more common below the wrist or ankle. Furthermore, dizziness, headache, tinnitus, and irritability can exist in some cases. If the disease is not treated or is improperly treated, the ipsilateral limbs will gradually become stiff with muscle and tendon spasm, and even deformity.

2. Clinical Signs   On the ipsilateral limbs, reduced muscle strength, hypoesthesia or disappearance of the sensation can be demonstrated. The nasolabial fold becomes less distinct, while the corner of the mouth droops because of paralyzed facial muscles. Patients are not able to blow a whistle and blow out their cheeks. Deep reflexes, such as that of the biceps, triceps, radial periosteal, knee, and ankle, are hyperactive. Superficial reflexes, such as the abdominal reflex, is decreased. Pathological reflex, including Babinski's sign and Hoffmann's sign are positive, while the patellar clonus can be induced.

3. Examinations

(1) *Head CT scan*: High density lesions may be visible in the cerebral parenchyma among patients suffering from hemorrhagic stroke, while low density lesions may be visible among those with ischemic stroke.

(2) *MRI of the brain*: MRI Examination can clearly show conditions such as early ischemic infarction, infarction of brainstem and cerebellum, and cerebral sinus thrombosis. Moreover, MRI can detect small amount of bleeding of the brainstem or cerebellum in patients with cerebral hemorrhage that cannot be confirmed by CT.

(3) *Digital subtraction angiography (DSA)*: DSA can be used to detect cerebral aneurysm, cerebral arteriovenous malformations and vasculitis.

Note:

Stroke should be differentiated from traumatic brain injury and brain tumor.

▶ Treatment

1. Purpose   Unblocking the meridians, regulating and harmonizing qi and blood, promoting functional recovery.

2. Treatment Principles   Calming the liver, extinguishing wind, invigorating blood, moving qi, relaxing the sinews, unblocking the collaterals, lubricating and benefiting joints. The disease can be treated with *tuina* at early stage, usually two weeks after the stroke when the blood pressure is stable.

3. Acupoints and Areas   *Tiān zōng* (SI 11), *gé shù* (BL 17), *gān shù* (BL 18), *dǎn shù* (BL 19), *shèn shù* (BL 23), *huán tiào* (GB 30), *yáng líng quán* (GB 34), *wěi zhōng* (BL 40), *chéng shān* (BL 57), *fēng shì* (GB 31), *fú tù* (ST 32), *xī yǎn* (EX-LE 5), *jiě xī* (ST 41), *bì nào* (LI 14), *chǐ zé* (LU 5), *qū chí* (LI 11), *shǒu sān lǐ* (LI 10), *hé gǔ* (LI 4), *tài yáng* (EX-HN 5), *jīng míng* (BL 1), *jiǎo sūn* (SJ 20), *fēng chí* (GB 20), *fēng fǔ* (DU 16) and *jiān jǐng* (GB 21). The back portion of the bladder meridians, both sides of the neck and nape, and the upper and lower limbs of the ipsilateral side.

4. Maneuvers   Rolling, pressing, kneading, foulage, scrubbing, grasping, twirling, rotation, smearing, and sweep-scattering.

5. Basic Operations

(1) Ask the patient to lie in a prone position. Apply the press-kneading method to work on the first line of both sides of bladder meridians top to bottom two to three times with focus on *tiān zōng* (SI 11), *gé shù* (BL 17), *gān shù* (BL 18), *dǎn shù* (BL 19) and *shèn shù* (BL 23) for about 5 minutes.

(2) Perform the rolling maneuver along both sides of the spine, work down to the buttocks, and posterior aspect of the thigh and the calf. Focus more on the the lumbar region of both sides, *huán tiào* (GB 30), *wěi zhōng* (BL 40), *chéng shān* (BL 57) and Achilles tendon. At the same time, coordinate with passive extension of the lumbar and the ip-

silateral limbs for about five minutes. Then, use horizontal scrubbing method to the lumbo-sacral region until the area feels warm.

(3) Ask the patient to lie a supine position. Perform the rolling method on the affected lower limb from the anterior superior iliac spine down to the knee and dorsal side of the foot along the anterior aspect of the thigh, focusing on *fú tù* (ST 32), *xī yǎn* (EX-LE 5) and *jiě xī* (ST 41). At the same time, coordinate passive flexion and extension of the hip, knee and ankle, and passive internal rotation of the whole lower extremity for about five minutes.

(4) Apply the grasping method on the affected lower limb, *wěi zhōng* (BL 40) and *chéng shān* (BL 57), with focus on the medial thigh and around the knee for two to three minutes. Next, perform the foulage method to the lower limbs top to bottom two to three times.

(5) Have the patient lie in a lateral position with the affected limb on top. Apply the rolling method on its lateral aspect top to bottom for three to four minutes, and the press-kneading method on *jū liáo* (GB 29), *fēng shì* (GB 31), *yáng líng quán* (GB 34) and *jiě xī* (ST 41) for one minute at each point.

(6) Ask the patient to be seated. Operate around the ipsilateral shoulder and both sides of the neck with the rolling method, and coordinate with passive posterior rotation, and abduction and adduction to the affected limb for three to five minutes. Next, apply the rolling method from the medial upper arm to the forearm of the ipsilateral side with the focus on the elbow and the surrounding area. At the same time, coordinate with passive elbow flexion and extension for three to five minutes. Then, perform the rolling method to the wrist, palm and fingers, coordinating with time with passive flexion and extension of the wrist and interphalangeal joints for two to three minutes.

(7) Use the press-kneading method on acupoints such as *chǐ zé* (LU 5), *qū chí* (LI 11), *shǒu sān lǐ* (LI 10) and *hé gǔ* (LI 4) for two to three minutes. Next, apply the twirling method to finger joints, three times for each finger.

(8) Perform the grasping method from the shoulder to the wrist back and forth for three to four times. Next, apply the rotation method counterclockwise on the shoulder, elbow, and wrist for three times each joint. Then, use the foulage method from the shoulder to the wrist back and forth two to three times.

(9) Apply the split-smearing method from *yìn táng* (EX-HN 3) to *tài yáng* (EX-HN 5) four to five times, coordinating with press-kneading method on *jīng míng* (BL 1) and *tài yáng* (EX-HN 5) 30 times at each point. Next, perform the sweep-scattering method along the head portion of the gallbladder meridians from the anterosuperior to the posterior-inferior aspect 20 to 30 times on each side, coordinating with the method of press-kneading on *jiǎo sūn* (SJ 20) 30 times.

(10) Use the press-kneading method on both sides of the neck, *fēng chí* (GB 20), *fēng fǔ* (DU 16) and *jiān jǐng* (GB 21) for two to three minutes. Then, apply the grasping *fēng chí* (GB 20) and *jiān jǐng* (GB 21) 20 to 30 times each.

6. Modifications Based on Symptoms

(1) *Speech difficulty*: Apply the press-kneading maneuver on *lián quán* (RN 23, 廉泉), *tōng lǐ* (HT 5, 通里) and *fēng fǔ* (DU 16) for one minute at each acupoint.

(2) *Deviated mouth and eyes*: Use the push-smearing method gently in the affected side of the face gently for three to five minutes, and the press-kneading maneuver on *quán liáo* (SI 18, 颧髎), *tóng zǐ liáo* (GB 1, 瞳子髎), *dì cāng* (ST 4) and *jiá chē* (ST 6), for one minute at each point.

(3) *Drooling*: Apply the press-kneading method in the face and *dì cāng* (ST 4) of the affected side and push-rubbing on *chéng jiāng* (RN 24), for one minute at each point.

Note:

In treating sequalae of apoplexy, the *tuina* maneuvers applied should be gentle, while the passive movements should be carried out within the patient's tolerance range to prevent iatrogenic injury.

▶ Precautions

1. *Tuina* is fairly beneficial in treating sequalae of apoplexy, while the recovery of the body and limbs is directly related to the time delay before treatment begins. Therefore, it is better begin treatment promptly, generally two weeks after the stroke when the blood pressure is stable.

2. The patient should keep emotional stability, follow a regular life routine, stop smoking, and avoid alcohol, strong stimulations, and food high in animal fat.

3. When the condition improves and the limbs can move, patients should be encouraged to engage in self recovery exercises actively to restore the functions of the body and limbs. At the same time, avoid being exhausted.

Note:

Along with *tuina* treatment, herbal medicine such as modified *Bǔ Yáng Huán Wǔ Tāng* (Yang-Supplementing and Five-Returning Decoction, 补阳还五汤) can also be taken orally. In addition, body and scalp acupuncture can also be used to enhance the treatment efficacy.

XI. Facial Paralysis

Facial paralysis is a disease characterized by symptoms of deviated mouth and eyes. Facial paralysis can be divided into two subtypes including peripheral facial paralysis and central facial paralysis. Peripheral facial paralysis is caused by acute non-purulent facial neuritis in the foramen stylomastoideum; whereas central facial paralysis is mainly caused by ischemia and bleeding owing to intracranial lesions, often accompanied by hemiplegia. In this section, we will only discuss peripheral facial paralysis caused by facial neuritis. Peripheral facial paralysis, is also known as Bell's palsy or facial neuritis. The disease can occur at any age, while it is more common in adults between the age of 20 and 40, affecting more men than women. It mostly occurs on one side of the face without obvious seasonality. In Chinese medicine, it pertains to the scope of "wry mouth and eyes".

Note:

Chinese medicine believes that the original cause of facial paralysis is the deficiency of the healthy qi and emptiness of the meridians. Thus, the wind-cold or wind-heat pathogen is able to enter the body, causing qi blockages in *shaoyang* and *yangming* meridians. Since the meridian sinews and muscles are not nourished and become lax, the disease occurs.

▶ Diagnosis

1. Clinical Symptoms   The disease has a sudden onset. Many patients wake up in the morning and notice that one side of their face was tense, numb, and paralyzed with deviated mouth, drooling of saliva, one eye not able to close, tearing, and unable to chew. In the early stage, a small number of patients may have pain behind and below the ear, and in the face.

2. Clinical Signs   The forehead wrinkles of the patient disappear, while on the ipsilateral side of the face, the nasolabial fold is shallow or even disappears and the eyelid cannot close completely. A patient is unable to wince, frown, show teeth, puff cheeks, or whistle. The corner of the mouth is skewed to the contralateral side. In severe cases, the patient may experience hearing impairment, and the taste sense of the front 2/3 of the tongue may diminish or disappear on the ipsilateral side. Herpes may be seen in the auricula, auricular tube, and eardrum. Some may experience dysfunctional sweating.

3. Examinations

(1) *Blood test*: Mostly normal or increased of lymphocyte ratio.

(2) *EMG examination*: During onset, the pathological potential and exercise potential of the facial muscles are decreased.

Note:

Peripheral facial paralysis should be differentiated from central facial paralysis, multiple root neuritis of acute infectious type, neuropathic Lyme disease, mumps and parotid gland tumors.

▶ Treatment

1. Purpose   Improving local circulation, reducing facial nerve edema and inflammation, promoting the recovery of the nerve function.

2. Treatment Principles   Relaxing the meridians, unblocking the collaterals, invigorating blood, and dissolving stasis

3. Acupoints and Areas   Acupoints include *yìn táng* (EX-HN 3), *jīng míng* (BL 1), *yáng bái* (GB 14), *yíng xiāng* (LI 20), *xià guān* (ST 7), *jiá chē* (ST 6), *dì cāng* (ST 4), *fēng chí* (GB 20) and *hé gǔ* (LI 4). The facial area is to be treated with more focus on the ipsilateral side and less focus on the contralateral aspect.

4. Maneuvers   Thumb pushing, pressing, kneading, scrubbing, and grasping.

5. Basic Operations

(1) Ask the patient to be seated. Apply the thumb-pushing method repeatedly for about five minutes along the route of *yìn táng* (EX-HN 3), *yáng bái* (GB 14), *jīng míng* (BL 1), *sì bái* (ST 2, 四白), *yíng xiāng* (LI 20), *xià guān* (ST 7), *jiá chē* (ST 6) and *dì cāng* (ST 4).

(2) First, perform the press-kneading method on the affected side of the face, then the contralateral side of it for about five minutes.

(3) Gently apply the scrubbing method on the affected side of the face until the area feels warm.

(4) Perform the thumb-pushing method on *fēng chí* (GB 20) and the nape for three to five minutes.

(5) Apply the press-kneading method on *fēng chí* (GB 20) for one minute.

(6) Perform the grasping method on *fēng chí* (GB 20) and *hé gǔ* (LI 4) for one to two minutes.

Note:

In the early stage of facial paralysis, the maneuvers applied to the ipsilateral side should be gentle. Avoid strong stimulation to prevent aggravating the damage of the local nerves.

▶ Precautions

1. If the patient receives prompt *tuina* treatment, the treatment is more effective and the recovery is faster.

2. Patients should keep the face warm, avoid stimulation of wind-cold and fatigue from overstrain. If the eyelid cannot close, apply aureomycin ointment to the eye o   r wear goggles to protect the cornea from being damaged.

3. For home care, use a wet towel or warm water bottle under the affected ear. When the function of the facial nerve begins to recover, the patient should practice the voluntary movements of the paralyzed facial muscles in front of a mirror.

Note:

Patients with facial paralysis can apply the push-kneading method on their own to points such as *xià guān* (ST 7), *jiá chē* (ST 6) and *dì cāng* (ST 4), for a minute at each point, and use the palmar scrubbing method on the affected side of the face bottom up gently 30 times, once a day.

XII. Chronic Cholecystitis

Chronic cholecystitis is one of the most common inflammatory gallbladder diseases. The disease can either manifest with symptoms including indigestion, pain on the upper abdomen, discomfort or persistent dull pain on the right hypochondrium, or be clinically asymptomatic. The disease affects more women than men, and can occur at any time of the year. The disease is within the scope of "hypochondriac pain" in Chinese medicine.

Note:

Chinese medicine believes that the disease is mainly associated with the liver, gallbladder, spleen and stomach. The excess patterns of the disease, characterized by "pain due to blockages", are usually caused by qi stagnation, blood stasis, and damp-heat, while in deficient pattern, it is often the result of liver yin deficiency.

▶ Diagnosis

1. Clinical Symptoms

(1) *Abdominal pain:* The pain is located in the right upper quadrant of the abdomen, radiating to the back, persistent for a few hours before it eases. The occurrence is usually associated with high fat and high protein diet.

(2) *Indigestion:* belching, fullness, bloating, nausea and so on.

2. Clinical Signs Chronic cholecystitis patients have tenderness in the right upper quadrant of the abdomen, and will produce a positive Murphy's sign. A few cases can have tenderness to the side of the 8th to 10th thoracic vertebrae on the right side.

3. Examinations

(1) *Ultrasound:* Visible rough gallbladder wall or gallstones.

(2) *X-ray:* Showing signs of gallstones, and calcification and gallbladder and gallbladder expansion. Gallbladder angiography can detect stones, shrinkage or deformation of the gallbladder, and contraction and bile concentration dysfunction of the gallbladder.

(3) *CT and MRI:* Help to rule out other diseases.

Note:

Chronic cholecystitis should be differentiated from diseases such as peptic ulcer, chronic gastritis, chronic hepatitis, and chronic pancreatitis.

▶ Treatment

1. Purpose Resolving spasm, relieving pain, and easing symptoms of biliogenic dyspepsia.

2. Treatment Principles Soothing the liver, promoting gallbladder function, moving qi, and relieving pain.

3. *Acupoints and Areas* Gé shù (BL 17), gān shù (BL 18), dǎn shù (BL 19), ashi point, zhāng mén (LR 13), qī mén (LR 14), yáng líng quán (GB 34), dǎn náng (EX-LE 6, 胆囊), zú sān lǐ (ST 36), sān yīn jiāo (SP 6), tài chōng (LR 3), xíng jiān (LR 2), the back portion of the bladder meridians and the hypochondria.

4. Maneuvers Precision pressing, pressing, thumb-pushing, scrubbing, spontaneous torquing, kneading, and foulage.

5. Basic Operations

(1) Ask the patient to lie in a prone position. Apply precision pressing or pressing on *gé shù* (BL 17), *gān shù* (BL 18), *dǎn shù* (BL 19) and *ashi* point, with force until each point feels sore.

(2) Perform the thumb-pushing method on the back portion of the bladder meridians for three minutes followed by scrubbing method to make the area feel thoroughly warm.

(3) Perform the shoulder spontaneous torquing maneuver, or the maneuver of elbow-pressing thoracic reduction in a supine position.

(4) Ask the patient to lie a supine position. Apply the finger-pressing method on *zhāng mén* (LR 13) and *qī mén* (LR 14) for one minute at each point.

(5) Perform the foulage and scrubbing on both hypochondria until the areas are thoroughly warm.

(6) Ask the patient to lie in a supine position. Use the methods of precision-pressing or pressing on *zhī gōu* (SJ 6), *yáng líng quán* (GB 34), *dǎn náng* (EX-LE 6, 胆囊), *zú sān lǐ* (ST 36), *sān yīn jiāo* (SP 6), *tài chōng* (LR 3) and *xíng jiān* (LR 2), for one minute at each point.

6. Modification Based on Pattern Differentiation Extend the treatment time on *tài chōng* (LR 3), *zhāng mén* (LR 13) and *qī mén* (LR 14) for a qi stagnation excess pattern. For blood stasis excess pattern, extend the treatment time on *gé shù* (BL 17), *gān shù* (BL 18) and *dǎn shù* (BL 19). The modification for the deficient pattern is to apply the thumb-pushing, pressing and kneading methods on *qì hǎi shù* (BL 24), *guān yuán* (RN 4) and *sān yīn jiāo* (SP 6).

> **Note:**
>
> The patient should be referred to the ER for comprehensive treatment including anti-infection therapies or removal of stones if the disease presents with an acute onset accompanied by severe abdominal pain, jaundice, vomiting and other symptoms.

▶ Precautions

1. *Tuina* has obvious effect in relieving biliary colic pain. It is, however, still necessary to conduct further relevant examinations to clarify the cause and treat the underlying cause accordingly after the pain is alleviated with *tuina*.

2. Patients should maintain a pleasant mood, and avoid depression and irritability. Stay away from oily, greasy and spicy food, avoid overeating, eat more food rich in fiber to benefit defecation, and pay attention to personal hygiene to prevent ascariasis.

> **Note:**
>
> Patients with chronic cholecystitis can apply self *tuina* procedures with the application of the press-kneading maneuver on *rì yuè* (GB 24, 日 月), *yáng líng quán* (GB 34), *dǎn náng* (EX-LE 6), *xíng jiān* (LR 2) and *tài chōng* (LR 3), for one minute at each point, once in the morning and once in the evening.

XIII. Gout

Gout refers to a purine metabolic disorder causing the continuous increase of serum uric acid and damage to tissues and organs. Clinically, gout is characterized by hyperuricemia, recurrent acute arthritis, and deposition of urate crystals. Chronic gouty arthritis can often implicate the kidneys. The disease tends to occur in middle-aged or older people, about 95% of the cases are male. The disease pertains to the "*bi* pattern" in Chinese medicine, which is similar to the symptoms of "heat *bi*", "multiple joint *bi*", and "white tiger multi-joint *bi*".

> **Note:**
>
> Chinese medicine believes that the disease is due to lack of healthy qi, plus external contraction of wind cold and dampness, or gluttony of sea food, food with strong smell and food inducing excessive heat. When wind cold and dampness pathogens invade the body, flow to the meridians, stay in the joints, and obstruct qi and blood, the results can lead to *bi* disease.

▶ Diagnosis

1. Clinical Symptoms

(1) *Acute gouty arthritis*: The disease often has a sudden onset, mainly affecting the big toe and its first metatarsophalangeal joints. The lesion is usually red, swollen, painful, and burning, often with exudate in the joint cavity. Gout may be accompanied by systemic symptoms such as fever, chills, headache and fatigue, and acute lesions can also be seen in ankles, knees, heel and other lower limb joints. After symptoms are relieved a pigmentation can remain on the skin on where the lesion was located. During the remission period, there is no symptoms at all; yet, the disease relapses in majority of the patients after six months. In some cases, gout never recurs after the initial attack. Factors inducing the initial attack of acute gouty arthritis include exposure to cold, fatigue due to overstrain, alcohol consumption, eating food high in purines, trauma, surgery and intake of drugs that impact uric acid excretion.

(2) *Chronic arthritis and tophi*: There is visible joint deformity and bone defects in the area. Urate crystal deposits in the tendon,

tendon sheath and connective tissue of the skin near the joints, forming different sizes of tophi that are commonly found in the toes, fingers, elbows, helix and antihelix.

(3) *Gouty kidney disease*: During the early stage, there is only intermittent
proteinuria with decreased specific gravity of urine. Along with the progression
of the disease, continuous proteinuria can occur, hypertension can gradually increase, blood urea nitrogen and serum creatinine can increase, and renal insufficiency can be life-threatening. Some patients may also experience renal colic caused by urinary tract stones or hematuria with discharge of stones.

2. Clinical Signs   During an acute attack, the joint is red, swollen, burning and painful, with exudate in the joint cavity, especially in the first metatarsophalangeal of the big toe. In the stage of chronic arthritis, joint deformity can be seen, along with different sizes of tophi in the toes, fingers, elbows, helix or antihelix.

3. Examinations

(1) *Serum uric acid levels*: Men > 420μmol/L, women > 350μmol/L (uricase method).

(2) *Blood analysis*: During the acute stage of gout attack, white blood cells and erythrocyte sedimentation rate are increased.

(3) *Synovial fluid examination*: Birefringent needle-shaped urate crystals in leukocytes can be found in puncture fluid of the intra-articular bursa, often with increased polymorphonuclear leukocytosis.

(4) *Content examination of the tuberculum arthriticum*: A patient suffering from gout can have urate crystals in ruptured tuberculum arthriticum or puncture fluid, while the urinary tract stones discharged can be confirmed as urate with lab analysis.

(5) *X-ray examination*: Round or irregular chisel-like translucent bone damage and narrowed joint space can be found adjacent to the osteochondral margin of the affected joints. Some patients can have bone destruction between the size of 2 mm to 5 mm, and irregular or lobular depression of the bone near the tuberculum arthriticum.

▶ Treatment

1. Purpose   Promoting local blood circulation to dissipate urate crystals and achieve the effects of dissolving inflammation and relieving pain.

2. Treatment Principles   Regulating and harmonizing qi and blood, unblocking the collaterals, and relieving pain.

3. Acupoints and Areas   *Gōng sūn* (SP 4), *tài xī* (KI 3), *sān yīn jiāo* (SP 6), *tài chōng* (LR 3), *guāng míng* (GB 37, 光明), *pí shù* (BL 20), *shèn shù* (BL 23), *guān yuán shù* (BL 26), *páng guāng shù* (BL 28, 膀胱俞), *zhōng wǎn* (RN 12), *zhāng mén* (LR 13), *liáng mén* (ST 21, 梁门), *tiān shū* (ST 25), *dà héng* (SP 15), *guān yuán* (RN 4) and the affected joints.

4. Maneuvers   Rubbing, rolling, precision-pressing, pushing, and kneading.

5. Basic Operations

(1) Ask the patient to lie in a supine position. Apply the rubbing and rolling methods on the first metatarsophalangeal joints and the affected joints for about one minute. Then, perform precision-pressing on *yǒng quán* (KI 1), *gōng sūn* (SP 4), *tài chōng* (LR 3), *tài xī* (KI 3), *sān yīn jiāo* (SP 6), *guāng míng* (GB 37) of the affected side, for one minute at each point. Next, use the grasp-kneading method on *yáng líng quán* (GB 34) and *yīn líng quán* (SP 9) for a total of one minute.

(2) Ask the patient to lie in a prone position. Perform the pushing method on the
back portion of the bladder meridians for two minutes. Then, apply the precision-pressing maneuver on *pí shù* (BL 20), *shèn shù* (BL 23), *guān yuán shù* (BL 26) and *páng guāng shù* (BL 28) for a total of three minutes.

(3) Ask the patient to lie in a supine position. Use the three-finger kneading method to gently operate on *zhōng wǎn* (RN 12) for a minute. Next, place one palm on top of the other, and apply the double-palmar-rubbing method on the abdomen for two minutes. Then, use the middle finger to perform the precision-kneading maneuver to *zhāng mén* (LV 13), *liáng mén* (ST 21, 梁门), *tiān shū* (ST 25), *dà héng* (SP 15) and *guān yuán* (RN 4) for a total of two minutes.

Note:

In a severe attack of gout, have the patient take colchicine and non-steroidal anti-inflammatory drugs to alleviate the condition of the disease under the guidance of a specialist.

▶ Precautions

1. In the acute stage, patients should rest in bed and raise the affected limb. Choose low purine foods, limit the total calorie intake, and avoid alcohol. A reasonable diet is low in protein and fat with adequate carbohydrates, vitamins and minerals.

2. Do more aerobic exercises, such as walking, cycling, and swimming. Walking once or twice a day for at least 30 minutes a time to induce slight sweat. However, avoid strenuous exercise.

Note:

Instruct patients suffering from gout to perform *tuina* by themselves with the press-kneading maneuver on *yīn líng quán* (SP 9), *tài xī* (KI 3), *sān yīn jiāo* (SP 6), *fēng lóng* (ST 40) and *qū chí* (LI 11), for one minute at each point, once in the morning and once in the evening.

IX. Hyperlipidemia

Hyperlipidemia refers to the abnormal increase of one or more lipid components in the blood, such as hypercholesterolemia and hypertriglyceridemia. Hyperlipidemia is an important pathogenic risk factor of atherosclerosis and coronary heart disease, which can significantly increase the morbidity and mortality of cardiovascular and cerebrovascular diseases. In recent years, due to the life style changes, the incidence of this disease has gradually increased among middle-aged populations. The disease is in the "phlegm turbidity" category defined in Chinese medicine.

Note:

Chinese medicine believes that firstly, the disease is closely related to uncontrolled diet with excessive intake of fatty, greasy and rich food, causing the failure of the transportation and transformation of the spleen and stomach system. It further results in endogenous phlegm and cohesion of fat turbidity that flow into the meridians. Secondly, hyperlipidemia may have spleen damage due to excessive thinking, or liver damage owing to stagnant anger transforming to liver fire, so that liquid is concentrated to accumulated phlegm dampness. The third reason is because of qi transformation failure of the kidney, leading to fluid metabolic disorders that further results in endogenous phlegm dampness concentrating into fat.

▶ Diagnosis

1. Clinical Symptoms   Normally, most patients do have no obvious symptoms. Many patients discover that their plasma lipoprotein level is elevated in a biochemical test of blood. Most patients have life history of eating oily and greasy food, are often obese, and have a family history of hyperlipidemia. Lipid deposition in the dermis causes visible yellow lipomyoma around the eyelid, and in fewer cases, the face, neck, torso and limbs.

2. Chinese Medicine Pattern Differentiation

(1) *Phlegm turbidity constraint*: The clinical manifestations are obesity, fatigue, addicted to fat, greasy and rich food, dizziness, heavy headedness, chest tightness, abdominal distension, nausea, vomiting, and cough with sputum. The tongue is pale with thick and greasy coating, while the pulse is wiry and slippery.

(2) *Transportation and transformation failure*

due to spleen deficiency: Obesity, general heaviness sensation, weak limbs, dizziness, heavy headedness, loss of appetite, epigastric obstruction, bloating, loose stools, and nausea. The tongue is pale, swollen with teeth marks on the edge, while the coating is white and greasy. The pulse is wiry and thready or soggy and moderate.

(3) *Stagnation of liver qi*: Dizziness, headache, chest tightness, sense of suffocation, chest and hypochondriac pain, belching, and sighing. Sometimes the pain in the hypochondriac area can radiate to the neck and shoulder with hand tremor and limb numbness. The pulse is wiry.

(4) *Qi transformation failure of the kidney*: Obesity, dizziness, tinnitus, pale face, bloating, loss of appetite, abdominal distension, aching and weak waist and knees, cold limbs, edema, oliguria, and turbid and even scanty and painful urine. The tongue is pale with thin and white coating, while the pulse is thin or slow.

3. Clinical Signs Generally, there is no special sign, although some patients can have yellow lipomyoma, early corneal arcus and hyperlipidemia fundus.

4. Examination Serum total cholesterol (TC) $\geqslant$ 6.22 mmol/L, LDL-C $\geqslant$ 4.14 mmol/L, high density lipoprotein cholesterol (HDL-C) < 1.04 mmol/L, and triglyceride (TG) $\geqslant$ 2.26 mmol/L.

▶ Treatment

1. Purpose Regulating dyslipidemia, preventing and treating cardiovascular and cerebrovascular diseases.

2. Treatment Principles Fortifying the spleen, boosting the kidney, soothing the liver, and invigorating blood.

3. Acupoints and Areas *Shàng wǎn* (RN 13), *zhōng wǎn* (RN 12), *xià wǎn* (RN 10, 下脘), *guān yuán* (RN 4), *zhōng jí* (RN 3, 中极), *gé shù* (BL 17), *gān shù* (BL 18), *pí shù* (BL 20), *shèn shù* (BL 23), *nèi guān* (PC 6), *yīn líng quán* (SP 9), *fēng lóng* (ST 40), *zú sān lǐ* (ST 36), *sān yīn jiāo* (SP 6), *tài chōng* (LR 3) and the four limbs.

4. Maneuvers Thumb-pushing, rubbing, press-kneading, precision pressing, vibration, grasping, rolling, pushing, and tapping.

5. Basic Operation

(1) Ask the patient to lie in a supine position. Apply the palmar rubbing method to the entire abdomen, both clockwise and counterclockwise for a total of three minutes.

(2) Perform the thumb pushing maneuver along the abdominal portion of *ren mai*, the spleen meridian and the stomach meridian for about three minutes.

(3) Use clockwise palmar kneading method on the entire abdomen for two minutes.

(4) Apply the press-kneading maneuver on *zhōng wǎn* (RN 12), *qì hǎi* (RN 6), *guān yuán* (RN 4) and *zhōng jí* (RN 3), for about a minute at each point. Then, apply the precision-pressing method with the middle finger on *zhōng wǎn* (RN 12) and *tiān shū* (ST 25), each point for half a minute. Next, perform the lift-grasping method several times on the abdomen with a level of force that is tolerable to the patient.

(5) Perform the vibration method to the lower abdomen for one minute.

(6) Apply the grasp-kneading method with both hands to the three yin and three yang meridians from the thigh to the ankle four to five times along each meridian. Next, perform the precision-pressing to *yīn líng quán* (SP 9), *fēng lóng* (ST 40), *zú sān lǐ* (ST 36), *sān yīn jiāo* (SP 6) and *tài chōng* (LR 3), for half a minute at each point.

(7) Ask the patient to lie in a prone position. Perform the rolling maneuver over the first and second lines of the bladder meridian for three to four minutes.

(8) Apply the palmar-scrubbing method horizontally to the lumbar area until it is thoroughly warm.

(9) Perform the precision-pressing maneuver to *gé shù* (BL 17), *gān shù* (BL 18), *pí shù* (BL 20) and *shèn shù* (BL 23) for half a minute at each point. Then, apply the tapping method on the first and second lines of the bladder meridian for three times each.

(10) Ask the patient to be seated. Use the grasping method along the three yin and three yang meridians of both arms according to their circulation directions, moving along each meridian three to five times.

(11) Perform precision-pressing on *nèi guān*

(PC 6), *shǒu sān lǐ* (LI 10) and *qū chí* (LI 11), for half a minute at each point.

4. Modification Based on Pattern Differentiation

(1) *Phlegm-turbidity constraint*: Use thumb-pushing method on *fēng lóng* (ST 40), *zú sān lǐ* (ST 36) and *zhōng wǎn* (RN 12), for two minutes at each point.

(2) *Failure of the deficient spleen to transport*: Apply the press-kneading method on *pí shù* (BL 20) and *wèi shù* (BL 21), each point for a minute. Then, perform the thumb-pushing method on *jiàn lǐ* (RN 11, 建里) and *zú sān lǐ* (ST 36), for two minutes at each point .

(3) *Liver qi stagnation*: Perform the press-kneading maneuver on *gān shù* (BL 18), *dǎn shù* (BL 19), *zhāng mén* (LR 13) and *qī mén* (LR 14), for one minute at each point.

(4) *Qi transformation failure of the kidney*: Apply the thumb-pushing method to *qì hǎi* (RN 6), *guān yuán* (RN 4), *tài xī* (KI 3) and *fù liū* (KI 7, 复溜), at each point for one to two minutes.

Precautions

1. The patient's diet should contain very little animal fat, animal organs, or seafoods such as squid and shellfish. At the same time, limit the excessive intake of carbohydrates, and eat more fresh fruits, vegetables, lean meat, fish and beans.

2. Patients should participate in appropriate amount of physical activity, balance work and rest, maintain psychological wellbeing, ease mental tension, and keep emotional stability.

XV. Obesity

Obesity is a chronic metabolic disease associated with excessive accumulation and/or abnormal distribution of body fat and significant weight gain caused by interaction of multiple factors, including genetic and environmental factors. Generally, when more calories are eaten than calories burned, the excess calories will be stored in the form of fat. Obesity occurs when the amount of caloric intake exceeds the normal physiological requirements. Simple obesity is defined when there is no obvious causal mechanism, whereas secondary obesity can be associated with a specific disease. Obesity can be seen at any age, although it is more common between the age of 40 and 50, and affects more women than men. Obesity and diseases associated with it can impair the physical and mental health, cause deterioration in the quality of life and shorten the life expectancy of a patient. In this section we will focus on the treatment of simple obesity with *tuina*.

▶ Diagnosis

1. Clinical Symptoms　Obese, body fat evenly distributed. The fat is generally distributed in the neck and torso areas, especially more in the abdomen, and less in limbs among males. On the other hand, more fat is distributed in the waist, buttocks and limbs with moist and tightened skin among women. In addition, obesity is often accompanied by symptoms such as shortness of breath, profuse sweating, aversion to heat, abdominal distension, chest tightness, fatigue, drowsiness, dizziness, palpitation, and low libido and sexual dysfunction.

2. Chinese Medicine Pattern Differentiation

(1) *Phlegm-dampness pattern*: Obesity, a history of eating high fat diet and consuming alcohol excessively, abundant sputum, nausea, vomiting, sense of heaviness, weakness, abdominal distension, fullness and discomfort, and walking difficulty. The tongue is pink with white, glossy and greasy coating, while the pulse is soggy and slippery.

(2) *Qi deficiency pattern*: Obesity, edema, lethargy, shortness of breath, unwillingness to engage in movement and talking, and sweating while moving. The tongue is pale with white, moist and glossy coating, while the pulse is deep and weak.

(3) *Water-dampness pattern*: Obesity, mental and physical fatigue, drowsiness, unwillingness to move, swelling, and soreness in the lumbar and knee area. The tongue is pale with white, moist and glossy coating, while the pulse is deep and weak.

(4) *Stomach heat pattern*: Obesity, excessive eating, getting hungry easily, dry mouth,

bad breath, and constipation. The tongue is red with yellow and greasy coating, while the pulse is slippery.

(5) *Qi stagnation pattern*: Obesity, emotional depression, irritability, chest and hypochondriac pain and distension, irregular menstruation, and sighing all the time. The tongue is red with white and greasy coating, while the pulse is wiry.

3. Clinical signs   The patient is considered obese when his or her weight exceeds the standard weight for gender, age and height by 20%, and the body mass index (BMI) $\geq$ 25. The formula of standard body weight is: male (kg) = height (cm) - 105, and female (kg) = height (cm) -100, while BMI is calculated as: weight (kg) / height (m) ^{2}. In addition, when male waist $\geq$ 85 cm, or female waist $\geq$ 80 cm, it is considered as abdominal obesity or central obesity. Some patients have black spots, pink spots, or pigmentation on area such as face, areola, abdomen, and legs.

4. Examinations

(1) *CT or MRI*: When scanning the abdomen at the level of the 4th to the 5th lumbar intervertebral disc in calculating the area of visceral fat, take the intra-abdominal fat area $\geq$ 100 cm^2 as the cut-off point to identify the increase of fat.

(2) Other examinations used to determine the total body fat include body density measurement, bioelectrical impedance analysis, and dual-energy X-ray absorptiometry (DXA).

▶ Treatment

1. Purpose   Losing weight to eventually restore weight to the standard range.

2. Treatment Principles   Fortifying the spleen, eliminating dampness, dissolving phlegm, and dispersing the phlegm.

3. Acupoints and Areas   *Zhōng wǎn* (RN 12), *tiān shū* (ST 25), *qì hǎi* (RN 6), *qū chí* (LI 11), *yīn líng quán* (SP 9), *fēng lóng* (ST 40), *tài chōng* (LR 3), the entire abdomen, the upper limbs and the lower limbs.

4. Maneuver   Rubbing, rolling, grasp-kneading, foulage, scrubbing, and shaking.

5. Basic Operations

(1) Ask the patient to lie in a supine posi-

tion. Apply the palmar rubbing method on the entire abdomen clockwise and counter-clockwise for a total of three minutes.

(2) Perform the thumb pushing method along the abdominal portion of the *ren mai*, the spleen meridian and the stomach meridian for three minutes.

(3) Perform the palmar kneading maneuver on the entire abdomen clockwise for two minutes.

(4) Apply the press-kneading method to *zhōng wǎn* (RN 12), *qì hǎi* (RN 6), *guān yuán* (RN 4), and *zhōng jí* (RN 3), each point for a minute. Then, use the middle finger to apply the precision-pressing on *zhōng wǎn* (RN 12) and *tiān shū* (ST 25)for half a minute each point. Next, perform the lift-grasping on the abdomen several times to the extent that the patient can tolerant.

(5) Perform the shaking method on the lower abdomen for one minute.

(6) Ask the patient to lie in a prone position. Use both palms alternately to push the *du mai* and the first and second lines of the bladder meridian for five to ten times each.

(7) Perform the precision-pressing method on *jiā jǐ* (EX-B 2, 夹脊) and the back-*shu* points, for half a minute each.

(8) Apply the pinching *jǐ* (spine) method along the spine bottom up five to seven times.

(9) Ask the patient to lie in a supine position. Use one hand to hold one of the patient's upper limbs, and the other hand to apply the grasp-kneading method to the three hand yin meridians and three hand yang meridians of the same limb. Perform the same procedure on both sides three to five times on each side.

(10) Use both hands to perform the grasp-kneading method to the three foot yin meridians and three foot yang meridians of one of the patient's lower limbs. Apply the same maneuver on both side three to five times on each side.

6. Modification Based on Pattern Differentiation

(1) *Phlegm-dampness*: Apply the press-kneading method on *zhōng wǎn* (RN 12), *fēng lóng* (ST 40), *yīn líng quán* (SP 9) and *yǐn bái* (SP 1,

隐白), for one to two minutes at each point.

(2) *Qi deficiency*: Apply the press-kneading method on *qì hǎi* (RN 6), *guān yuán* (RN 4) and *zú sān lǐ* (ST 36), for one to two minutes at each point.

(3) *Water-dampness*: Apply the press-kneading method on *shuǐ dào* (ST 28, 水道), *pí shù* (BL 20) and *guān yuán* (RN 4), for one to two minutes at each point. Then, apply the palmar-scrubbing method horizontally on *shèn shù* (BL 23) and *mìng mén* (DU 4) until the area feels thoroughly warm.

(4) *Stomach heat*: Apply the press-kneading method on *nèi tíng* (ST 44, 内庭), *qū chí* (LI 11) and *shàng jù xū* (ST 37, 上巨虚), for one to two minutes at each point.

(5) *Qi stagnation*: Apply the press-kneading method on *tài chōng* (LR 3), *qī mén* (LR 14) and *tài yáng* (EX-HN 5), for one to two minutes at each point.

▶ Precautions

1. Patients should be on reasonable diet, restrain from greasy food, sugar, and carbonated drinks, eat more vegetables and coarse grains, and have small dinners.

2. Adjust life routine, sleep adequately, and maintain a good mood. In addition, engage in more physical exercises by increasing the amount of aerobic activity, such as outdoor activities including jogging, cycling, swimming, climbing, and playing ball.

XVI. Diabetes Mellitus

Diabetes mellitus is a group of chronic metabolic disorders characterized by abnormally high blood glucose (a.k.a. blood sugar) levels due to impaired ability of the body to produce or react to insulin. Diabetes mellitus is mainly manifested by increased thirst and hunger plus increased urine output. Clinically, many patients may report fatigue while some clients may be asymptomatic. Long-term metabolic disorders like diabetes mellitus can cause multiple organ damage and chronic progressive lesions, dysfunction or even failure of the eyes, kidneys, nerves, heart, blood vessels and other tissues and organs. When the disease condition is serious, there can be diabetic ketoacidosis or hyperosmolar comas. Diabetes can have serious negative impacts by reducing the quality of life, shortening life expectancy, and increasing mortality. In Chinese medicine, the disease pertains to the scope of "*xiāo kě* (wasting-thirst, 消渴)".

▶ Diagnosis

1. Clinical Symptoms   The disease has a slow onset, often without obvious symptoms in the early stage or mild cases, so that it is quite often discovered in a routine urine examination. Typical symptoms are fatigue, increased urine output, thirst, increased water intake, increased hunger and appetite. Consequently, polyuria, polydipsia, polyphagia, and weight loss are the four main signs of diabetes.

2. Chinese Medicine Pattern Differentiation

(1) *Xiāo kě of the upper jiao (dryness and heat damage of the lung)*: Thirst, polydipsia, dry mouth and throat, easy to be hungry, polyphagia, polyuria, and dry stool. The tongue is red with thin yellow coating, while the pulse is rapid.

(2) *Xiāo kě of the middle jiao (stomach dryness with fluid damage)*: Swift digestion with rapid onset of hunger, constipation, dry mouth with desire to drink, and weight loss. The tongue is red with yellow coating, while the pulse is slippery.

(3) *Xiāo kě of the lower-jiao (kidney yin deficiency)*: Frequent and turbid urine, dizziness, tinnitus, blurred vision, dry lips and mouth, insomnia and vexation.The tongue is red with no coating, while the pulse is wiry, thready and rapid.

3. Clinical Signs   Edema, and paresthesia of skin of the four extremities, including asense of formication (insects crawling on the skin), numbness, tingling, and itching.

4. Examinations

(1) Plasma glucose at any time ≥ 11.1 mmol/L (200 mg/dL), fasting blood glucose ≥ 7.0 mmol/L (126 mg/dL), or two hours postprandial blood glucose ≥ 11.1 mmol/L (200 mg/dL). Need to repeat the examination to confirm the diagnosis.

(2) For patients with no diabetic symptoms

but the blood glucose test reaches the diagnostic criteria for diabetes, the test result must be confirmed on a different day to confirm the diagnosis. If the second test results did not meet the diagnostic criteria for diabetes, the patient should be tested regularly.

(3) Other examinations may include urine glucose, specific urine gravity, glucose tolerance test, glycosylated hemoglobin, fructosamine determination, plasma insulin test, insulin release test, and C-peptide test.

▶ Treatment

1. Purpose   Helping to correct metabolic disorders of blood glucose to improve the quality of life of the patient.

2. Treatment Principles   Nourishing yin, clearing heat, boosting qi, and supplementing the kidney. For patients with dryness and heat damage of the lung, supplementing the treatment with methods to relieve dryness and moist the lung, while clearing stomach dryness and engendering fluids for patients suffering from stomach dryness with fluid damage. For patients with kidney yin deficiency, it is necessary to add treatment methods to nourish yin and consolidate the kidney.

3. Acupoints and Areas   *Gé shù* (BL 17), *yí shù/wèi wǎn xià shù* (EX-B 3, 胰俞 / 胃脘下俞), *gān shù* (BL 18), *dǎn shù* (BL 19), *pí shù* (BL 20), *wèi shù* (BL 21), *shèn shù* (BL 23), *mìng mén* (DU 4), *sān jiāo shù* (BL 22), *dà zhuī* (DU 14), *zhōng wǎn* (RN 12), *liáng mén* (ST 21), *qì hǎi* (RN 6), *guān yuán* (RN 4), *shén què* (RN 8), *qū chí* (LI 11), *zú sān lǐ* (ST 36), *sān yīn jiāo* (SP 6), *yǒng quán* (KI 1) and the abdomen.

4. Maneuvers   Rolling, thumb-pushing, pressing, kneading, precision-pressing, scrubbing, pushing, and vibration.

5. Basic Operation

(1) Ask the patient to lie in a prone position Apply the rolling method to work on the first line of the bladder meridian for five minutes.

(2) Perform the thumb-pushing maneuver between *gé shù* (BL 17) and *shèn shù* (BL 23) for seven minutes.

(3) Apply the press-kneading method on *gé shù* (BL 17), *yí shù* (EX-B 3), *gān shù* (BL 18), *dǎn shù* (BL 19), *pí shù* (BL 20), *wèi shù* (BL 21) and *shèn shù* (BL 23) with the focus on *yí shù* (EX-B 3) for three minutes and other points for one minute each. Then, perform the thumb-kneading method on *dà zhuī* (DU 14) for one minute.

(4) Apply the hypothenar-scrubbing maneuver along the *du mai* and both sides of the first line of the bladder meridian, and the horizontal scrubbing method on the areas where *shèn shù* (BL 23) and eight *liáo* (BL 31 ~ BL 34) are located until both areas are warm thoroughly.

(5) Ask the patient to lie in a supine position. Use thumb-pushing method to work on *zhōng wǎn* (RN 12), *qì hǎi* (RN 6) and *guān yuán* (RN 4), for one minute at each point.

(6) Perform the palmar-shaking method over *shén què* (RN 8) for a minute. Next, apply the rubbing method to the entire abdomen for three minutes. Then, apply the flat pushing maneuver to both the hypochondria for three minutes until the areas are thoroughly warm.

(7) Perform the press-kneading maneuver to both *qū chí* (LI 11) for one minute.

(8) Perform the precision-pressing method on *zú sān lǐ* (ST 36) and *sān yīn jiāo* (SP 6) to the degree that the points have the soreness *de*-qi sensation.

(9) Apply the scrubbing method to *yǒng quán* (KI 1) until the area is thoroughly warm.

6. Modification Based on Pattern Differentiation

(1) *Dryness and heat damage of the lung*: Add the press-kneading method on *fèi shù* (BL 13), *zhōng fǔ* (LU 1), *yún mén* (LU 2), and *kù fáng* (ST 14, 库房), at every point for one minute. Next, perform the scrubbing method straightly on *dàn zhōng* (RN 17) until it is thoroughly warm. Then, apply the press-kneading maneuver on *shǒu sān lǐ* (LI 10) and *shào shāng* (LU 11, 少商), and the grasping method to *jiān jǐng* (GB 21) for five to ten times until the patient feels the *de*-qi and soreness sensation.

(2) *Stomach dryness with fluid damage*: Add the press-kneading method on *jiàn lǐ* (RN 11), *xuè hǎi* (SP 10), *qī mén* (LR 14), *zhāng mén* (LR 13), *zhōng wǎn* (RN 12) and *liáng mén* (ST 21), each point for one minute. Then, apply

the scrubbing method to the hypochondria for one minute until the area is thoroughly warm.

(3) *Kidney yin deficiency*: Add press-kneading on *zhì shì* (BL 52, 志室), *rán gǔ* (KI 2), *tài xī* (KI 3) and *yǒng quán* (KI 1), for one minute at each point. Next, apply scrubbing on *fù liū* (KI 7) and *jiāo xìn* (KI 8, 交信) until the points are thoroughly warm.

▶ Precautions

1. The patient should be on a light diet, never over-eat, and avoid spicy, pungent, fatty, greasy and sweet food. Stop smoking and alcohol, participate in physical exercise and work. In addition, it is not appropriate to lie down right after meals or sit all day long.

2. During treatment, always make sure that the patient is relaxed, maintain a good mood, and avoid over-exertion. Patients should be moderate while engaging in sexual intercourse.

XVII. Chronic Fatigue Syndrome

Chronic fatigue syndrome (CFS) is characterized by chronic, recurrent and extreme fatigue lasting more than half a year, accompanied by symptoms of low grade fever, headache, muscle and joint ache, insomnia and various mental symptoms. The disease was officially named by the U.S. Centers for Disease Control and Prevention in 1987. At present, the exact mechanism of this disease is not clear, while most people think that it may be related to factors such as mental stress, bad life habits, mental and physical over-exertion and viral infection, leading to disorders of the neuroendocrine-immune regulatory network. In recent years, the incidence of CFS has gradually increased, mainly among the 20 to 50-year old population with more women being affected. In Chinese medicine, the disease is in categories such as "deficiency-consumption (*xū láo*, 虚 劳)" and "the five kinds of consumptive diseases (*wǔ láo*, 五劳)".

▶ Treatment

1. Clinical Symptoms

(1) The patient suffers from persistent or recurrent serious fatigue for no identifiable reason lasting for several months. The fatigue cannot be alleviated after rest. In addition, the patient experiences significantly decreased professional, academic, life and social ability and engagement compared to that of the patient prior to the illness.

(2) At the same time, the patient has at least four of the following eight conditions ① loss of memory or shorter attention span; ② sore throat; ③ stiff neck or swollen axillary lymph nodes; ④ muscular pain; ⑤ multiple joint pains; ⑥ recurrent headache; ⑦ poor sleep quality and not relaxed while getting up; ⑧ muscle ache after work.

2. Clinical Signs   Generally, there is no specific positive signs.

3. Examinations   There is no specific examination for chronic fatigue syndrome. Clinically, other diseases causing the persistent fatigue need to be ruled out by relevant examinations.

▶ Treatment

1. Purpose   Improve the symptoms of fatigue and general malaise, improve and restore the quality of life.

2. Treatment Principles   Supplementing and boosting qi and blood, and regulating qi movement.

3. Acupoints and Areas   *Bǎi huì* (DU 20), *sì shén cōng* (EX-HN 1, 四神聪), *tài yáng* (EX-HN 5), *fēng chí* (GB 20), *fèi shù* (BL 13), *xīn shù* (BL 15), *gān shù* (BL 18), *pí shù* (BL 20), *shèn shù* (BL 23), the head, back and lumbar area.

4. Maneuvers   Rubbing, rolling, pressing, kneading, grasping, finger-tapping, pushing, scrubbing, and patting.

5. Basic Operations

(1) Ask the patient to lie in a supine position. Apply press-kneading method to *bǎi huì* (DU 20), *sì shén cōng* (EX-HN1), *tài yáng* (EX-HN 5) and *fēng chí* (GB 20) for five minutes.

(2) Perform the grasping the five meridians on the head and the sweep-scattering maneuvers for one minute each. Then, apply the five-finger tapping to the head for another minute.

(3) Ask the patient to lie a prone position. Apply the palmar-pushing method top down

along the back portion of the first and second bladder meridian lines for three to five times. Next, perform the palmar-kneading or rolling maneuver along both sides of the erector spine muscles of the back up and down and back and forth for five minutes.

(4) Perform the pressing method on *fèi shù* (BL 13), *xīn shù* (BL 15), *gān shù* (BL 18), *pí shù* (BL 20), *shèn shù* (BL 23), one minute each point until the point is sore and the *de*-qi sensation has been obtained.

(5) Use the vertical hypothenar-scrubbing method to operate along *du mai* and horizontally on *mìng mén* (DU 4) until the areas are thoroughly warm.

(6) Perform the spinal-pinching method from the caudal vertebra up to *dà zhuī* (DU 14) for five to seven times.

(7) Perform the palmar-patting on the waist and the back along the erector spinemuscles of both sides from top to bottom for about two minutes on each side.

▶ Precautions

1. Dietary therapy, vitamins and minerals can be used to supplement the treatment.
2. Maintain an optimistic mood, avoid mental trauma, balance work and rest, and actively participate in physical exercises.

Section 3   Gynecologic Diseases

I. Dysmenorrhea

Dysmenorrhea refers to a common gynecologic disease characterized by pain, sometimes unbearable, in the lower abdomen and lumbar areas that women experience before, during or after menstrual period. Other symptoms that may accompany dysmenorrhea can include pale face, cold sweat on the head and face, cold limbs, nausea and vomiting. In Western medicine, the disease can be divided into two categories: primary dysmenorrhea and secondary dysmenorrhea. The former, indicating an onset without any obvious organic diseases, is also known as functional dysmenorrhea, and is commonly seen in unmarried women. The latter can be secondary to organic diseases of the reproductive system, such as endometriosis of the pelvis, adenomyosis, and chronic pelvic inflammation. It is easier to cure functional dysmenorrhea, whereas, dysmenorrhea caused by organic diseases has a relatively long course of disease, is refractory and difficult to cure. In Chinese medicine, dysmenorrhea belongs to the category of "abdominal pain due to menstrual period".

▶ Diagnosis

1. Clinical Manifestation   Periodic lower abdominal pain before, during or after each menstrual period that is sometimes severe and unbearable, and often accompanied by vomiting, sweating, cold limbs, and even fainting. Pain can radiate to the lumbosacral, anal and both sides of the thigh areas.

2. Chinese Medicine Pattern Differentiation

(1) *Qi stagnation and blood stasis*: Menstrual or premenstrual lower abdominal pain, distention of the hypochondria and breasts, dark and scanty menstrual flow with blood clots, and pain eased after discharge of the clots. The tongue is purplish or with dark spots at the edge, while the pulse is deep and wiry.

(2) *Cold-damp stagnation*: Premenstrual or menstrual cold pain of the abdomen that sometimes radiates to the erector spine muscles of the lumbar area. The pain is eased with heat. The menstrual flow is light, blood is dark with clots. The patient has a greenish pale facial complexion, low tolerance to cold, and loose stool. The tongue color is dull with white coating, while the pulse is deep and tight.

(3) *Qi and blood deficiency*: Lower abdomen has continuous pain during or after menstrual period, which can be reduced by pressing the abdomen. The color of the discharged blood is light red and the texture is thin. The patient has a pale facial complexion and is mentally fatigue. The tongue is pale with thin coating, while the pulse is thready and weak.

3. **Clinical Signs**   The patient is apparently in pain, and even in lying position with hands pressing on lower abdomen. In

physical examination of the abdomen, local tenderness can be found, but without muscle tension and rebound tenderness. Generally, there are no abnormal lesions of the genitalia in the pelvis, although there might be uterine dysplasia, stenosis of the cervical orifice, prolonged cervical canal with stenosis, or excessive uterine curvature.

4. Examinations

(1) *Menstrual prostaglandin determination*: Test is currently a major objective clinical indicator, in which an increased PCF index reveals abnormality.

(2) *Pelvic blood flow examination*: Poor pelvic blood flow.

(3) *Ultrasound*: Abnormalities cannot be found in patients with primary dysmenorrhea.

▶ Treatment

1. Purpose   Invigorating blood and unblocking the collaterals.

2. Treatment Principles   Unblocking and regulating qi and blood, harmonizing the collaterals, relieving pain. For qi stagnation and blood stasis, rectify qi, invigorate blood, dissolve stasis, and relieve pain. For blood stasis due to congealing cold, warm the meridians, dissipate cold, dispel stasis, and relieve pain. For qi and blood deficiency, supplement qi, nourish blood, harmonize the center and relieve pain.

3. Acupoints and Areas   *Qì hǎi* (RN 6), *guān yuán* (RN 4), *zhāng mén* (LR 13), *qī mén* (LR 14), *zú sān lǐ* (ST 36), *shèn shù* (BL 23), eight *liáo* (BL 31 ~ BL 34), *gān shù* (BL 18), *pí shù* (BL 20), *gé shù* (BL 17) and *wèi shù* (BL 21).

4. Maneuvers   Thumb-pushing, rubbing, rolling, pressing, kneading and scrubbing.

5. Basic Operations

(1) Ask the patient to lie in a supine position. Apply clockwise palmar rubbing on the patient's abdomen for five minutes.

(2) Perform the thumb pushing method on *qì hǎi* (RN 6), *guān yuán* (RN 4), on each point for about two minutes.

(3) Ask the patient to lie in a prone position. Apply the rolling maneuver on both sides of the lumbar spine and the sacral area

for five minutes.

(4) Perform the press-kneading maneuver on *shèn shù* (BL 23), eight *liáo* (BL 31 ~ BL 34), for one to two minutes at each point.

(5) Apply the palmar-scrubbing method horizontally on eight *liáo* (BL 31 ~ BL 34) to obtain a sense of warmth.

6. Modification Based on Pattern Differentiation

(1) *Qi stagnation and blood stasis*: Apply the press-kneading method on *zhāng mén* (LR 13), *qī mén* (LR 14), *gān shù* (BL 18) and *gé shù* (BL 17), for one minute at each point. Then, perform the grasping method on *xuè hǎi* (SP 10) and *sān yīn jiāo* (SP 6) to induce both soreness and a *de-qi* sensation.

(2) *Congealed cold-damp*: Perform the palmar-scrubbing method along the back portion of *du mai* and horizontally on *shèn shù* (BL 23) and *mìng mén* (DU 4) until the areas are thoroughly warm. Next, apply the press-kneading maneuver on *xuè hǎi* (SP 10) and *sān yīn jiāo* (SP 6), for one minute at each point.

(3) *Qi and blood deficiency*: Apply the palmar-scrubbing method along the back portion of *du mai* and horizontally on the left side of the back until the areas are warm thoroughly. Then, perform the finger-kneading maneuvers on *zhōng wǎn* (RN 12) for two to three minutes. Next, apply the press-kneading on *pí shù* (BL 20), *wèi shù* (BL 21) and *zú sān lǐ* (ST 36) for one minute at each point.

▶ Precautions

1. Patients suffering from dysmenorrhea should keep warm, avoid overworking, and maintain a good personal hygiene during menstrual period.

2. Maintain emotional stability prior to the period, avoid anger or melancholy, maintain healthy eating habits, and avoid spicy, cold, and raw food.

II. Irregular Menstruation

Irregular menstruation refers to a group of disorders that affect the menstrual cycle, menstruation duration, and color, volume, and quality of menstrual blood. Irregular menstruation is often accompanied by other symptoms. Clinically, it can be divided into early menstruation, delayed menstruation, and irregular menstruation based on changes in the cycle. According to changes in blood, it can be divided into menorrhagia (i.e. profuse menstruation), and scanty menstruation. Usually, early menstruation is associated with menorrhagia, while delayed menstruation has a higher correlation with scanty period.

▶ Diagnosis

1. Clinical Symptoms   Patients can experience abnormal menstrual cycle, duration of menstruation, menstrual flow, and texture of the menses, while other symptoms can include backache, discomfort, distention and pain of the lower abdomen, breast and hypochondria distention and pain, headache, nausea, vomiting, and abnormal urination or bowel movement.

2. Chinese Medicine Pattern Differentiation

(1) *Early menstruation*: The period comes earlier in a cycle, or even twice in a given month. ① *Excess heat*: Purplish and sticky menses with large amount, chest oppression, irritability, dry stool. The tongue is red with thin and yellow coating, while the pulse is floating and rapid. ② *Yin deficiency and blood heat*: Scanty and red menses, red cheeks and lips, heat sensation in the palmar side of the hands and feet. The tongue is red with yellow coating, while the pulse is thready and rapid. ③ *Heat due to liver qi stagnation*: Clots in the menses, irritability, bitter taste in the mouth, dry throat, and distention and pain in the hypochondria, breasts and lower abdomen prior to the period. The tongue is red with yellow coating, while the pulse is wiry and rapid.   ④ *Qi deficiency*: Pale, thin and scanty menses, lumbar and knee soreness and weakness, mental fatigue, shortness of breath, palpitations. The tongue is pale with thin coating, while the pulse is thready.

(2) *Delayed menstruation*:   ① *Excess cold*: Delayed menstruation with small amount of dark red blood and clots, cold pain with resistance to press that eases with heat, and

aversion to cold with cold limbs. The tongue coating is thin and white, while the pulse is deep and tight. ② *Deficient cold*: Pale face, and scanty menses with light color, dull abdominal pain that is relieved with heat. The tongue is pale with white coating, while the pulse is deep, slow and weak. ③ *Qi stagnation*: Scanty menses with dark color, distended abdominal pain, depressed, and chest oppression and discomfort that slightly relieves by blowing out air. The tongue coating is yellow and the pulse is wiry and choppy. ④ *Blood deficiency*: Empty pain of the abdomen, sallow complexion, dry skin, dizziness, and palpitations. The tongue is pale with thin coating, while the pulse is deficient and thready.

(3) *Irregular menstrual cycle*: ① *Liver constraint*: Early or delayed menstrual period, sluggish flow, distended pain of the hypochondria, breasts and lower abdomen, mentally depressed, chest tightness and discomfort, intention of sighing from time to time, belching, and decreased appetite. The pulse is wiry. ② *Kidney deficiency*: Small amount of menstrual discharge in light color and thin texture, dull complexion, dizziness, tinnitus, lumbar and knee pain, and nocturia. The tongue is pale with thin coating, while the pulse is deep and thready.

3. Clinical Symptoms   Generally there are no special signs. Gynecological examination can determine whether the development of the uterus and ovaries is normal.

4. Examinations   Ultrasound is used to determine the size, shape of the uterus, any neoplasm in the uterine cavity, or thickness of the endometrium. Diagnostic curettage and hysteroscopy could further clarify the lesion and endometrial pathology. Ovarian function tests can also help to confirm the diagnosis.

▶ Treatment

1. Purpose   Regulating the meridian and treating the root cause.

2. Treatment Principles   Regulate and harmonize qi and blood is the main principle. ① *Blood heat*: Clear heat and cool the blood; ② *Qi deficiency*: Supplement qi to contain the blood and regulate menses; ③ *Blood cold*: Warm the channel, dissipate cold, and regulate menses. ④ *Blood deficiency*: Nourish the blood and regulate menses; ⑤ *Liver constraint*: Soothe the liver, rectify qi, resolve the constrain and regulate menses; ⑥ *Kidney deficiency*: Supplement kidney and regulate menses.

3. Acupoints and Areas   *Zhōng wǎn* (RN 12), *guān yuán* (RN 4), *qì hǎi* (RN 6), *zhōng jí* (RN 3), *zhāng mén* (LV 13), *qī mén* (LV 14), *pí shù* (BL 20), *gān shù* (BL 18), *shèn shù* (BL 23), *mìng mén* (DU 4), eight *liáo* (BL 31 ~ BL 34), *zú sān lǐ* (ST 36), *sān yīn jiāo* (SP 6), *xuè hǎi* (SP 10) and *yīn líng quán* (SP 9).

4. Maneuvers   Thumb pushing, rubbing, pressing, kneading, pinching, and grasping.

5. Basic Operation

(1) Ask the patient to lie in a supine position. Use the thumb-pushing method on *zhōng wǎn* (RN 12), *qì hǎi* (RN 6), *guān yuán* (RN 4), and *zhōng jí* (RN 3), for one to two minutes at each point .

(2) Apply the palmar rubbing maneuver in a clockwise direction on the lower abdomen for five minutes.

(3) Perform the grasp-kneading method on *zú sān lǐ* (ST 36), *sān yīn jiāo* (SP 6), *xuè hǎi* (SP 10) and *yīn líng quán* (SP 9), for one to two minutes at each point.

(4) Ask the patient to lie in a prone position. Apply the thumb-pushing method on both the first lines of the back portion of the bladder meridians, focusing on *pí shù* (BL 20), *gān shù* (BL 18), *shèn shù* (BL 23) repeatedly for five minutes.

(5) Use the press-kneading maneuver on *mìng mén* (DU 4) and eight *liáo* (BL 31 ~ BL 34), for one to two minutes at each point.

(6) Perform the spinal-pinching method from sacrum to cervical vertebrae three times.

6. Modification Based on Pattern Differentiation

(1) *Blood heat*: Apply the press-kneading method on *dà zhuī* (DU 14) for one to two minutes, the palmar-scrubbing maneuver on *dà zhuī* (DU 14) until the point feels thoroughly warm, the press-kneading method on *qū chí* (LI 11) and *shén mén* (HT 7) for one

minute each point, and the scrubbing method on *yǒng quán* (KI 1) for one minute.

(2) *Congealed cold*: Apply the grasping method to *jiān jǐng* (GB 21) for five to ten times. Perform the split palmar pushing method to the abdomen at the navel level until the area is thoroughly warm.

(3) *Qi deficient*: Perform clockwise abdominal rubbing for five minutes and the palmar vibration to *guān yuán* (RN 4) for one to three minutes.

(4) *Blood deficient*: Apply the press-kneading method on points such as *pí shù* (BL 20), *wèi shù* (BL 21), *zú sān lǐ* (ST 36), *sān yīn jiāo* (SP 6) and *xuè hǎi* (SP 10) for one minute at each point.

(5) *Qi stagnation*: Perform the press-kneading method on *dàn zhōng* (RN 17) for one minute, and *zhāng mén* (LV 13) and *qī mén* (LV 14) for one to two minutes. Then, apply scrubbing on both hypochondria until the areas are thoroughly warm.

(6) *Kidney deficiency*: Perform the straight scrubbing method on the back portion of *du mai* and both sides of the bladder meridians for five to seven times, and horizontal scrubbing on *shèn shù* (BL 23), *mìng mén* (DU 4), *bái huán shù* (BL 30) and the eight *liáo* (BL 31 ~ BL 34) until these areas are thoroughly warm. Then, apply palmar-pressing on *guān yuán* (RN 4) for three to five minutes until the heat penetrates to the deeper level of the abdomen. Then, use the thumbs to knead both *yǒng quán* (KI 1) points continuously for one minute. Lastly, apply the palmar-scrubbing method repetitively along the longitudinal axis of the sole until the frictional heat is felt.

▶ Precautions

1. Patients should rest well and not be involved in strenuous exercise causing physical fatigue. Adjust to an appropriate diet, avoid raw, cold, or spicy food and drinks.

2. Pay attention to menstrual hygiene, wear appropriate clothing according to the change of weather, keep warm, and stay away from wind-cold contraction. In addition, maintain a good mood and avoid excessive emotional turbulence.

III. Perimenopausal Syndrome

Perimenopausal syndrome refers to autonomic dysfunction and metabolic disorders of mid-aged women before and after menopause due to decreased estrogen levels as the result of gradual decline or loss of ovarian function, also known as menopause syndrome. In Chinese medicine, the disease falls into the categories of "visceral agitation" or "patterns before or after menopause".

▶ Diagnosis

1. Clinical Symptoms Menstrual disorders, agitation, irritability, hot flashes with sweating, dizziness, tinnitus, palpitations, insomnia, fatigue, and memory loss.

2. Chinese Medicine Pattern Differentiation

(1) *Kidney yin deficiency*: Dizziness, tinnitus, backache, weakness of the legs, hot flashes with sweating, five centered heat, memory loss, insomnia, excessive dreaming; or itchiness, and irregular menstruation with fluctuating menses or continuous spotting of blood with purplish-red color. The tongue is red with little coating, while the pulse is thready and rapid.

(2) *Kidney yang deficiency*: Dizziness, tinnitus, cold abdomen, uterine prolapse, cold limbs, lower back pain, dull facial complexion, mental fatigue; light colored menstrual blood in large amount, scanty or spotting continuously. The tongue is pale with white and glossy, while the pulse is deep, slow and weak.

3. Signs The disease involves multiple systems, therefore, there are no characteristic signs.

4. Examinations

(1) *Endocrine hormonal assay*: Decreased estradiol (E_2), and increased follicle stimulating hormone (FSH), and luteinizing hormone (LH).

(2) *DEXA, CT or MRI*: Rapid loss of bone calcium owing to low level of estrogen that can lead to postmenopausal osteoporosis.

▶ Treatment

1. Purpose Harmonizing yin and yang.

2. Treatment Principles Supplementing the kidney and calming the mind. For patients with kidney yin deficiency, it is appropriate to enrich kidney, boost liver yin, foster yin and subdue yang. For patients suffering from kidney yang deficiency, the proper treatment principle should be warm the kidney, strengthen yang, supplement essence and nourish blood.

3. Acupoints and Areas *Dàn zhōng* (RN 17), *zhōng wǎn* (RN 12), *qì hǎi* (RN 6), *guān yuán* (RN 4), *zhōng jí* (RN 3), *jué yīn shù* (BL 14, 厥阴俞), *gé shù* (BL 17), *gān shù* (BL 18), *pí shù* (BL 20), *shèn shù* (BL 23), *mìng mén* (DU 4), *fēng chí* (GB 20), *tài yáng* (EX-HN 5), *cuán zhú* (BL 2), *sì bái* (ST 2), *yíng xiāng* (LI 20), *bǎi huì* (DU 20), *jiān jǐng* (GB 21), the first line of the back portion of the bladder meridian, the forehead, orbits, both sides near the nasal wings, nape, vertex, epigastric area and the lower abdomen.

4. Maneuvers Thumb-pushing, knead-rubbing, press-kneading, kneading, rolling, scrubbing, grasping, and smearing.

5. Basic Operations

(1) Ask the patient to lie in a supine position. Apply the thumb-pushing method on points such as *dàn zhōng* (RN 17), *zhōng wǎn* (RN 12), *qì hǎi* (RN 6), *guān yuán* (RN 4), and *zhōng jí* (RN 3), for one to two minutes at each point.

(2) Perform the rubbing method clockwise on the epigastric area and the lower abdomen, for five minutes on each area.

(3) Apply the horizontal scrubbing using the hypothenar eminence on *qì hǎi* (RN 6) until the area is thoroughly warm.

(4) Ask the patient to lie in a prone position. Perform the rolling method on both the first lines on the back portion of the bladder meridian from top to down repeatedly for about five minutes.

(5) Perform the press-kneading maneuver on *fèi shù* (BL 13), *xīn shù* (BL 15), *gé shù* (BL 17), *gān shù* (BL 18), *dǎn shù* (BL 19), *shèn shù* (BL 23), *páng guāng shù* (BL 28) and *cì liáo* (BL 32), for one to two minutes at each acupoint.

(6) Perform the scrubbing method horizontally on the lumbosacral area with the hypothenar eminence until the area is thor-

oughly warm.

(7) Ask the patient to be seated. Apply the five-finger grasping method to the top of the head from the front hairline to back hairline for five to 10 times. Then, perform the grasping method to *fēng chí* (GB 20) of both sides and the nape for two minutes.

(8) Perform the kneading method on the forehead using the thenar eminence for three to five minutes.

(9) Use the pad of the thumb to apply the smearing maneuver on the forehead, orbits and both sides of the nose for five to ten times.

(10) Apply the press-kneading method on *tài yáng* (EX-HN 5), *cuán zhú* (BL 2), *sì bái* (ST 2), and *yíng xiāng* (LI 20), for half a minute at each point.

(11) Use the press-kneading method with the thumb on *bǎi huì* (DU 20) for half a minute, and the grasping method on *jiān jǐng* (GB 21) for five to ten times.

6. Modification Based on Pattern Differentiation

(1) *Kidney yin deficiency*: Additional methods include: (a) Precision-pressing on *zhì shì* (BL 52), *xuè hǎi* (SP 10), *yīn líng quán* (SP 9), *sān yīn jiāo* (SP 6), and *tài xī* (KI 3), each point for half a minute; and (b) Pushing on both *qiáo gōng* (bridge arch) points twenty times on each side.

(2) *Kidney yang deficiency*: Additional maneuvers include (a) Palm-vibration on *guān yuán* (RN 4) and horizontal scrubbing on the eight *liáo* (BL 31~34) until the area is warm thoroughly; (b) Press-kneading on *qū chí* (LI 11), *hé gǔ* (LI 4), *xuán zhōng* (GB 39) and *wěi zhōng* (BL 40), for half a minute at each point; and (c) Scrub-foulage on *yǒng quán* (KI 1).

▶ Precautions

1. Keep doing regular physical exercises, increase exposure time to the sun, and have adequate intake of protein and calcium-rich foods.

2. Maintain a happy mood, balance work and rest, engage more with family and friends, increase time going out or traveling, and maintain a proper sex life. Lastly, have necessary gynecological examination regularly.

IV. Hypogalactia

Hypogalactia, occurring often 12 to 15 days after delivery and commonly in primiparous women, is the postpartum condition of reduced or even no milk secretion, so that the needs of the infant growth and development cannot be met. In a normal situation though, a temporary lack of milk within one week after the delivery is considered normal physiologically due to the loss of qi and blood. When qi and blood of the body recover, the milk should soon be produced and secreted.

Hypogalactia is defined in Chinese medicine as "insufficient postpartum milk" or "milk secretion disability".

▶ Diagnosis

1. Clinical Symptoms   Low or even no milk supply during lactation period in postpartum women; or the milk was normal, but suddenly becomes deficient after emotional overstimulation.

2. Chinese Medicine Pattern Differentiation

(1) *Qi and blood deficiency*: Reduced or no postpartum milk supply, pale face, mental fatigue, tender breasts without distention and/or pain, and poor appetite. The tongue is pale with little coating, while the pulse is deficient and thready.

(2) *Liver constraint and qi stagnation*: Reduced or no postpartum milk supply, depressed, unhappy, chest and hypochondriac distention, reduced appetite, and sometimes a mild fever may be present. The tongue coating is thin and yellow, while the pulse is wiry and thready.

3. Clinical Signs   If the palpation found that the breasts are soft with no sense of fullness, and excretion of thin and clear milk, it is mostly a deficient pattern. On the other hand, if the breasts are tender with palpable knots, or if the breasts are painful while trying to squeeze the milk out with difficulty and the milk is thick, it is mostly an excess pattern.

4. Examination   Relevant laboratory tests

can be performed if necessary.

▶ Treatment

1. Purpose   Supplementing qi and blood and unblocking the mammary ducts.

2. Treatment Principles   Fortifying the spleen, engendering blood, unblocking the collaterals, and promoting lactation.

3. Acupoints and Areas   *Dàn zhōng* (RN 17), *rǔ gēn* (ST 18), *nèi guān* (PC 6), *shào zé* (SI 1, 少泽), *qī mén* (LR 14), *gān shù* (BL 18), *pí shù* (BL 20), *wèi shù* (BL 21), *zú sān lǐ* (ST 36), *tài chōng* (LR 3), and the breasts.

4. Maneuvers   Pressing, precision-pressing, pushing, five-finger smear-scraping, kneading, and grasping.

5. Basic Operations

(1) Ask the patient to lie in a supine position. Apply precision-pressing on *dàn zhōng* (RN 17), *nèi guān* (PC 6), *shào zé* (SI 1) and *zú sān lǐ* (ST 36) with gradually increasing force for one to two minutes at each point.

(2) Perform straight-pushing from *tiān tū* (RN 22) to *dàn zhōng* (RN 17) for one to two minutes.

(3) With the fingers separated as comb-shaped, apply the smear-scraping from the outer ring of the breasts towards the middle repeatedly for three to five minutes.

(4) Apply the grasp-kneading maneuver to both breasts for five to seven minutes.

(5) Ask the patient to lie in a prone position. Perform precision-pressing on *gān shù* (BL 18), *pí shù* (BL 20), and *wèi shù* (BL 21), for one to two minutes at each point.

(6) Apply the press-kneading maneuver on *zú sān lǐ* (ST 36) and *tài chōng* (LR 3), for one to two minutes at each point.

6. Modification Based on Pattern Differentiation

(1) *Qi and blood deficiency*: Additional methods include thumb-pushing on *qì hǎi* (RN 6), *guān yuán* (RN 4) and *xuè hǎi* (SP 10) for two minutes at each point, and horizontal scrubbing with the palm on *shèn shù* (BL 23) and *mìng mén* (DU 4) until the area is thoroughly warm.

(2) *Liver constraint and qi stagnation*: Additional maneuvers include thumb-pushing on *zhāng mén* (LR 13) and *qī mén* (LR 14) for two to three minutes at each point, and oblique scrubbing with the palm on both sides of the hypochondria until the areas are thoroughly warm.

▶ Precautions

1. Pay attention to postpartum nutrition, eat more protein-rich foods and fresh vegetables, drink sufficient fluids, avoid impatience, and maintain a pleasant state of mind.

2. Consult with a certified lactation consultant. Master the correct breast-feeding methods, have adequate rest, exercise properly, keep qi and the blood in harmony and unblocked to benefit the secretion of milk.

Part **Three**

Pediatric *Tuina*

Chapter **Ten**

Maneuvers of Pediatric *Tuina*

Section 1 Basic Maneuvers

I. Pushing

The pushing maneuver is to perform a one-way, and linear or circular move with the pad of the thumb, the index or the middle finger as the origin of the force on a certain acupuncture point or the affected area of an infant.

Specific Operations

1. Straight Pushing (Figure 10-1) Use one hand to hold the affected limb of the infant, with the other hand's thumb naturally flexed and the finger pad or radial margin as the origin of the force and perform unidirectional linear pushing. An alternative is to use the extended index and middle fingers with the finger pads as the origin of the force, with the frequency at 220 to 280 times per minute.

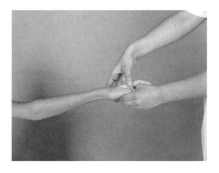

Figure 10-1 Straight Pushing

2. Circular Pushing (Figure 10-2) With the thumb pad as the origin of the force on an acupoint, perform clockwise circular movements, with the frequency at 160 to 200 times per minute.

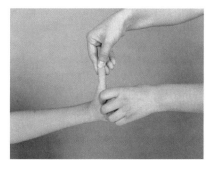

Figure 10-2 Circular Pushing

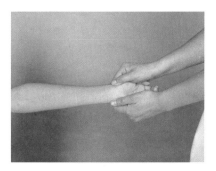

Figure 10-3 Bilateral Outward-pushing

3. Bilateral Outward-pushing (Figure 10-3) With the pad or radial margin of both thumbs, or with both palms as the origins of force, perform outward linear pushing to both sides (←   →) from the acupuncture point or the middle of the area.

4. Bilateral Inward-pushing The bilateral inward-pushing method is the opposite of the bilateral outward-pushing. With the thumb pads of both hands or the palms as the origins of the force, perform linear or arched pushing from the two sides of the acupoint or area towards the center.

Precautions

1. Do not damage the skin while performing the pushing maneuver.

2. According to the condition, location, and acupoint, pay attention to the reinforcing and reducing effects of the maneuver.

3. During treatment, the maneuver should not be sluggish.

Applicable Areas: The straight pushing method is best used for the linear or five-meridian acupoints in pediatric *tuina*, and more commonly used in the head, face, limbs, and the spine. Conversely, the circular pushing method is mostly used for the five-meridian points and arc-shaped-points of the hand. The bilateral outward-pushing maneuver is best used for the head, the face, the chest, the abdomen, the wrists, the palms, the shoulders and the scapulae, while the bilateral inward-pushing method is applicable for the head, the face, the chest, the abdomen, the wrist and the palm.

II. Kneading

The kneading method is performed using gentle and slow clockwise or counterclockwise circular movements with the tip or pad of the finger, the palm, the thenar eminence, or the palm heel as the origin of the force. Make sure that you connect to the treatment site or acupoint, and make the treatment site and its subcutaneous system to move together at the same time.

Specific Operations

1. Finger Kneading Use the pad or tip of the thumb, or the pads of the index, middle and ring fingers as the origin of the force and connect them firmly to the treatment site or acupoint, and perform gentle, slow, small-ranged, clockwise or counterclockwise circular kneading movements, causing the subcutaneous system to move along with it.

2. Thenar Kneading With the thenar eminence as the origin of the force on the operation site, use moderate power to apply the pressure, through the wrist joints force part of the treatment area to do gentle and mild, small, clockwise or counterclockwise actions of circular kneading moving so that the subcutaneous tissue rub together.

3. Palm-root Kneading Connect the root of the palm firmly to the treatment site with moderate downward pressure, and perform gentle, small-ranged and circular kneading maneuver in a clockwise or counterclockwise direction, making the subcutaneous tissue to move along with the kneading. The maneuver should also involve additional forces of the forearm and the wrist.

Precautions: When performing the kneading method, do not cause friction on the child's skin or apply excessive pressure.

Applicable Areas: The thumb or middle finger kneading method is applicable anywhere on the body or at any acupoints, while the two-finger kneading maneuver with the index and middle fingers rubbing method works best at acupoints such as *fèi shù* (BL 13), *pí shù* (BL 20), *wèi shù* (BL 21), *shèn shù* (BL 23) and *tiān shù* (ST 25). The three-finger kneading method is proper for the sterno-cleidomastoid, *qí* (umbilicus, 脐), and both sides of *tiān shù* (BL 25). Lastly, the thenar eminence kneading maneuver is appropriate for the head, face, chest, abdomen, hypochondria, and four limbs, while the palm-root kneading method is applicable for the back, lower back, abdomen and four limbs.

III. Pressing

The pressing maneuver can be performed with the root of the palm, or the tip or pulp of the thumb or the middle finger. Use any of these areas to connect firmly to an acupoint or treatment area of the child, apply gradual and downward pressure perpendicularly, retain the force for a moment, or press then relax right away.

Specific Operations

1. Finger Pressing Use the tip or pad of the thumb or the middle finger to apply perpendicular force firmly at an acupoint or the body area of the child to be treated, press down for a few seconds and then release the pressure. Repeat the sequence.

2. Palmar Pressing   Keep the wrist in dorsiflexion position, and five fingers relaxed and extended. Use the surface or the root of the palm to firmly connect to the area to be treated of the child, apply perpendicular continuous downward pressure for several seconds.

Precautions

1. Avoid the use of violent force during the pressing treatments so as to prevent tissue damage.

2. Upon completion of the pressing maneuver, it is not appropriate to abruptly withdraw the force. Rather, gradually reduce the pressure.

Applicable Areas: The finger-pressing method is applicable to all body areas, meridians and acupoints. The palmar pressing maneuver, on the other hand, is more appropriate to larger and flatter areas, such as the chest, abdomen, back and lower back.

IV. Rubbing

The rubbing method uses the pad of index, middle, ring or little finger, or the surface of the palm to perform a circular rhythmic stroking action at the treatment site.

Specific Operations

1. Finger Rubbing   Use the index finger, middle finger, ring finger, little finger or all four fingers together, connect to a certain part of the child's body surface or points, through the wrist joints and perform clockwise or counterclockwise circular motions.

2. Palmar Rubbing   Using the entire hand from the fingerprints to the palm of your hand, connect to a certain part of the child's body surface, and perform clockwise or counterclockwise circular motions.

Precautions: Same as mentioned in the rubbing maneuver for adults.

Applicable Areas: The finger rubbing and palmar rubbing methods are mainly applied to the chest and abdomen.

V. Nail-pressing

The nail-presing maneuver of using the nails to apply perpendicular pressing on the acupoint or the treatment area of the child.

Specific Operation: The physician should make an empty fist with the thumb straight and the thumb pad firmly connected to the radial margin of middle phalange of the index finger. Apply the force using the nail of the thumb to press steadily on the acupoint or the treatment area of the child and gradually increase the power to perform the pressing maneuver.

Precautions: The nail-pressing maneuver is a strong stimulation; therefore, it should not be used repeatedly for a long time to avoid damaging the skin. After performing the nail-pressing method, the kneading method is often applied to ease the stimulus and reduce the local pain or discomfort.

Applicable Areas: Suitable for head and face and hand and foot points.

VI. Pinching

The pinching maneuver is operated using one or both hands with the thumb or thumbs applying the force against the index and middle fingers, or against all four fingers, holding the child's skin and muscles, squeezing and then releasing while gradually moving from one site another. In pediatric *tuina*, the pinching method is mainly used over the spine, known as spinal pinching or pinching *jí* (spine).

Operations

1. The child should be in a prone position and expose the area to be pinched. Make two empty fists with the center of the palms facing down. Use the front 1/3 or the radial margin of the thumbs to firmly grab the skin next to *guī wěi* (turtle's tail, tailbone, 龟尾), apply the force with the force of the index and middle fingers to pinch the skin, and lift it up slightly. Perform the pinching method with both hands alternating with each other from the tailbone all the way to *dà zhuī* (DU 14) (Figure 10-4).

2. The child should be in a prone position or sit with the upper body leaning forward on a massage chair. Make two empty fists with the center of the palms facing down. Have the index finger be in half-flexion position with the radial and dorsal margin and of its middle phalange connected firmly to the skin of *guī wěi* (the tailbone) area. Use the force of the thumb and index finger at the same time to pinch the skin and lift it up slightly. Perform the pinching method with both hands alternating with each other from the tailbone to *dà zhuī* (DU 14) (Figure 10-5)

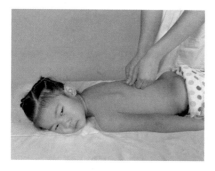

Figure 10-4   Pinching (1)

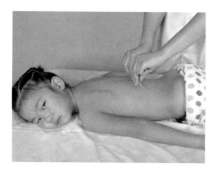

Figure 10-5   Pinching (2)

Precautions

1. Use the pad instead of the tip of the finger while performing the pinching method. Do not twist the skin or the muscle, or apply pressure to them with the nails to avoid pain.

2. Do not grab too little or too much skin and muscle while performing the pinching method. The former makes moving forward sluggish, while the latter makes it easy to slip. Excessive force leads to pain, while insufficient force does not have treatment effect.

3. When moving forward along the spine, the pinching should stay on a straight line.

4. The pinching method does not show the effect instantly. Therefore, the method needs to be performed persistently.

Applicable Area: The spine.

VII. Revolving Method

The revolving method uses the pad of the thumb, index finger, or middle finger to perform a circular or arc-shaped movement on the body surface of an infant.

Operations: Hold the child's arm with one hand, use the pad of the thumb, index finger or middle finger as the surface of the force to the treatment area or the acupoint, make arc-shaped movement from the starting area or acupoint to another area or acupoint (Figure 10-6). Alternatively, perform continuous circular movement with the speed of 60 to 120 times a minute.

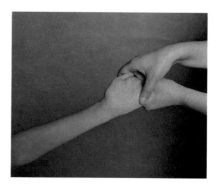

Figure 10-6   Thumb-revolving Method

Precautions: A lubricant can be used as to protect the child's skin during the operation.

Applicable Areas: Mainly used on arc or circular-shaped pediatric acupoints.

Section 2   Compound Maneuvers

I. Saving the Moon from the Bottom of the Water (Circular Pushing While Blowing Air)

Operations: The child should be in a sitting or supine position. The physician should sit in front and slightly to the side, hold four fingers of the child with the child's palm facing up, and drop some cold water into the center of the palm. Next, firmly place the pad of the other thumb on the child's palm center to perform the circular pushing maneuver and blow air to the palm center simultaneously. Continue to do the operation for three to five minutes (Figure 10-7).

Action and Applications: The technique acts a cooling method that can clear heart heat, reduce high body temperature, and drain fire. It can be used to treat excessive heat pattern with manifestations such as high fever with unconsciousness, heat entering *ying*-blood, agitation, restlessness, and constipation.

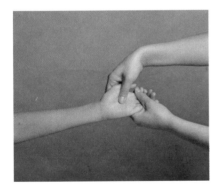

Figure 10-7   Saving the Moon from the Bottom of the Water

II. Wasp Entering the Cave (Finger-kneading the Nasal Wall)

Operations: The child should be sitting with the physician sitting in front and to the side. Gently insert of the tip of a finger to the child's nose and perform the kneading maneuver (Figure 10-8).

Action and Applications: Promoting sweat and releasing the exterior. It can be applied to treat externally contracted pathogens in children, failure of the interstitial space to diffuse qi, and fever without sweat.

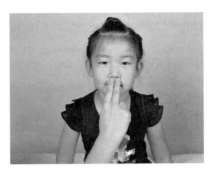

Figure 10-8   Wasp Entering the Cave

III. Celestial Gate Entering to the Tiger's Mouth

Operation: The child should either be sitting or in a supine position. Use one hand to hold the four fingers of the child with the radial aspect of the index finger facing up, while the radial side pad of the other thumb is used to apply the force. Dip the thumb in the spring onion ginger water, push directly from the radial side tip of the child's index finger where the life pass is located to the *hǔ kǒu* (tiger's mouth, *hé gǔ* [LI 4], 虎口). Then, apply the pinching kneading method using the tip of the thumb on the *hǔ kǒu* several dozen times (Figure 10-9)

Action and Applications: Fortifying the spleen, promoting digestion, normalizing qi, and engendering blood. It is applicable in treating problems including deficiency of the spleen and stomach, disharmonized qi and blood, distention of the abdomen, diarrhea, and food accumulation.

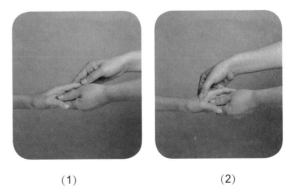

(1)   (2)

Figure 10-9   Celestial Gate Entering to the Tiger's Mouth

IV. Moving Water to Earth

Operation: The child should be in a sitting or supine position. Hold the four fingers with one hand, the palm facing up, and use the lateral aspect of the thumb as the origin of the force. Apply the push-revolving method for 100 to 300 times from the *shèn shuǐ* (kidney water, 肾水) acupoint at the tip of the little finger, push along the margin of the palm, pass the transverse palmar creases and *xiǎo tiān xīn* (minor celestial heart, 小天心), and reach the *pí tǔ* (spleen earth, 脾土) acupoint at the tip of the thumb (Figure 10-10).

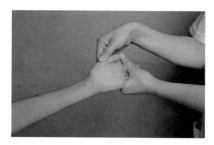

Figure 10-10   Moving Earth to Water

Action and Applications: Fortifying the spleen, improving the function of stomach, nourishing dryness, and promoting defecation. The method treats ailments caused by deficiency patterns of the spleen and stomach including indigestion, poor appetite, constipation, abdominal distention, diarrhea, dysentery, and malnutrition with food accumulation.

V. Moving Earth to Water

Operation: The child should be in a sitting or supine position. Hold the four fingers with one hand, palm facing up, and use the lateral aspect of the thumb as the origin of the force. Apply the push-revolving method for 100 to 300 times from *pí tǔ* (spleen earth) at the tip of the thumb, push along the margin of the palm, pass *xiǎo tiān xīn* (minor celestial heart) and *zhǎng xiǎo héng wén* (small crease of the palm, 掌小横纹), and reach *shèn shuǐ* (kidney water) at the tip of the little finger (Figure 10-11).
Action and Applications: Nourishing kidney yin, clearing damp-heat of the spleen and

stomach, improving urination, and arresting diarrhea. It is applicable in treating diseases such as dark, scanty, and frequent urination, distention of the lower abdomen, diarrhea and dysentery.

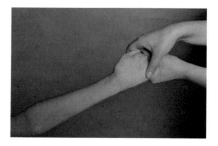

Figure 10-11   Moving Water to Earth

VI. Pressing the Rib and Applying Foulage and Rubbing

Operation: The child should be in a sitting position or have the parent hold the child. The child's arms should be crossed and hands placed on opposite shoulders. Sit facing the child, use both palms as the origins of the force, attach them on each side of the hypochondria, apply the foulage-rubbing method symmetrically 50 to 500 times top down on *dù jiǎo* (abdominal corner, 肚角) of both sides (Figure 10-12).
Action and Applications: Rectifying qi, dissolving phlegm, fortifying the spleen, and promoting digestion. It is used to treat problems such as phlegm accumulation, cough, panting, chest obstruction, abdominal pain, abdominal distension, food accumulation and stagnation, and hepatosplenomegaly.

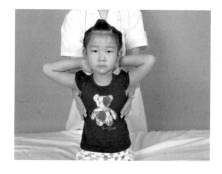

Figure 10-12   Pressing the Rib and Applying Foulage and Rubbing

VII. Opening *Xuán Jī* (Rotary Gear, 璇玑)

Operation: Apply bilateral outward-pushing top down using both thumbs along the ribs starting from *xuán jī* (RN 21) to the hypochondria of the child. Next, perform straight pushing from *jiū wěi* (RN 15) to the navel area and push-rubbing both sides of the abdomen area of the child. Then, apply straight pushing from the navel area to the lower abdomen. Lastly, perform the pushing *qī jié gǔ* (seven segmental bones, 七节骨) maneuver. Each maneuver should be performed 50 to 100 times (Figure 10-13).

Action and Application: Diffusing qi, enhancing qi movement, promoting digestion, and dissolving phlegm. Opening *xuán jī* is applicable to situations including phlegm block, chest tightness, cough, shortness of breath, food accumulation, bloating, abdominal pain, vomiting, diarrhea, fever due to external contraction, fainting, and convulsions.

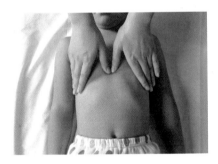

Figure 10-13 Opening *Xuán Jī*

VIII. Kneading *Qí* (Umbilicus), *Guī Wěi* (Turtle's Tail), and Scrubbing *Qī Jié Gǔ* (Seven Segmental Bones)

Operation: The child should be in a supine position. Use the pad of the middle finger or the index, middle and index fingers together to perform the kneading method on *qí* (umbilicus). Then, with the child in a prone position, use the pad of the middle finger or the thumb to knead the *guī wěi* (turtle's tail). Finally, use the pad of the thumb or the palm to perform the pushing method to *mìng mén* (DU 4) for supplementing purpose, or from *mìng mén* (DU 4) to push down to *guī wěi* (the tailbone) for draining pur-

pose, each for 100 to 300 times [Figure 10-14 (1), Figure 10-14 (2), Figure 10-14 (3)].

Action and Application: Freeing and regulating *ren mai* and *du mai*, regulating and rectifying the bowels, arresting diarrhea, and removing stagnation. It can be used for treating diseases including diarrhea, dysentery, and constipation.

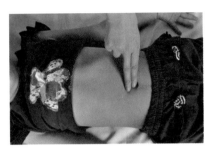

(1)

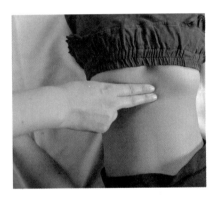

(2)

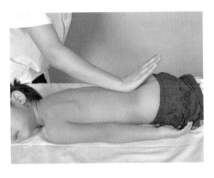

(3)

Figure 10-14 Kneading *Qí* and *Guī Wěi*, and Scrubbing *Qī Jié Gǔ*

IX. Driving the Horse to Cross the Celestial River

Operation: The child should be in a sitting or supine position. Use one hand to hold the four fingers of the child with the palm facing up, use the pad of the middle finger to perform the revolving method to *láo gōng* (PC 8). Next, use the index, middle and ring fingers together and beat the child's arm from *zǒng jīn* (total tendons, 总筋) to *hóng chí* [same as *qū chí* (LI 11), 洪池] along *tiān hé shuǐ* (celestial river water, 天河水). The same action can also be performed by using the index and middle fingers to flick along *tiān hé shuǐ* (celestial river water) until reaching the elbow. The beating or flicking should be repeated 20 to 30 times (Figure 10-15).

Action and Application: Clearing heat, unblocking the collaterals, moving qi and invigorating blood. It is applicable to situations of the excess heat pattern such as high fever, irritability, unconsciousness, delirious speech, and numbness and convulsions of the upper limbs.

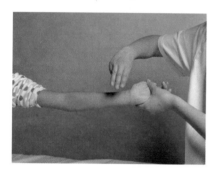

Figure 10-15　Driving the Horse to Cross the Celestial River

X. General Closure

Operation: The child should be in a sitting position. Use the pad of the index or middle finger as the origin of the force, pinch first, then perform the press-kneading method to the child's *jiān jǐng* (GB 21). At the same time, use the thumb, index, and middle fingers to hold the index and ring fingers of the child, flex and extend, and rotate the child's upper limb for 20 to 30 times (Figure 10-16).

Action and Applications: Refreshing the mind, moving qi and unblocking blood of the whole body. It is applicable for physical weakness owing to chronic illness, internal injuries, external pathogenic contraction, and an ending procedure of pediatric *tuina*.

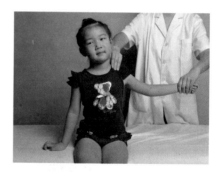

Figure 10-16　General Closure

Chapter **Eleven**

Common Acupoints Used in Pediatric *Tuina*

Section 1   Head, Facial and Neck Acupoints

I. *Gāo Gǔ* (Prominent Bone, 高骨)

Location: At the posterior hairline, in the depression inferior to the mastoid process. It is also known as *ěr hòu gāo gǔ* (prominent bone behind the ear, 耳后高骨) (Figure 11-1).

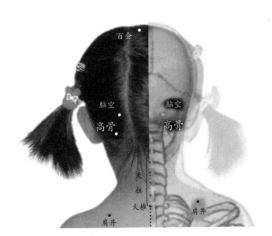

Figure 11-1   Head and face points (1)

Operation: Use the tip of the thumb or middle finger to knead, usually 30 to 50 times. Or, use both thumbs to perform the revolving maneuver on each side, usually 30 to 50 times.

Action and Application: Kneading *gāo gǔ* disperses wind and release the exterior. It is used to treat problems such as cold and headache, often combined with maneuvers such as pushing *cuán zhú* (gathering bamboo, 攒竹),

pushing *kǎn gōng* (kan trigram palace, 坎宫) and kneading *tài yáng* (EX-HN 5). The method also has the effect of calming the mind and eliminating irritability, so that it is applicable in treating loss of consciousness and agitation.

II. *Cuán zhú* (Gathering Bamboo, 攒竹) or *Tiān Mén* (Celestial Gate, 天门)

Location: The straight line between the middle of the eyebrows and the front hairline (Figure 11-2).

Operation: Use both thumbs alternately to perform straight pushing bottom down along *tiān mén* (celestial gate) 30 to 50 times, which is called pushing *cuán zhú* (gathering bamboo) or opening *tiān mén*. If the physician pushes from the glabella to the fontanelle 30 to 50 times, known as "grand opening of *tiān mén*".

Action and Applications: The actions of opening *tiān mén* are dispersing wind, releasing the exterior, opening the orifices, awakening the brain, and calming the mind. It is commonly used in fever and headache due to external contraction, often combined with pushing *kǎn gōng* (kan trigram palace) and *tài yáng* (EX-HN 5). If there is fright, restlessness, and irritability, the physician can add maneuvers such as clearing *gān jīng* (liver meridian, 肝经) and press-kneading *bǎi huì* (DU 20). The maneuver should be used with caution among children having a weak constitution with profuse sweating, or those suffering from rickets.

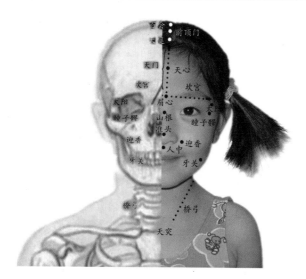

Figure 11-2   Head and face points (2)

III. *Kǎn Gōng* (*Kan* Trigram Palace, 坎宫)

Location: The straight line from the glabella to the lateral end of each eyebrow (Figure 11-2).

Operation: Pushing *kǎn gōng* (*kan* trigram palace) uses both thumbs to perform bilateral outward-pushing from the glabella to the lateral ends of the eyebrows 30 to 50 times.

Action and Applications: Actions of pushing *kǎn gōng* include dispersing wind, releasing the exterior, awakening the brain, brightening the eyes, and arresting headache. It is commonly used in fever and headache due to external pathogenic attack, often combined with pushing *cuán zhú* (gathering bamboo) and kneading *tài yáng* (EX-HN 5). When it is used to treat red and painful eyes, it is often combined with clearing *gān jīng* (liver meridian), pinch-kneading *xiǎo tiān xīn* (minor celestial heart), and clearing *tiān hé shuǐ* (celestial river water).

IV. *Shān Gēn* (Root of the Hill, 山根)

Location: The midpoint between the two inner canthi of the eyes, at the depression of nose bridge (Figure 11-2).

Operation: Using the thumbnail to pinch three to five times is called pinching *shān gēn* (root of the hill).

Action and Applications: Pinching *shān gēn* has the effect of opening the orifices,

awakening the eyes and calming the mind. It is applicable in treating infantile convulsions, coma, and spasm, often used in combination with pinching *shuǐ gōu* (DU 26) and *lǎo lóng* (senior dragon, 老龙).

V. *Tiān Zhù* (Celestial Pillar, 天柱) / *Tiān Zhù Gǔ* (Celestial Pillar Bone, 天柱骨)

Location: On the neck, the straight line between the middle of the posterior hair line and *dà zhuī* (DU 14) (Figure 11-1).

Operation: Pushing *tiān zhù* (celestial pillar) method uses the pads of the thumb, or the index and middle fingers to push along a straight line from top to bottom for 100 to 300 times. In addition, the scraping *tiān zhù* method uses a tool such as a spoon by dipping it into water from time to time to scrape top down until slight marks showing up on the skin.

Action and Applications: Pushing and scraping *tiān zhù* are effective in sending counterflow downwards, arrest vomiting, dispelling wind and dissipating cold, so that they are applicable in treating nausea and vomiting and often combined with pushing from the wrist crease to *bǎn mén* (board gate, 板门) and kneading *zhōng wǎn* (RN 12). To treat fever, stiff neck and neck pain owing to external contraction, combine this maneuver with the grasping *fēng chí* (GB 20) and pinch-kneading *èr shàn mén* (two-panel door, 二扇门). The scraping *tiān zhù* method, is applicable in treating sunstroke and contraction of summer-heat, and employs a tool such as a spoon by dipping it into ginger or cool water to scrape top down until slight marks appear on the skin.

VI. *Qiáo Gōng* (Bridge Arch, 桥弓)

Location: The straight line along the sternocleidomastoid muscle on each of the side of the neck (Figure 11-2).

Operation: Perform the kneading method on *qiáo gōng* (bridge arch) 30 times, smearing 50 times, and grasping three to five times.

Action and Applications: Kneading, smearing and grasping of *qiáo gōng* (bridge arch) has the action of invigorating blood, dissolving stasis, and eliminating swelling.

It is therefore used to treat pediatric muscle torticollis, often in combination with the neck rotation method.

Section 2 Acupoints on the Upper Extremities

I. *Pí Jīng* (Spleen Meridian, 脾经)

Location: The thumb pad of a child (Figure 11-3).

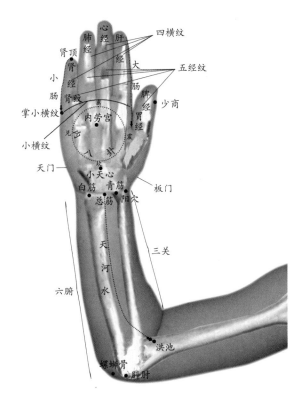

Figure 11-3 Acupoints of the Upper Extremity (1)

Operation: There are several methods available that can be used for clearing *pí jīng* (spleen meridian), supplementing *pí jīng*, and even supplementing and draining *pí jīng*. Collectively the methods are known as the pushing *pí jīng* method.

1. Supplementing *Pí Jīng* Stabilize the thumb of the child with one hand, and perform the circular pushing method on *pí jīng*.

Another way is to have the child's thumb in a flexed position, and the practitioner uses the tip of his or her thumb to push from the radial aspect of the child's thumb tip directly to the root of the thumb. The maneuver needs to be performed 100 to 500 times.

2. Clearing *Pí Jīng* Hold the child's thumb in an extended position, and push directly from the root of the thumb to the tip 100 to 500 times.

3. Even Clearing and Supplementing *Pí Jīng* Pushing *pí jīng* back and forth.

Action and Applications: The supplementing *pí jīng* method is used to fortify the spleen and stomach, boost qi and blood, and is often used to treat spleen and stomach deficiency, loss of appetite owing to insufficient qi and blood, emaciation and indigestion. The method is often performed in combination with maneuvers such as supplementing *wèi jīng* (stomach meridian, 胃经), kneading *zhōng wǎn* (RN 12), rubbing the abdomen and press-kneading *zú sān lǐ* (ST 36). The clearing *pí jīng* method, is effective in clearing heat, draining dampness, dissolving phlegm and arrest vomiting. The method is also applicable to excess patterns manifested with damp-heat jaundice, nausea, vomiting, diarrhea, dysentery and food accumulation. It is often used in conjunction with methods such as clearing *wèi jīng* (stomach meridian), kneading *bǎn mén* (board gate), clearing *dà cháng* (large intestine, 大肠), kneading *zhōng wǎn* (RN 12) and kneading *tiān shū* (ST 25). The even clearing and supplementing *pí jīng* method has the actions of harmonizing the stomach, promoting digestion, and increasing appetite, so that it is commonly used in the treatment of fullness and distention of the stomach, acid swallowing, loss of appetite, diarrhea and nausea caused by food stagnation and disharmony of the spleen and stomach. It is normally combined with methods including revolving *nèi bā guà* (inner eight trigram), kneading *bǎn mén* (board gate) and bilateral outward-pushing *fù yīn yáng* (abdominal yin yang, 腹阴阳).Since the system of the spleen and the stomach is weaker among infants and small children, it is not appropriate to use excessive draining methods. Rather, a supplementing method is more applicable while the clearing method is used for children with strong physical constitution and in excess disease patterns.

II. *Wèi Jīng* (Stomach Meridian, 胃经)

Location: The palmar side of the first proximal phalange of the thumb (Figure 11-3).

Operation: Supplementing *wèi jīng* (stomach meridian) and clearing *wèi jīng*, are collectively known as the method of pushing *wèi jīng*.

1. Supplementing *Wèi Jīng* Perform circular pushing on *wèi jīng* 100 to 500 times.

2. Clearing *Wèi Jīng* Push from the root of the thumb toward the end of the proximal phalange of the thumb of the child 100 to 500 times.

Action and Applications: The method of supplementing *wèi jīng* fortifies the spleen and stomach and promotes transportation and transformation. Therefore, it is commonly used in treating spleen and stomach deficiency, indigestion, abdominal distension and loss of appetite while often combining with supplementing *pí jīng* (spleen meridian), kneading *zhōng wǎn* (RN 12), rubbing the abdomen, and press-kneading *zú sān lǐ* (ST 36). Additionally, the clearing *wèi jīng* method has effects of clearing the damp-heat of the middle *jiao*, harmonizing the stomach, descending qi counterflow, draining stomach fire, eliminating irritability and dissolving thirst, treating illnesses of excess pattern such as nausea and vomiting owing to qi counterflow, abdominal distension and fullness, fever, thirst, constipation, loss of appetite and nose bleed. It is often used in combination of maneuvers of clearing *pí jīng* (spleen meridian) and *dà cháng* (large intestine), pushing *tiān zhù* (celestial pillar), pushing *liù fǔ* (six *fu*-organs, 六腑) and pushing *qī jié gǔ* (seven segmental bones) downwards.

III. *Gān Jīng* (Liver Meridian, 肝经)

Location: The pad of the index finger (Figure 11-3).

Operation: Supplementing *gān jīng* (liver meridian) and clearing *gān jīng* are collective-

ly known as the pushing *gān jīng* method.

1. Supplementing *Gān Jīng* Use the thumb pad to perform circular pushing on the pad of the index finger of the child 100 to 500 times.

2. Clearing *Gān Jīng* Use the tip of the thumb to push directly from the tip to the root of the child's index finger 100 to 500 times.

Action and Applications: The clearing *gān jīng* method is effective in calming the liver, draining fire, extinguishing wind, suppressing fright, resolving constraint, and eliminating vexation. It is appropriate to clear *gān jīng* rather than supplementing it. If there is evidence of liver deficiency, clearing method should be performed after supplementing it, or replace it by supplementing *shèn jīng* (kidney meridian, 肾经), known as "nourishing the kidney to foster the liver". The method of clearing *gān jīng* is commonly used in treating convulsions, spasm, restlessness, and heat of the five centers if they are of the excess pattern. In addition, it is often combined with pinching *shuǐ gōu* (DU 26), *lǎo lóng* (senior dragon) and *shí xuān* (EX-UE 11), and kneading *xiǎo tiān xīn* (minor celestial heart).

IV. *Xīn Jīng* (Heart Meridian, 心经)

Location: The pad of the middle finger (Figure 11-3).

Operation: Both the supplementing *xīn jīng* (heart meridian) and clearing *xīn jīng* methods are known collectively as the pushing *xīn jīng* method.

1. Supplementing *Xīn Jīng* Perform the circular pushing method on the pad of the middle finger 100 to 500 times.

2. Clearing *Xīn Jīng* Push from the tip to the root of the middle finger of the child 100 to 500 times.

Action and Applications: Clearing *xīn jīng* is effective in clearing heat and eliminating heart fire; therefore, it is used to treat problems such as high fever, loss of consciousness, red face, mouth ulcer, and scanty urine of the heart fire flaring up pattern. The clearing method is often performed in conjunction with the method of clearing *tiān hé shuǐ* (celestial river water) and *xiǎo cháng* (small intestine, 小肠). Conversely, the supplementing *xīn jīng* maneuver is rarely used, because it can stir up the heart fire. If the child suffers from qi and blood deficiency with symptoms of vexation, restlessness, and exposing sclera while asleep, clearing method should be added after the supplementing method, or replace it with the supplementing *pí jīng* (spleen meridian).

V. *Fèi Jīng* (Lung Meridian, 肺经)

Location: The pad of the ring finger (Figure 11-3).

Operation: Supplementing *fèi jīng* (lung meridian) and clearing *fèi jīng* methods are known collectively as the pushing *fèi jīng* method.

1. Supplementing *Fèi Jīng* Perform the circular pushing method on the pad of the ring finger 100 to 500 times.

2. Clearing *Fèi Jīng* Push from the tip to the root of the ring finger of the child 100 to 500 times.

Action and Applications: The supplementing *fèi jīng* method is effective in boosting lung qi, often used in treating cough, enuresis, spontaneous sweating, and night sweats if the patient displays deficient pattern. It is usually combined with the methods such as supplementing *pí jīng* (spleen meridian), kneading *èr mǎ* (two horses, 二马) and pushing *sān guān* (trigate, 三 关) upwards. The method of clearing *fèi jīng*, with actions of diffusing lung qi, clearing heat, dispersing wind, releasing the exterior, arresting cough, and resolving phlegm, are often applied to treat cough owing to organ heat, fever owing to common cold and constipation that are showing excess pattern. It is often used in combination with the clearing *tiān hé shuǐ* (celestial river water), pushing *liù fǔ* (six *fu*-organs), push-kneading *dàn zhōng* (RN 17) and revolving *nèi bā guà* (inner eight trigram, 内八卦).

VI. *Shèn Jīng* (Kidney Meridian, 肾经)

Location: The pad of the little finger (Figure 11-3).

Operation: The supplementing *shèn jīng* (kidney meridian) and clearing *shèn jīng* methods are known collectively as the pushing *shèn jīng* method.

1. Supplementing *Shèn Jīng* Perform the circular pushing method on the pulp of the little finger 100 to 500 times.

2. Clearing *Shèn Jīng* Push from the tip to the root of the little finger of the child 100 to 500 times.

Action and Applications: Actions of the supplementing *shèn jīng* method include tonifying the kidney, benefiting the brain, warming and nourishing kidney qi. Therefore, it is often used to treat conditions such as congenital deficiency, deficiency due to chronic illness, chronic diarrhea owing to kidney deficiency, polyuria, enuresis, deficient sweating, and wheezing. Additionally, the method is often used in combination with supplementing *pí jīng* (spleen meridian) and *fèi jīng* (lung meridian), kneading *shèn shù* (BL 23), scrubbing *mìng mén* (DU 4) and pinching *jí* (spine, 脊). The clearing *shèn jīng* method also has the effect of clearing and unblocking damp-heat of the lower *jiao*, so that it is applicable to clinical conditions such as accumulated heat in the bladder, scanty and dark urine and diarrhea due to damp-heat. Consequently, it is often used in conjuction with pinch-kneading *xiǎo tiān xīn* (minor celestial heart), clearing *xiǎo cháng* (small intestine) and pushing *jī mén* (dustpan entrance, 箕门). Clinically, the supplementing method is used more commonly on *shèn jīng*, while the clearing method on *shèn jīng* is often replaced by clearing *xiǎo cháng* (small intestine).

VII. *Sì Héng Wén* (Four Horizontal Creases, 四横纹)

Location: On the palmar aspect, the creases of first interphalangeal joints of the index, middle, ring and little fingers (Figure 11-3).

Operation: There are two types of maneuvers that can applied at *sì héng wén* (four horizontal creases): Pinching *sì héng wén* and pushing *sì héng wén*. The first method is to pinch each of the four creases three to five times using the thumb nail working the index, middle, ring and little finger in order. The second method is to have the four fingers closed together, and push from the crease of the index finger to the little finger using the thumb pad 100 to 300 times.

Action and Applications: The pinching *sì héng wén* method can reduce fever, eliminate vexation and disperse stasis and masses, while the actions of the pushing *sì héng wén* method are regulating the center, moving qi, harmonizing qi and blood, and clearing fullness and distention. In treating chest suppression, wheezing owing to phlegm, methods including revolving *nèi bā guà* (inner eight trigram), pushing *fèi jīng* (lung meridian) and pushing *dàn zhōng* (RN 17) are usually added. For children suffering from food accumulation and malnutrition, abdominal distention, disharmony of qi and blood and indigestion, pinching *sì héng wén* can often be combined with supplementing *pí jīng* (spleen meridian) and kneading *zhōng wǎn* (RN 12). As a primary acupoint in treating food accumulation and malnutrition, one can also use a regular acupuncture or a three-edged needle to puncture *sì héng wén* and get a few drops of blood.

VIII. *Xiǎo Héng Wén* (Minor Horizontal Creases, 小横纹)

Location: On the palm, the transverse creases on the joints between the palm and proximal phalanges of the index, middle, ring and little fingers (Figure 11-3).

Operation: The methods can either be pinching or pushing *xiǎo héng wén* (minor horizontal creases). The first is done by pinching each of the four creases three to five times using the thumb nail with the index, middle, ring and little finger in order. The second is to have the four fingers closed together, and push from the crease of the index finger all the way to the little finger with the radial aspect of the thumb 100 to 300 times.

Action and Applications: Push-pinching *xiǎo héng wén* can reduce fever, dissolve bloating and dissipate masses. The pushing *xiǎo héng wén* method is designated for treating dry rales of the lung, while pinching *xiǎo héng wén* method treats heat accumulation of the spleen and stomach, cracked lips, ulcerous mouth and bloating. If the bloating is of deficient spleen pattern, add the method

of supplementing *pí jīng* (spleen meridian), while maneuvers such as kneading *qí* (umbilicus), clearing and supplementing *pí jīng* (spleen meridian), revolving *nèi bā guà* (inner eight trigram) can be added for patients with food damage. In addition, it is often combined with the method of clearing *pí jīng* (spleen meridian), *wèi jīng* (stomach meridian) and *tiān hé shuǐ* (celestial river water) for children having cracked lips, sore tongue and ulcerous mouth.

IV. *Dà Cháng* (Large Intestine, 大肠)

Location: The straight line on radial margin connecting the tip of the index finger to *hǔ kǒu* (tiger's mouth, *hé gǔ* [LI 4]) (Figure 11-3).

Operation: The supplementing *dà cháng* (large intestine) and clearing *dà cháng* methods are known collectively as the pushing *dà cháng* method.

1. Supplementing *Dà Cháng* Push directly along *dà cháng* from the tip of the index finger to *hǔ kǒu* using the pad of the thumb 100 to 500 times.

2. Clearing *Dà Cháng* Push from *hǔ kǒu* to the tip of the index finger of the child 100 to 500 times.

Action and Applications: The actions of the supplementing *dà cháng* method include astringing the intestines, rescuing the intestines from desertion, warming the center and arresting diarrhea, commonly used in diarrhea due to deficient cold pattern and rectal prolapse. Supplementinng *dà cháng* is often performed in conjunction with methods including supplementing *pí jīng* (spleen meridian), pushing *sān guān* (trigate), supplementing *shèn jīng* (kidney meridian), kneading *qí* (umbilicus), bilateral outward-pushing *fù yīn yáng* (abdominal yin yang) and pushing *qī jié gǔ* (seven segmental bones) upwards. Conversely, the treatment effects of the clearing *dà cháng* method can include clearing intestine heat, eliminating damp-heat, and guiding out digestive stagnation and accumulation. Therefore, the method is commonly used in clearing intestinal bowel, clearing damp-heat, and stagnation. The clearing *dà cháng* maneuver is commonly used in treating damp-heat, food accumulation, digestive stagnation, body ache owing to heat, constipation and dysentery mixed with blood and pus. It is often combined with maneuvers such as clearing *tiān hé shuǐ* (celestial river water), pushing *liù fǔ* (six *fu*-organs) downwards, bilateral outward-pushing *fù yīn yáng* (abdominal yin yang), clearing *pí jīng* (spleen meridian), clearing *fèi jīng* (lung meridian), pushing *qī jié gǔ* (seven segmental bones) downwards, and kneading *guī wěi* (turtle's tail). *Dà cháng* is also known as the *triple gate* and can be used as part of the observation diagnostic routine in pediatric clinic.

X. *Xiǎo Cháng* (Small Intestine, 小肠)

Location: The straight line between the tip and the root on the ulnar aspect of the little finger (Figure 11-3).

Operation: The supplementing *xiǎo cháng* (small intestine) and clearing *xiǎo cháng* methods are known collectively as the pushing *xiǎo cháng* method.

1. Supplementing *Xiǎo Cháng* Push directly with the pad of the thumb along *xiǎo cháng* from the tip of the little finger to its root 100 to 500 times.

2. Clearing *Xiǎo Cháng* Push directly with the pad of the thumb along *xiǎo cháng* from the root to the tip of the little finger 100 to 500 times.

Action and Applications: The effects of supplementing *xiǎo cháng* are warming and tonifying the lower-*jiao*, so that it can be used in problems including polyuria, enuresis, if they show evidence of deficient cold of the lower-*jiao* pattern. The method is often combined with supplementing *pí jīng* (spleen meridian), *fèi jīng* (lung meridian) and *shèn jīng* (kidney meridian), kneading *dān tián* (elixir field, 丹田) and *shèn shù* (BL 23), and scrubbing the lumbo-sacral area. Conversely, the actions of the clearing *xiǎo cháng* method include clearing damp-heat of the lower-*jiao*, separating the clear from the turbid, and is therefore, used to treat problems such as dark, scanty and difficult urination, urinary retention, and watery diarrhea. If there is heat in the heart meridian being transferred

to the small intestine, the method can be used in conjuncton with clearing *tiān hé shuǐ* (celestial river water) to enhance the effect of clearing heat and to benefit urination.

XI. *Shèn Dǐng* (Kidney Apex, 肾顶)

Location: The tip of the little finger of a child (Figure 11-3).

Operation: Kneading *shèn dǐng* (kidney apex) 100 to 500 times.

Action and Applications: Kneading *shèn dǐng* has the effects of restraining original qi, consolidating the exterior and arresting sweating. The method is commonly used in treating conditions such as spontaneous sweating, night sweating or profuse sweating. In treating night sweating, it is often combined with kneading *shèn jīng* (kidney meridian) and *èr mǎ* (two horses), and supplementing *fèi jīng* (lung meridian). In treating spontaneous sweating owing to yang deficiency, combine the kneading *shèn dǐng* with supplementing *pí jīng* (spleen meridian).

XII. *Zhǎng Xiǎo Héng Wén* (Minor Crease of the Palm, 掌小横纹)

Location: The palmar aspect of the crease at the ulnar side, under the root of the little finger (Figure 11-3).

Operation: Kneading 100 to 500 times.

Action and Applications: The actions of kneading *zhǎng xiǎo héng wén* (minor crease of the palm) include clearing heat, dissipating masses, opening the chest, diffusing lung qi, dissolving phlegm and relieving cough. As a key acupoint in treating pertussis, pneumonia and wet lung rales, the method of kneading *zhǎng xiǎo héng wén* can often be used for wheezing, cough, mouth ulcers and tongue sores. For the treatment of wheezing and coughing, the method is often used in combination of clearing *fèi jīng* (lung meridian), pushing *liù fǔ* (six *fu*-organs) and opening *xuán jī* (rotary gear). When the method is applied to treat moutth sores, it is often used in combination of methods of clearing *xīn jīng* (heart meridian), *wèi jīng* (stomach meridian) and *tiān hé shuǐ* (celestial river water).

XIII. *Bǎn Mén* (Board Gate, 板门)

Location: The surface of the thenar eminence (Figure 11-3).

Operation: The methods applied at this location include kneading *bǎn mén* (board gate), pushing from *bǎn mén* to the wrist crease and pushing from the wrist crease to *bǎn mén*. Kneading *bǎn mén*, also known as revolving *bǎn mén*, should be performed 50 to 100 times. The method of pushing from *bǎn mén* to the wrist crease or vice versa should be performed 100 to 300 times.

Action and Applications: The method of kneading *bǎn mén*, is used for fortifying the spleen, harmonizing the stomach, promoting digestion and dissolving stagnation and is often used to treat milk and food stagnation and accumulation, loss of appetite, belching, bloating, diarrhea and vomiting. The method should be combined with the five *jīng* (*gān jīng*, *xīn jīng*, *pí jīng*, *fèi jīng* and *shèn jīng*) and pushing *xiǎo héng wén* (minor horizontal creases). The method of pushing from *bǎn mén* to the wrist crease is used for fortifying the spleen and arresting diarrhea and is often combined with maneuvers of pushing *pí jīng* (spleen meridian), pushing *dà cháng* (large intestine) and pushing *qī jié gǔ* (seven segmental bones) upwards. The pushing from wrist crease to *bǎn mén* method can treat vomiting, because it reverses rebellious stomach qi, and is often combined with the clearing *wèi jīng* (stomach meridian) method.

XIV. *Nèi Bā Guà* (Internal Eight Trigram, 内八卦)

Location: On the palmar side of the hand, take two thirds of the distance from the center of the palm to the crease on the root of the middle finger as the radius, and make an imaginary circle. The positions of *nèi bā guà* (internal eight trigram) are located on this circle. The eight palaces are *qián* (乾), *kǎn* (坎), *gèn* (艮), *zhèn* (震), *xùn* (巽), *lí* (离), *kūn* (坤) and *duì*, representing eight directions. Facing *xiǎo tiān xīn* (minor celestial heart) is the *kǎn* (坎) palace (i.e. point), while the one facing the middle finger is the *lí* (离) palace. The

zhèn palace is located on the upper half of the circle, halfway between *lí* and *kǎn*, while *duì* is right at the middle point dividing the circle to half near the little finger (Figure 11-3).

Operation: There are three ways to perform the revolving *nèi bā guà* (internal eight trigram) method. The in-sequence revolving *nèi bā guà* maneuver starts from *qián*, revolves to the direction of *kǎn* and ends at the *duì* palace, while the reverse revolving *nèi bā guà* method is the opposite, starting from *duì*, revolving to *kūn* and continuing to end at the *qián* palace. Both maneuvers should be repeated 100 to 500 times. In the third variant, the route of the method is separated into different segments, according to the symptoms, and each segment can receive the revolving maneuver 100 to 200 times.

Action and Applications

1.*In-sequence revolving nèi bā guà maneuver* The method has the actions of loosening up the chest, rectifying qi, arresting cough, dissolving phlegm, moving stagnation and promoting digestion, and is applicable in treating cough owing to phlegm masses, internal damage due to milk and food, chest tightness, abdominal distension, vomiting and loss of appetite. In treating these problems, the method can often be combined with other maneuvers such as pushing *pí jīng* (spleen meridian) and *fèi jīng* (lung meridian), and kneading *bǎn mén* (board gate) and *zhōng wǎn* (RN 12).

2.*Reverse revolving nèi bā guà maneuver* The method has the actions of redirecting counterflow of qi and calming panting, therefore can treat panting due to phlegm and vomiting. The reverse revolving method is often combined with maneuvers including supplementing *pí jīng* and *fèi jīng*, and pushing *sān guān* (trigate), *tiān zhù gǔ* (celestial pillar bone) and *dàn zhōng* (RN 17).

3.*Segmental maneuvers* Revolving from the *qián* to the *zhèn* palace calms the ethereal soul, *xùn* to *duì* palace brings peace to the corporeal soul, *lí* to *qián* arrests cough, and *kūn* to *kǎn* clears heat. In addition, revolving from the *kǎn* to the *xùn* palace eliminates diarrhea, and *gèn* to *lí* promotes sweating. Lastly, the reverse revolving method from the *kǎn* to the *xùn* palace arrests vomiting.

XV. *Xiǎo Tiān Xīn* (Minor Celestial Heart, 小天心)

Location: In the depression where the thenar and the hypothenar eminences meet (Figure 11-3).

Operation: The operations at this point include kneading, pinching, and pounding. The kneading method on *xiǎo tiān xīn* (minor celestial heart) requires holding the four fingers of the child with one hand, having the child's palm facing up, while the pinching *xiǎo tiān xīn* method uses the thumb nail to pinch three to five times. The pounding method on *xiǎo tiān xīn*, uses the tip or the flexed interphalangeal joint of the middle finger at the point 10 to 30 times.

Action and Applications: Kneading *xiǎo tiān xīn* has the effect of clearing heat, suppressing fright, promoting urination and improving eyesight. Therefore, it is applicable in conditions such as red, painful and swollen eyes, aphtha, tongue sore, restlessness owing to fright, or scanty and dark urination due to heart heat being transferred to the small intestine. The technique is often combined with methods of clearing *xīn jīng* (heart meridian), *tiān hé shuǐ* (celestial river water) and *gān jīng* (liver meridian), and press-kneading *jīng níng* (essence calming, 精宁). In addition, this method can be used for newborn scleroderma, jaundice, enuresis, edema and incomplete eruption of pox rash. The pinching or pounding *xiǎo tiān xīn* maneuvers are often used for convulsions, night crying, hypervigilance and restlessness. If there are symptoms such as infantile convulsions, sanpaku eyes (sclera visible above or below the iris) and strabismus, combine the method with maneuvers of pinching *lǎo lóng* (senior dragon) and *shuǐ gōu* (DU 26), and clearing *gān jīng* (liver meridian). If the eyeballs turn to the top, pinch or pound downwards. For right strabismus, pinch or pound to the left; otherwise, for left strabismus, pinch or pound to the right.

XVI. *Dà Héng Wén* (Major Transverse Crease, 大横纹)

Location: On the palmar aspect, the transverse crease of the wrist. The portion under the thumb is called *yáng chí* (yang pond, 阳池), while the portion under the little finger is *yīn chí* (yin pond, 阴池).

Operation: The methods of outward-pushing *yīn yáng* and inward-pushing *yīn yáng* are used at this point. Hold the child's palm with the thumbs placed below the center of *dà héng wén*, push outward at the same time from *zǒng jīn* (total tendons) 30 to 50 times. The method is called the bilateral outward-pushing *dà héng wén* maneuver, but is also known as the outward-pushing *yīn yáng* method. When using the thumbs to push from each side of the wrist crease to *zǒng jīn* 30 to 50 times, the method is referred to as bilateral inward-pushing *dà héng wén* or inward-pushing *yīn yáng*.

Action and Applications: Outward-pushing *yīn yáng* can balance yin and yang, harmonize qi and blood, move stagnation and promote digestion. The method is, therefore, often used with maneuvers of opening *tiān mén* (celestial gate), bilateral outward-pushing *kǎn gōng* (*kan* trigram palace), kneading *tài yáng* (EX-HN 5) and pinching *zǒng jīn* to treat irritability, milk and food stagnation, bloating, diarrhea and vomiting if the problems are the result of disharmony of yin and yang, or qi and blood. If the disease pattern is of excess heat, an accelerated bilateral outward-pushing *yáng chí* maneuver is performed, while an escalated lateral outward-pushing *yīn chí* maneuver is done for deficienct cold pattern. The inward-pushing *yīn yáng* method has the effects of dissolving phlegm and dissipating masses, is often combined with manauvers of clearing *tiān hé shuǐ* (celestial river water) and kneading the kidney crease of the *sì héng wén* (four horizontal creases), and is usually used in treating cough due to phlegm masses and chest tightness.

XVII. *Zǒng Jīn* (Total Tendons, 总筋)

Location: On the palmar aspect, the midpoint of the transverse wrist crease (Figure 11-3).

Operation: The operations at this point can include kneading *zǒng jīn* method and pinching *zǒng jīn* method. The former is performed by holdinng the four fingrs of the child, and usinng the tip of the thumb to press-knead *zǒng jīn* 100 to 300 times, while the latter is using the thumb nail to pinch *zǒng jīn* three to five times.

Action and Applications: Kneading *zǒng jīn* clears heat in the heart meridian, dissipates masses, arrests convulsions and regulates qi of the whole body. It is commonly used to treat mouth and tongue sores, hot flashes, night crying due to excess heat, and is often employed in combination with the method clearing *tiān hé shuǐ* (celestial river water) and *xīn jīng* (heart meridian). The pinching *zǒng jīn* method calms fright and arrests convulsions. The method is therefore applicable in treating infantile convulsions and tics, often in combination with methods such as pinching *shuǐ gōu* (DU 26), grasping *hé gǔ* (LI 4) and pinching *lǎo lóng* (senior dragon).

XVIII. *Sān Guān* (Trigate, 三关)

Location: A straight line between *yáng chí* (yang pond) and *qū chí* (LI 11) on the radial aspect of the forearm. *Yáng chí* (yang pond) is the same as *tài yuān* (LU 9) (Figure 11-3).

Operation: Hold the child's palm with one hand, and use the radial aspect of the thumb or the pad of the index and middle fingers to push from the wrist crease to the elbow along *sān guān* (trigate) 100 to 500 times. The method is known as the method of pushing *sān guān*. An alternative method, known as the major pushing *sān guān* method is to push from the lateral aspect of the thumb to the elbow with the child's thumb flexed.

Action and Applications: The pushing *sān guān* method warms yang, dissipates cold, moves qi, boosts qi, promotes sweating and releases the exterior, so that it is appropriate for any conditions demonstrating deficienct cold pattern. It is commonly used in the treating problems owing to qi and blood deficiency, *mìng mén* (life gate, 命门) fire failure, or deficient cold of the lower origin, such as extreme cold of the four limbs, pale or sallow

facial complexion, loss of appetite, malnutrition, food accumulation, vomiting and diarrhea. It is often performed in combination with the following maneuvers: supplementing *pí jīng* (spleen meridian) and *shèn jīng* (kidney meridian), kneading *dān tián* (elixir field), pinching *jí* (spine) and rubbing *fù* (abdomen). In treating common cold due to wind-cold, aversion to cold with absence of sweat, and incomplete eruption of measles, it is usually used with methods of clearing *fèi jīng* (lung meridian), pushing *cuán zhú* (gathering bamboo) and pinch-kneading *èr shàn mén* (two-panel door).

IXX. *Tiān Hé shuǐ* (Celestial River Water, 天河水)

Location: On the forearm, a straight line between *zǒng jīn* (total tendons) and *hóng chí* [same as *qū chí* (LI 11)] (Figure 11-3).

Operation: The clearing or pushing *tiān hé shuǐ* method involves holding the child's hand with one hand, and pushing along *tiān hé shuǐ* (celestial river water) with the pads of the index and middle fingers 100 to 500 times .

Action and Applications: The effects of clearing *tiān hé shuǐ* are clearing heat, releasing the exterior, draining fire and relieving vexation. As a mild cooling method, the clearing heat effect is gentle and appropriate for clearing heat at the *wei* (defensive) or qi level without damaging yin. When applied in conjunction with maneuvers of clearing *xīn jīng* (heart meridian) and pushing *liù fǔ* (six *fu*-organs), it is appropriate for all kinds of heat patterns, frequently used in treating illnesses such as five center vexation and heat, dry mouth, dry throat, lip and tongue sores and night crying. For common cold, fever, headache, aversion to wind, slight sweating and sore throat as the result of externally contracted wind-heat, the method should be combined with pushing *cuán zhú* (gathering bamboo), pushing *kǎn gōng* (*kan* trigram palace) and/or kneading *tài yáng* (EX-HN 5).

XX. *Liù Fǔ* (Six *Fu*-organs, 六腑)

Location: The straight line between *yīn chí*

(yin pond) and the elbow crease on the ulnar side of the forearm (Figure 11-3).

Operation: Retreating *liù fǔ* or pushing *liù fǔ* involves holding the child's wrist in one hand to stabilize it, and pushing along *liù fǔ* 100 to 500 times with the pads of the thumb or the index and middle fingers.

Action and Applications: Retreating *liù fǔ* has the effect of clearing heat, cooling blood and dissolving toxins, and is applicable for all excess heat patterns. Specific diseases treatable with the method include warm pathogens entering the *ying*-blood level, accumulated and stagnant heat constraint of *zang-fu* organs, high fever with thirst and vexation, mumps and swollen glands owing to toxicity. For arresting sweating, combine with the supplementing *pí jīng* (spleen meridian) maneuver. The method can be used to balance yin and yang, clear heat without damaging the healthy qi and prevent the child from being hurt by excess cold or heat while combined with the pushing *sān guān* (trigate) method. In situations of cold-heat complex, if the heat is the major factor, it can be performed by repeating the procedure of pushing *liù fǔ* three times and *sān guān* once. Conversely, if cold is the major factor, then the ratio should be to repeat the procecure of pushing *sān guān* three times and *liù fǔ* once. Please note that the method should be used with caution in children suffering from spleen deficient diarrhea.

XXI. *Lǎo Lóng* (Senior Dragon, 老龙)

Location: 0.1 cun below the center of the nail base of the middle finger (Figure 11-4).

Operation: Pinching *lǎo lóng* is performed by holding the child's hand with one hand and pinching *lǎo lóng* (senior dragon) point with the thumb nail of the other hand three to five times, or until the child revives.

Action and Applications: The effects of the pinching *lǎo lóng* method are reviving the consciousness and opening the orifices. It is used as a first aid measure, treating acute infantile convulsions, high fever, spasm and unconsciousness. In sudden attack, if the child reacts to the pain caused by the pinch-

ing *lǎo lóng* method, the treatment is easier. If the child does not react to the pinching pain and remains silent, the condition is generally considered refractory.

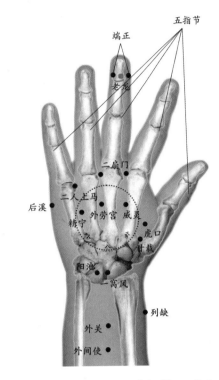

Figure 11-4 Acupoints of the Upper Extremity (2)

XXII. *Duān Zhèng* (Straighten-up, 端正)

Location: On the lateral side of the nail base of the middle finger where the margin of the red and white converges. The one on the radial aspect is the left *duān zhèng* (Straighten-up), while the one on the ulnar side is the right *duān zhèng* (Figure 11-4).

Operation: To perform the pinch-kneading *duān zhèng* method, hold the hand of the child with one hand, and pinch *duān zhèng* using the thumb nail or to knead with the pad of the thumb of the other hand 50 times.

Action and Applications

1. Kneading the right *duān zhèng* has the effect of directing qi counterflow down and arresting vomiting. The method is often used

to treat nausea and vomiting due to rebellious stomach qi. Kneading the right *duān zhèng* is commonly applied in combination with methods such as clearing *wèi jīng* (stomach meridian) and pushing from the wrist crease to *bǎn mén*.

2.Kneading the left *duān zhèng* has the action of lifting the center qi to arrest diarrhea and can treat watery diarrhea and dysentery. Kneading the left *duān zhèng* is often combined with maneuvers such as pushing *pí jīng* (spleen meridian) and *dà cháng* (large intestine).

3.Pinching *duān zhèng* has the actions of reviving consciousness, opening orifices and arresting bleeding. The method is used to treat infantile convulsions and is usually combined with pinching *lǎo lóng* (senior dragon) and clearing *gān jīng* (liver meridian) methods.

4. Tying around *duān zhèng*: Use a piece of thread to tie around (avoid being too tight) the transverse crease, including both *duān zhèng* points, of the distal interphalangeal joint of the middle finger. The method is used to stop bleeding, such as nosebleed.

XXIII. *Èr Shàn Mén* (Two-panel Door, 二扇门)

Location: On the dorsal side of the hand, in the depression of the base of the middle finger (Figure 11-4).

Operation: The maneuver includes pinching and kneading *èr shàn mén* (two-panel door). In the kneading variant, hold the child's hand with one hand, and use the other hand to perform the kneading method on both *èr shàn mén* using the index and middle fingers respectively 100 to 500 times. The pinching *èr shàn mén* maneuver though, is performed by holding the child's wrist firmly with one hand, having the child's palm facing down, pinching *èr shàn mén* both sides with both thumb nails respectively. Then, knead the points for a little while, and repeat three to five times.

Action and Applications: The pinching and kneading *èr shàn mén* method, is used as a key sweat-inducing maneuver, can promote sweating, vent the exterior, eliminate the fe-

ver and calm asthma. In treating frail patients with externally pathogenic attack, the method is often combined with kneading *shèn dǐng* (kidney apex), supplementing *pí jīng* (spleen meridian) and supplementing *shèn jīng* (kidney meridian). The kneading *èr shàn mén* method, often used in treating an external attack of wind-cold, should be performed relatively faster with intermediate power.

XXIV. *Wēi Líng* (Powerful Spirit, 威灵)

Location: On the dorsum of the hand, between the second and third metacarpal bones (Figure 11-4).

Operation: Pinching *wēi líng* (powerful spirit) is performed by holding the four fingers of the child with the dorsum facing up, and pinching the point five times or until the child revives. Finish the technique by kneading the point.

Action and Applications: The effects of pinching *wēi líng* are opening the orifices and reviving consciousness. The method is mainly used to treat acute infantile convulsions, unconsciousness and coma that may lead to death. It is often applied in conjunction with the pinching *jīng níng* (essence calming) to strengthen the effect of opening the orifices and resuscitation.

XXV. *Jīng Níng* (Essence Calming, 精宁)

Location: On the dorsum of the hand, between the fourth and the fifth metacarpal bones (Figure 11-4).

Operation: The pinching *jīng níng* (essence calming) method is performed by holdinng the four fingers of the child with the dorsum facing up, and pinching *jīng níng* five times or until the child revives. Finish the technique by kneading the point. .

Action and Applications: The effects of pinching *jīng níng* are moving qi, breaking masses and dissolving phlegm. The method is often used for phlegm accumulation, rough breathing, wheezing with phlegm, malnutrition and food accumulation. It is usually used in combination with methods of supplementing *pí jīng* (spleen meridian), pushing *sān guān* (trigate) and pinching *jí* (spine). Be cautious when using this method on patients with weak physical constitution.

XXVI. *Yī Wō Fēng* (Rushing Wind, 一窝风)

Location: The depression in the middle of the wrist crease on the dorsum of the hand (Figure 11-4).

Operation: Kneading *yī wō fēng* (rushing wind) is performed by holding the child's hand and kneading the point 100 to 300 times.

Action and Applications: The effects of the kneading *yī wō fēng* method are warming the center, moving qi, relieving pain owing to *bì* pattern and benefiting the joints, so that it is often applied to treat abdominal pain owing to externally contracted cold, food accumulation, or *bì* pain due to cold stagnation in meridians and collaterals. It is generally used in combination with methods of grasping *dù jiǎo* (abdominal corner), pushing *sān guān* (trigate) and kneading *zhōng wǎn* (RN 12).

Section 3 Thoracic and Abdominal Acupoints

I. *Xié Lèi* (Hypochondrium, 胁肋)

Location: The lateral sides of the torso from the armpit to *tiān shū* (ST 25) on both sides (Figure 11-5).

Operation: The child should be sitting in upright position and apply the foulage-rubbing method along *xié lèi* (hypochondrium) 50 to 100 times. The method is also known as the maneuver of pressing the rib and applying foulage and rubbing.

Action and Applications: The method breaks up masses and accumulations, smoothens qi, dissolves phlegm and relieves chest tightness, therefore, it treats pediatric conditions such as chest oppression and abdominal distension owing to food accumulation, phlegm congestion and qi counterflow. If it is applied in treating hepatosplenomegaly, it should be performed repeatedly for many sessions. Conversely, the maneuver

should be used with caution among children suffering from sunken center qi or with failure of the kidney to grasp qi.

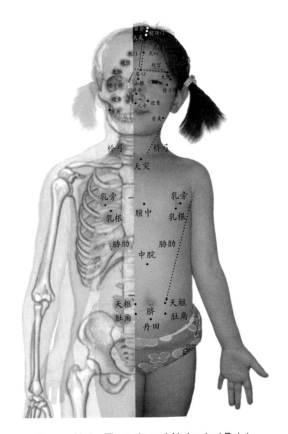

Figure 11-5 Thoracic and Abdominal Points

II. *Fù* (Abdomen, 腹)

Location: The abdomen (Figure 11-5).

Operation: The child should be a supine position. Rubbing *fù* (abdomen) and bilateral outward-pushing *fù yīn yáng* (abdominal yin yang) are the two common maneuvers for the *fù* pediatric point. The former method is performed by using the surface of the palm or the four fingers to rub *fù* for five minites. Clockwise rubbing is considered supplementing and counterclockwise is draining. Rubbing *fù* back and forth is considered an even supplementing and draining maneuver. On the other hand, the bilateral outward-pushing *fù yīn yáng* method is performed from the edges of the ribs or both sides of *zhōng wǎn*

(RN 12) to *qí* (umbilicus) 100 to 200 times using the tip of the thumbs.

Action and Applications

1. *Rubbing fù*   The method promotes digestion, rectifies qi, sends the counterflow of qi downward. It treats stagnation of milk and food, nausea and vomiting due to rebellious stomach qi, and abdominal distension. The method is often combined with revolving *nèi bā guà* (internal eight trigram), pushing *pí jīng* (spleen meridian) and press-kneading *zú sān lǐ* (ST 36). In treating pediatric anorexia, rubbing *fu* is often used in conjunction with methods such as kneading *bǎn mén* (board gate), revolving *nèi bā guà* and pinching *jí* (spine). The supplementing method can fortify the spleen and arrest diarrhea, which is often used in diarrhea related to a spleen deficiency or damp-cold pattern. Conversely, the draining method of rubbing *fù* promotes digestion, guides out food stagnation and improves defecation, so that it can be used to treat constipation, abdominal distension, anorexia, and diarrhea due to food and milk damage. It is often applied in combination with the method of bilateral outward-pushing *fù yīn yáng*.

2. *Bilateral outward-pushing fù yīn yáng*   The treatment effects of this method include fortifying the spleen, harmonizing the stomach, rectifying qi and promoting digestion. It is often combined with the draining method applied on *fù* which is rubbing the area counterclockwise.

3. *Even supplementing and draining maneuver for fù*   The even supplementing and draining method can harmonize the stomach. It can be used as a common preventative method in pediatric *tuina* with the effect of promoting digestion and strengthening the health in general, it should be performed for an extended period. In this case, the method is often combined with maneuvers of supplementing *pí jīng*, pinching *jí* and press-kneading *zú sān lǐ* (ST 36).

III. *Qí* (Umbilicus, 脐)

Location: The center of the navel (Figure 11-5).
Operation: The two methods applied on the *qí* point (umbilicus) are kneading and rubbing. The child should lie in a supine position. The kneading *qí* maneuver uses the tip of the middle finger or root of the palm to knead 100 to 300 times. As an alternative, use the thumb, the index and the middle fingers to grasp the navel and perform shake-kneading 100 to 300 times. The rubbing *qí* method is operated with the palm or fingers.

Action and Applications: Both the kneading and rubbing *qí* methods can warm yang, dissipate cold, replenish qi, nourish blood, fortify the spleen, harmonize the stomach, promote digestion and guide out food stagnation that are common issues in pediatric medicine. Kneading and rubbing *qí* can therefore be used to treat diarrhea, constipation, abdominal pain, food accumulation and malnutrition. Both method can be used in combination with rubbing *fù* (abdomen), pushing *qī jié gǔ* (seven segmental bones) upwards and kneading *guī wěi* (turtle's tail).

IV. *Dān Tián* (Elixir Field, 丹田)

Location: On the lower abdomen, between two and three cun below the umbilicus (Figure 11-5).
Operation: The two techniques that are applied at the *dān tián* (elixir field) are rubbing and kneading. The child should be in a supine position. The rubbing *dān tián* method employs the palm to rub the point for two to three minutes, while using the thumb or the tip of the middle finger to knead the point 100 to 300 times is the kneading *dān tián* maneuver.

Action and Applications: The treatment effects of kneading and rubbing *dān tián* are strengthening the kidney to secure the life foundation, warming and supplementing the kidney qi, and raising the clear and directing the turbid downward. Both methods are used to treat pediatric illnesses such as hernia, enuresis, rectal prolapse, congenital deficiencies, and abdominal pain due to congealed-cold in lower abdomen. The kneading and rubbing *dān tián* methods are often used in conjunction with supplementing *shèn jīng* (kidney meridian), pushing *sān guān* (trigate) and kneading *wài láo gōng* (EX-UE 8). In treating urinary retention, the two methods can be applied in combination with pushing *jī mén* (dustpan entrance) and clearing *xiǎo cháng* (small intestine).

V. *Dù Jiǎo* (Abdominal Corner, 肚角)

Location: The tendon two *cun* lateral from *shí mén* (RN 5, 石门), which is two *cun* below *qí* (umbilicus) (Figure 11-5).

Operation: The grasping *dù jiǎo* (abdominal corner) method employs the thumb, the index and the middle fingers to grasp deeply three to five times, whereas the method of pressing *dù jiǎo* is employing the tip of a finger to press three to five times.

Action and Applications: Both the methods of rubbing and kneading *dù jiǎo* are key maneuvers of relieving abdominal pain, especially pain induced by cold pathogen and food damage. The method is used for fortifying the spleen, harmonizing the stomach, rectifying qi and guiding out food stagnation. Due to the strong stimulation of both maneuvers, avoid doing these more than three to five times. After carrying out either one of the maneuvers, perform mild pushing, pulling, tightening and relaxing once. Lastly, the method of grasping *dù jiǎo* should be done upon completion of all other procedures to prevent the child from crying, which would negatively affect the treatment.

Thoracic and abdominal points see figure 11-5.

Section 4   Acupoints on Upper Back, Lumbar and Sacrum Areas

I. *Qī Jié Gǔ* (Seven Segmental Bones, 七节骨)

Location: The straight line between the depression at the base of the fourth lumbar vertebra [*yāo yáng guān* (DU 3)] and the point below the end of caudal vertebrae [*cháng qiáng* (DU 1, 长强)] (Figure 11-6).

Alternative Location: The straight line between the depression at the base of the second lumbar vertebra [*mìng mén* (DU 4)] and the point below the caudal vertebrae [*cháng qiáng* (DU 1)].

Operation: The two methods applied to *qī jié gǔ* (seven segmental bones) are pushing upward and downward. The method of pushing *qī jié gǔ* upward uses the radial aspect of the thumb pad or the pads of the index and middle fingers as the surface to apply the force, and push directly from the lower to the upper end of the *qī jié gǔ* 100 to 300 times. The pushing *qī jié gǔ* downward though is to push directly 100 to 300 times from top to bottom along the point.

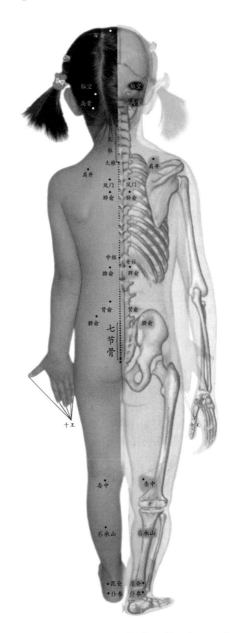

Figure 11-6 Acupoints on the Back and Lumbo-sacral Area

Action and Applications: The actions of pushing *qī jié gǔ* is to warm yang, arrest diarrhea, drain heat and promote defecation.

1. Pushing Qī Jié Gǔ Upwards   The method is often used in treating diarrhea due to yang deficiency or prolonged dysentery, while coordinating with press-kneading *bǎi huì* (DU 20) and kneading *dān tián* (elixir field). At the same time, pushing upwards also treats qi deficiency-related organ prolapse, enuresis and other illnesses. If the illness is of excess heat pattern, the method should not be performed to avoid abdominal distention or other transmuted pattern.

2. Pushing Qī Jié Gǔ Downwards   Pushing downwards treats constipation or dysentery of excessive heat pattern. If the child has diarrhea of deficient cold pattern, this maneuver cannot be used, avoiding rectal prolapse.

II. *Guī Wěi* (Turtle's Tail, 龟尾)

Location: *Guī wěi* (turtle's tail), a collateral acupoint of *du mai*, is located at the end of the coccyx with another name as *cháng qiáng* (DU 1). Although *cháng qiáng* is at the midpoint between the tip of the tailbone and anus in adults, it is customary to locate *guī wěi* at the end of the coccyx in pediatric *tuina* practice.

Operation: Kneading and pinching are the two maneuvers used on *guī wěi* (turtle's tail). The method of kneading *guī wěi* uses the tip of the thumb, index finger or middle finger to knead the point 100 to 300 times. The pinching *guī wěi* method is to use the thumb nail to pinch the point three to five times.

Action and Applications: With the actions of unblocking and regulating *du mai* and the large intestine, *guī wěi* can treat conditions such as diarrhea, constipation, rectal prolapse and bedwetting. The point is gentle in nature, it can either arrest diarrhea or promote defecation, and is often used in combination with methods of kneading *qí* (umbilicus) and pushing *qī jié gǔ* (seven segmental bones).

III. *Jí Zhù* (Spine, 脊柱)

Location: As an acupoint used in pediatric *tuina*, *jí zhù* (spine) or *jí* (spine, 脊) is the straight line between the first thoracic spinous process [*dà zhuī* (DU 14)] and the end of the coccyx [*guī wěi* (turtle's tail)] along the posterior midline. It is a line-shaped pediatric acupoint pertaining to the *du mai* (Figure 11-6).

Operation: There are three different maneuvers usually performed along *jí* that are pushing, pinching and pressing. The pushing *jí* method uses the pads of the index and middle fingers as the surface to apply the force and perform the straight pushing maneuver from top to bottom along *jí* about 100 to about 300 times. The pinching *jí* method, is performed by creating and opposing force between the thumb and the index and the middle fingers to pinch and release the tissue along *jí* starting from *guī wěi* to *dà zhuī* three to seven times. In addition, the method of pressing *jí* uses the pad of the thumb to perform press-kneading *jí zhù* from *dà zhuī* to *guī wěi* three to five times.

Action and Applications: The actions of *jí zhù* include regulating yin and yang, harmonizing *zang-fu* organs, rectifying qi and blood and unblocking the meridians and collaterals. The methods are commonly used in the treatment of fever, infantile convulsions, night crying, food accumulation and malnutrition, diarrhea, abdominal pain, vomiting and constipation.

Jí zhù is on the path of *du mai*, which travels throughout the spine, pertains to the brain and networks with the kidney, governs yang qi and leads the vital essence and the original qi. Clinically, the pinching method of *jí* is often used in coordination with other maneuvers including supplementing *pí jīng* (spleen meridian) and *shèn jīng* (kidney meridian), pushing *sān guān* (trigate), rubbing *fù* (abdomen) and press-kneading *zú sān lǐ* (ST 36) to provide effective treatment of chronic diseases due to congenital and acquired deficiencies.

When used alone, the pinching *jí* therapy, treats not only infantile diarrhea, malnutrition and food accumulation, but also problems among adults such as insomnia, gastrointestinal disorders and irregular menstruation. During the operation of pinching *jí*, the bladder meridians can also be involved by lifting or press-kneading relevant *shu* points to enhance the treatment according to disease presentations. In summary then, pinching *jí* is used for general physical strengthening purpose and is also a common preventational measure in pediatric *tuina*.

The direction of the pushing *jí* method is from top to bottom, which has the effect of clearing heat and often used in combination with methods such as clearing *tiān hé shuǐ* (celestial river water), retreating *liù fǔ* (six *fu*-organs) and pushing *yǒng quán* (KI 1) to treat fever, convulsions and other diseases. Lastly, the pressing *jí* method, which treats illnesses including low back stiffness and pain, opisthotonos, and yang deficiency of the lower-*jiao*. The maneuver is often used in combination with methods of kneading *shèn shù* (BL 23), press-kneading *yāo shù* (DU 2, 腰俞) and grasping *wěi zhōng* (BL 40) and *chéng shān* (BL 57).

Acupoints on the back and lumbo-sacral area see figure 11-6.

Section 5   Acupoints on the Lower Extremities

I. *Jī Mén* (Dustpan Entrance, 箕门)

Location: *Jī mén* (dustpan entrance), also known as *zú páng guāng* (foot bladder, 足膀胱), is the straight line along the thigh, from the medial aspect of the patella to the groin. The left leg is *zú páng guāng* (foot bladder), while the right leg is considered the *zú mìng mén* (foot life gate, 足命门). As a line-shaped point used specifically in pediatric *tuina*, it is different from the dot-shaped *jī mén* (SP 11) of the food *taiyin* spleen meridian located six cun above *xuè hǎi* (SP 10) at the medial aspect of the sartorius (Figure 11-7).

Operation: There are two maneuvers for *jī mén* that are the pushing *jī mén* method and the grasping *jī mén* method. The first, also known as the pushing *zú páng guāng* method, uses the pads of the index and middle fingers as the surface to apply the force to push bottom up directly along *jī mén* 100 to 300 times. The second, the grasping *zú páng guāng* method, is performed with the thumb, the index finger and the middle finger to lift-grasp the tendon along *jī mén* three to five times.

Action and Applications: *Ji men* has the actions of promoting urination and clearing heat and is commonly used in the treatment of dribbling, blocked, dark and scanty urination, watery diarrhea, and flaccidity and weakness of the area. The effect of the pushing *jī mén* is gentle, is effective in promoting urination, and is often used in conjunction with maneuvers such as kneading *dān tián* (elixir field) and press-kneading *sān yīn jiāo* (SP 6) to treat conditions such as urinary retention. When combined with the clearing *xiǎo cháng* (small intestine), pushing *jī mén* is effective in treating red, scanty and inhibited urination due to heat in the heart meridian. If it is used to treat urinary retention, the direction of pushing should be top down. When the method is employed in the treatment of watery diarrhea with no urination, however, the direction of pushing should be bottom up, which promotes urination and arrests diarrhea. Lastly, the gentle grasping method applied to the muscles and tendons along *jī mén* treats pain, flaccidity and weakness on the medial aspect of the thigh.

II. *Bǎi Chóng* (Hundred Worms, 百虫)

Location: *Xuè hǎi* (SP 10) is another name for *bǎi chóng* (hundred worms), which is located between the knee muscles 2.5 cun above the medial aspect of the patella and belongs to the foot *taiyin* spleen meridian (Figure 11-7).

Operation: The maneuvers used on this point are press-kneading *bǎi chóng* and grasping *bǎi chóng*. The press-kneading *bǎi chóng* maneuver is performed with the tip of the thumb or the front one third of the thumb pad as the surface to apply the force 10 to 30 times. The grasping *bǎi chóng* method uses the tip of the thumb, the index and the middle fingers to apply the force and performs the lift-grasping maneuver three to five times.

Action and Applications: *Bǎi chóng* has the actions of unblocking the meridians, invigorating the collaterals, calming the liver and extinguishing wind, consequently this point is often used to treat seizures and crippling *wěi* (atrophy, 痿) of the lower extremities. It is usually applied with methods of grasping *wěi zhōng* (BL 40) and press-kneading *zú sān lǐ* (ST 36) in treating conditions such as paralysis and painful *bì* pattern of lower limbs. If it is used for convulsions or seizures, a stronger stimulation should be employed.

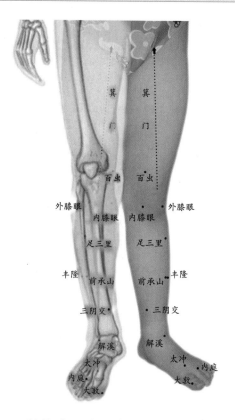

Figure 11-7 Acupoints of the Lower Extremeties

Chapter **Twelve**

Tuina Therapy for Common Pediatric Diseases

Section 1 Diarrhea

Diarrhea is a common pediatric condition characterized by increased stool frequency, thin or watery fecal material. The disease can occur throughout the year, with a higher occurrence especially in summer and autumn. There is a higher incidence among infants and young children, with especially high incidence among infants six months to two years of age. The disease is equivalent to diseases such as acute or chronic enteritis, and various gastrointestinal disorders in modern medicine.

Causes and Mechanism of the Disease

The main causes of diarrhea in children include externally contracted pathogens, damage due to improper eating and drinkinng, as well as weakness of the spleen and stomach. The main system affected by the disease is the spleen, while dampness is the main factor of disease mechanism, and deficiency of spleen, excess of dampness, transporting and transforming functional disharmony of the spleen and stomach are key factors in the occurrence of diarrhea. The stomach governs intake and decomposition of food and drinks, while the spleen is in charge of transportation and transformation dampness and decomposed food and drinks, consequently, if the spleen and stomach are diseased, these functions cannot be achieved. As a direct result of organ impairment, the separation of the clear and turbid is not accomplished and diarrhea occurs.

Clinical Manifestations

1. *Cold-damp Diarrhea*   The content of the diarrhea is clear and thin, and even watery, light-colored and generally devoid of odor. Associated symptoms can include stomachache, borborygmus, oppression of the stomach area, reduced food intake, aversion to cold, fever, nasal congestion, headache, and copious, clear urination. The tongue coating is thin white or greasy white, and the pulse is soggy and moderate, while the color of the finger venules are red.

2. *Damp-heat Diarrhea*   Watery or egg-drop-soup like feces with strong odor, and sometimes with a little mucus. The diarrhea can be urgent, pouring like water, or intermittent with spasmodically abdominal pain, loss of appetite or vomiting, and mental and physical fatigue. The child may also have fever, irritability, thirst, and reduced, dark urine. The tongue body is red with yellow greasy coating, while the pulse is slippery and rapid with purple finger venules.

3. *Food-damage Diarrhea*   Abdominal fullness and pain, borborygmus, belching with foul smell or vomiting, no desire to eat, restlessness at night, and thin watery stool with jello-like content or food residue that smells sour or like rotten eggs. The tongue coating is turbid, thick and greasy, or light yellow, while the pulse is slippery and excess with stagnant finger venules.

4. *Diarrhea Due to Spleen Deficiency*   Repeated bouts of light-colored diarrhea that alternate between loose and watery stool without much odor, frequently occurring after meals. Even a slightly careless diet would cause increased frequency of bowel movement, accompanied with undigested food. Other symptoms may include decreased appetite, abdominal distention and discomfort, pale facial complexion, lack of strength of limbs, fatigue, and emaciation. The tongue is pale in color with white coating, while there is moderate weak pulse with light finger venules.

Treatment

1. *Cold-damp Diarrhea*

(1) *Treatment Principles*: Dissipating cold, transforming dampness, warming the middle, and arresting diarrhea.

(2) *Prescription*: Perform pushing *sān guān* (trigate) and kneading the *wài láo gōng* (EX-UE 8, 外劳宫), 300 times each. Then, perform the supplementing *pí jīng* (spleen meridian) and *dà cháng* (large intestine) methods, 200 times each. Next, rub the abdomen, knead *guī wěi* (turtle's tail), 100 times each.

2. *Damp-heat Diarrhea*

(1) *Treatment Principles*: Clearing heat, draining dampness, and arresting diarrhea.

(2) *Prescription*: Perform the clearing *dà cháng* (large intestine) and retreating *liù fǔ* (six *fu*-organs) maneuvers, 300 times each. Then, perform the clearing *pí jīng* (spleen meridian) and *wèi jīng* (stomach meridian) methods, 200 times each. Next, push the *qī jié gǔ* (seven segmental bones) downwards, knead *guī wěi* (turtle's tail), 100 times each.

3. *Food-damage Diarrhea*

(1) *Treatment Principles*: Promoting digestion, guiding out stagnant food, assisting transportation of decomposed food, and arresting diarrhea.

(2) *Prescription*: Supplement *pí jīng* (spleen meridian), and revolve *nèi bā guà* (inner eight trigrams), 300 times each. Then, apply the maneuvers of clearing the stomach and *dà cháng* (large intestine), and retreating the *liù fǔ* (six *fu*-organs), 200 times each. Next, rub the abdomen, and knead *guī wěi* (turtle's tail), 100 times each.

4. *Diarrhea Due to Spleen Deficiency*

(1) *Treatment Principles*: Fortifying the spleen and boosting the *dà cháng* (large intestine), warming yang, and arresting diarrhea.

(2) *Prescription*: Supplement *pí jīng* (spleen

meridian) and *dà cháng* (large intestine), 300 times each. Then, knead *wài láo gōng* (EX-UE 8) 200 times. Next, rub the abdomen, push *qī jié gǔ* (seven segmental bones) upwards, and knead *guī wěi* (turtle's tail), 100 times each. At last, pinch the *jǐ* (spine, 脊) 20 times.

Prevention and Care

1. Pay attention to food hygiene, as food should be fresh and clean. Avoid cold, raw and spoiled food. Wash hands before eating and after using the restroom. The tableware needs to be clean. Avoid under- or over-feeding the child.

2. Encourage breastfeeding. It is not a good idea to stop breastfeeding during the summer or when the infant is sick. Comply with the common rules of adding solid food, and pay attention to reasonable feeding.

3. Increase outdoor activities, be aware of climate change, prevent externally contracted diseases, and last but not least, avoid exposure of abdomen to cold.

4. Control amount of the diet, and reduce the burden of the spleen and stomach system. Temporarily withdraw food from a child who suffers severe diarrhea with vomiting, or diarrhea due to improper eating. Later on, as the condition improves, gradually serve food in small increments to the child. Be cautious of giving greasy, raw, cold, and food that is difficult to digest.

5. Keep the skin of the kid clean and dry, and change diapers frequently. After each bowel movement, use warm water to clean the bottom of the infant, and apply toilet powder to prevent rashes.

6. Closely observe changes in the condition in order to detect transmutation of diarrhea into a more serious condition. Once the pattern has transmuted such that fever occurs, take immediate measures and have the child treated with Chinese or conventional medicine.

Section 2　Vomiting

Vomiting, as an instinctive visceral reflex,

is a common symptom of disorder within the spleen and stomach system, owing to rebellious stomach qi. The counterflowing stomach qi travels upward, and brings milk and other food out from the stomach, so that the child spits it. The disease is equivalent to biomedically defined diseases such as acute or chronic gastritis, indigestion, and gastrointestinal dysfunction.

Causes and Mechanism of the Disease

1. *Food-damage Vomiting* Improper feeding that leads to food retention in the stomach. The stomach qi fails to descend, so that turbid qi counterflow travels upwards, and causes vomiting of undigested food. Conversely, if the stomach is unable to decompose food, and the spleen fails to transport and transform food, the result is food retention and productive vomiting with sour milk and other food.

2. *Vomiting of Heat Pattern* Accumulated heat in the stomach leading to fire, which is the so-called: "all counterflow up-surging is ascribed to fire". When children present with this pattern, they will vomit immediately after eating any food.

3. *Vomiting of Cold Pattern* The occurrence of this pattern is mostly due to an insufficient congenital condition, such that the spleen and stomach system is of deficient-cold pattern. As a direct consequence, the spleen fails to spread yang qi and achieve its transporting and transforming ability, causing food retention and phlegm accumulation. In this pattern counter-flow of qi with vomiting occurs some time after eating.

In modern conventional medicine, vomiting is thought to be an instinctive reflex action that expels harmful substances in the stomach, and therefore plays a protective role to the body. It is, however, not the case in most situations, such as acute gastritis, and stomach cramps. In these settings, frequent and violent vomiting can interfere with the diet, leading to dehydration, electrolyte imbalance, acid-base balance disorders, nutritional disorders, causing more harm to the body.

Clinical Manifestations

1. *Food-damage Vomiting* Frequent vomiting with sour and foul odor, bad breath, chest suppression, anorexia, and abdominal distention and fullness. The stool may be odoriferous, loose or constipated. The tongue coating is thick and greasy, while the pulse is slippery and excess with stagnant finger venules.

2. *Vomiting of Heat Pattern* Productive, sour and foul vomiting immediatly after eating anything, general fever, thirst, irritability, odoriferous stool or constipation, and dark urine. The lips are redder and dry, while the tongue coating is yellow and greasy with purple finger venules.

3. *Vomiting of Cold Pattern* Vomiting undigested food that comes and goes after eating a little more than usual, pale facial complexion, cold limbs, abdominal pain that relieves with heat patches, and thin stool. The tongue is light colored with thin white coating, while the finger venules are red.

Treatment

1. *Food-damage Vomiting*

(1) *Treatment Principles*: Promoting digestion, guiding out food stagnation, harmonizing the middle, and descending qi counterflow.

(2) *Prescription*: Supplementing *pí jīng* (spleen meridian), rubbing *bǎn mén* (board gate, 板门), pushing from the wrist crease to *bǎn mén*, revolving *nèi bā guà* and *wài bā guà* 200 times each; kneading *zhōng wǎn* (RN 12), simultaneous parting pushing *fù yīn yáng* (abdominal yin yang), and press-kneading *zú sān lǐ* (ST 36) 100 times each.

2. *Vomiting of Heat Pattern*

(1) *Treatment Principles*: Clearing heat, harmonizing stomach, directing counterflow downward, and arresting vomiting.

(2) *Prescription*: Clearing *pí jīng* (spleen meridian) and *wèi jīng* (stomach meridian) methods, pushing *tiān zhù* (celestial pillar), and retreating *liù fǔ* (six *fu*-organs) 200 times each. Revolving *nèi bā guà* (inner eight trigrams) and *wài bā guà* (outer eight trigrams) and pushing from the wrist crease to *bǎn mén* 200 times each. Clearing *dà cháng* (large intestine) and

pushing the *qī jié gǔ* (seven segmental bones) downwards 100 times each.

3. *Vomiting of Cold Pattern*

(1) *Treatment Principles*: Warming the middle, dissipating cold, harmonizing the stomach, and directing counterflow downwards.

(2) *Prescription*: Supplementing *pí jīng* (spleen meridian), kneading *zhōng wǎn* (RN 12) 200 times each, pushing *tiān zhù* (celestial pillar), and pushing from the wrist crease to *bǎn mén* (board gate) 200 times each. Kneading the *wài láo gōng*(EX-UE 8, 外 劳 宫), and pushing *sān jiāo* (trigate) 100 times each.

Prevention and Care

1. If the vomiting is severe, temporarily stop feeding the child for four to eight hours. At the same time, feed the child ginger water or thin rice soup. If necessary, take the child to the hospital for intravenous infusion.

2. After temporary fasting, the child should eat easy-to-digest and light food, the quantity should be reduced, and the variety should be limited.

3. Keep a quiet atmosphere, and pay attention to the body position of the child to prevent inhaling of the vomiting content into the trachea.

4. Pay attention to aspects of proper feeding, including the amount of milk, concentration, and feeding posture while breastfeeding or bottle feeding an infant.

Section 3   Constipation

Constipation refers to difficulty in passing stool, passing hard stool, prolonged or sense of incomplete bowel movement, and hardship in emptying the bowel. The disease is equivalent to functional constipation in modern medicine.

Causes and Mechanism of the Disease

1. *Pathogen Retention in Large Intestine*   Causes such as yang deficient physical constitution, residual heat lingering after suffering from a febrile disease, lung heat or lung dryness that has moved to the large intestine, surfeit of strong flavored or spicy food, or overdose of medicine with heat nature can all result in accumulation of stomach heat that damages body fluids. Thus, the large intestine dries out, causing dry stool that is not easily passed, which is the so-called "heat constipation".

2. *Qi Deficiency and Fluid Consumption*   Deficient qi and yang can be caused by spleen and stomach damage because of irregular eating and exhaustion-fatigue, insufficient yang qi due to weak body constitution, deficiency owing to unrecovered healthy qi after being sick, damaged yang qi due to surfeit of cold and raw food, or consumption of yang qi because of improper use of bitter-cold medicinals. Deficient qi and yang cause weakness of the transporting function of the large intestine. Moreover, deficient yang fails to warm up the large intestine, resulting in accumulation of internal yin-cold, which further causes weakness in defecation and prolonged bowel movement, forming deficient constipation.

Clinical Manifestations

1. *Excess Constipation* Dry and hard stool, low food intake, abdominal distension and pain, dry mouth, bad breath, ruddy face, body fever, vexation, restlessness, profuse sweating, desire for cold beverage, and scanty dark urine. The tongue coating can be thick and yellow while the finger venules are purple. The combination of these symptoms indicate heat accumulation of stomach and intestines.

In a yin-cold accumulation and stagnation pattern, the stool is dry and is not easily passed, and there is a sense of fullness in the abdomen. The patient prefers warm environment, has an aversion to cold, and the four limbs are cool, sometimes hiccups or vomiting may also occur. The tongue coating is white, while the finger venules are light.

2. *Deficient Constipation* Qi defiency pattern: Having desire for bowel movement but difficulty in defecation, sweating, shortness of breath, fatigue, pale complexion, tiredness of spirit, tired limbs and lazy to speak, thin and white tongue coating, light finger venules.

Blood deficiency and fluid consumption pattern: Stool is very dry and difficult to defecate, pale complexion, dry mouth, vexation, hot flashes, night sweating.

Treatment

1. *Excess Constipation*

(1) *Treatment Principles*: Regulating and rectifying the spleen and stomach, dispersing food accumulation, and guiding out food stagnation.

(2) *Prescription*: Perform the clearing *dà cháng* (large intestine) maneuver 300 times. Clearing and supplementing *pí jīng* (spleen meridian), retreating *liù fǔ* (six *fu*-organs), revolving *nèi bā guà* (inner eight trigram), and press-kneading *bó yáng chí* (yang pond of the arm, 膊阳池), 200 times each. Press-kneading *zú sān lǐ* (ST 36), and pushing *qī jié gǔ* (seven segmantal bones) downwards 100 times at each acupoint. Rubbing the abdomen, foulage-rubbing the ribs, and pinching the spine 20 times on each area.

2. *Deficiency Constipation*

(1) *Treatment Principles*: Fortifying the spleen, boosting qi, enriching blood, and nourishing yin.

(2) *Prescription*: Supplement *pí jīng* (spleen meridian), push *sān guān* (trigate), and press-knead *zú sān lǐ* (ST 36) 300 times at each point. Rub *fù* (abdomen) maneuver and pinch *jí* (spine) 20 times each. Supplement *shèn jīng* (kidney meridian), clear *dà cháng* (large intestine), press-knead *bó yáng chí* (yang pool of the arm), and kneading *shàng mǎ* (riding horse) 200 times each.

Prevention and Care

1. For infants and young children fed mostly with milk formula, the concentration of the milk should be thinner than usual, and add an appropriate amount of fruit or vegetable juice to the diet. For weaning children, the main diet should not be too refined. Encourage the child to eat more fiber-rich vegetables , or fruit such as bananas, pears, and apples. Drink sufficient water.

2. Try not to eat too much pungent, warm, and spicy food, in order to prevent internal fire from flaring upwards.

3. Teach the child to develop regular bowel habits, and break bad habits such as reading a book while sitting on the toilet.

4. Encourage the child to exercise regularly and maintain adequate daily exercise.

5. Treat primary diseases timely, such as Hirschsprung's disease, and allergic colitis.

Section 4   Enuresis

Enuresis refers to unknowingly urinating while asleep, especially among children over the age of three. It is more common among children under 10 years of age.

Causes and Mechanism of the Disease

1. *Congenitally deficiency*   Bedwetting among children is mostly due to inborn kidney qi deficiency, causing deficient cold of the kidney system. The Kidney governs hiding and storing, controls urination and defecation, and opens at the two lower orifices. The kidney pairs with the bladder, forming an interior and exterior relationship. If both the kidney and bladder have qi deficiency, the water passage is not controlled, resulting in bedwetting.

2. *Acquired Failure of Nourishment*   When the spleen and lung are deficient, qi sinks and bedwetting can occur as the result. After food enters the stomach, it is decomposed, transformed as essence under the control of the spleen, and then distributed elsewhere in the body. The clear part is distributed to the lung system. Some goes to the water passage and goes down to the bladder to maintain normal function of urination. The lung, pertaining to the upper-*jiao*, serves as the upper source of water. The spleen, however, pertains to the middle-*jiao*. Qi deficiency of the spleen and lung leads to unrestricted water passage, so that bedwetting occurs.

Clinical Manifestations

1. *Qi Deficiency of the Lung and Spleen*   Bedwetting in the night, increased frequency of urination in the day, frequently associated with cold, dull facial complexion, mental and physical fatigue, poor appetite, and thin or watery stool. The tongue is light red with thin white coating, while the pulse is deep and weak.

2. Insufficient Kidney Yang Bedwetting during sleep, clear and lengthy urination, pale complexion, cold limbs, and decreased mental acuity compared to children of the same age. The tongue looks pale with white slippery coating, while the pulse is deep and weak.

3. Failure of the Heart and Kidney to Interact Bedwetting while dreaming, restless sleep, irritability, noisy, hard to stay quiet during the day, five-center fever, and emaciation. The tongue is red, lacking of moisture with thin coating. The pulse is thready and rapid.

4. Damp-heat of the Liver Meridian Bedwetting during sleep, scanty and dark urine, impatience, and dreaminess. The tongue is red with yellow greasy coating, while the pulse is slippery and rapid.

Treatment

1. Qi Deficiency of the Lung and Spleen
(1) *Treatment Principles*: Supplementing the spleen and stomach, strengthenig the containing force of the bladder.
(2) *Prescription*: Supplement *pí jīng* (spleen meridian) and *fèi jīng* (lung meridian), and push *sān guān* (trigate) 300 times at each point. Press-rub *bǎi huì* (DU 20, 百 会) 200 times. Knead *dān tián* (elixir field), and scrub the lumbosacral region, 100 times at each area.

2. Insufficient Kidney Yang
(1) *Treatment Principles*: Warming and supplementing kidney yang, consolidating the containing power of the bladder.
(2) *Prescription*: Supplement *shèn jīng* (kidney meridian), and push *sān guān* (trigate) 200 times each. Knead *wài láo gōng* (EX-UE 8), *dān tián* (elixir field), *shèn shù* (BL 23, 肾俞) and *mìng mén* (DU 4, 命 门) 200 times each. Scrub the lumbosacral area 200 times. Press-knead *bǎi huì* (DU 20) 100 times.

3. Failure of the Heart and Kidney to Interact
(1) *Treatment Principles*: Clearing the heart fire, enriching the kidney water, calming the mind, and strengthening the holding power of the bladder.

(2) *Prescription*: Clearing *xīn jīng* (heart meridian) and *xiǎo cháng* (small intestine) and supplementing *shèn jīng* (kidney meridian) 300 times each. Clearing *tiān hé shuǐ* (celestial river water), kneading *èr mǎ* (two horses), pounding *xiǎo tiān xīn* (minor celestial heart), kneading *wǔ zhǐ jié* (five finger creases, 五指节) and *páng guāng shù* (BL 28), and press-kneading *sān yīn jiāo* (SP 6, 三阴交), 200 times each. *Wǔ zhǐ jié* (five finger creases) is the collective name of a combined pediatric *tuina* points that are composed of the dorsal side creases of the five proximal interphalangeal joints.

4. Damp-heat of the Liver meridian
(1) *Treatment Principles*: Clearing and draining damp-heat of the liver meridian and arresting the bedwetting.
(2) *Prescription*: Clearing *gān jīng* (liver meridian), *xīn jīng* (heart meridian) and *xiǎo cháng* (small intestine), 300 times each. Clearing *tiān hé shuǐ* (celestial river water), kneading *èr mǎ* (two horses), *láo gōng* (PC 8), and *páng guāng shù* (BL 28), and press-kneading *sān yīn jiāo* (SP 6, 三阴交), 200 times each.

Precautions

1. Teach the child to develop a good urination habit and reasonable daily life routine, and do allow the child to get overly exhausted.

2. If bedwetting has already occurred, proactively take the child to a doctor for treatment, provide him or her with proper nutritional food, and put him or her to rest. Do not allow the child to drink water two hours before bedtime. Eat less food containing a large portion of liquid.

3. The parents should set a time to wake up the child for urination at night.

Section 5   Infantile Malnutrition with Accumulation

Some of the main clinical manifestations of infantile malnutrition with accumulation include mental fatigue, sallow facial complexion, underdeveloped muscles, withered and yellow hair, bulging abdomen, thicker veins, poor appetite, plus thin and watery stool.

Causes and Mechanism of the Disease

1. Spleen Damage due to improper diet Due to inadequate, excessive or irregular feeding, so that sometimes the child is hungry and other times, overeating. At the same time, the diet may be poor in nutritional content, overly sweet and greasy. Consequently, the spleen and stomach are damaged, causing food accumulation and stagnation. Spleen and stomach damage leads to the failure of food digestion, so that the spleen and stomach lose the ability to transform and transport food essence. Over time, it turns into infantile malnutrition.

2. Weakness of the Spleen and stomach Spleen deficiency is a common condition among children owing to food damage, chronic illness, or weaning. The weakness of the spleen and stomach leads to a failure of the organs to transform, transport and disseminate qi, blood and other essence from food and fluids, leading to infantile malnutrition with accumulation.

Clinical Manifestations

1. Spleen Damage Due to Accumulated Stagnation Emaciated physique, stagnant weight or poor weight gain, abdominal distention and fullness, poor appetite, sluggish, unable to sleep well, and abnormal defecation often with foul odor. The tongue coating is thick and greasy.

2. Qi and Blood Deficiency Sallow or pale complexion, withered and sparse hair, scrawny, sluggish or irritable, restless, low crying voice, limbs lacking of warmth, developmental disorders, sunken abdomen, and loose stool or diarrhea. The tongue is pale with thin coating, while the finger venules are light.

Treatment

1. Spleen Damage Due to Accumulated Stagnation

(1) *Treatment Principles*: Dissolving accumulation, guiding out stagnation, and regulating the spleen and stomach.

(2) *Prescription*: Kneading *bǎn mén* (board gate) and *zhōng wǎn* (RN 12), simultaneous parting-pushing *fù yīn yáng* (abdominal yin yang), and kneading *tiān shū* (ST 25) 300 times each. Pushing *sì héng wén* (four horizontal creases), and revolving the *nèi bā guà* (inner eight trigram) 200 times each. Supplementing *pí jīng* (spleen meridian) and kneading *zú sān lǐ* (ST 36) 100 times each.

2. Qi and Blood Deficiency:

(1) *Treatment Principles*: Warming the center, fortifying the spleen, and replenishing qi and blood.

(2) *Prescription*: Supplementing *pí jīng* (spleen meridian) 300 times. Revolving *nèi bā guà* (inner eight trigram) 200 times. Pinch-kneading *sì héng wén* (four horizontal creases) and kneading *wài láo gōng* (EX-UE 8) 200 times. Pushing *sān guān* (trigate) 300 times, kneading *zhōng wǎn* (RN 12) and *zú sān lǐ* (ST 36) 200 times each, and pinching *jǐ* (spine) 30 times.

Prevention and Care

1. Pay attention to health maintenance and follow the feeding principles that are liquid food before solid food, vegetables prior to animal products, small quantity before large quantity, and soft food prior to chewy food.

2. Focus on combinations of food in terms of nutritional content and calorific value.

3. If necessary, treat the patient with the approach of integrative medicine, especially for the primary, and consumptive disease.

Section 6 Fever

Pediatric basal body temperature refers to the normal range of body temperature:
- Rectal: $\leqslant 37.5\,^{\circ}\text{C}$
- Mouth: $\leqslant 37.2\,^{\circ}\text{C}$
- Axillary: $\leqslant 37.0\,^{\circ}\text{C}$.

The patient can be considered to have a fever is when the oral temperature is greater than $37.5\,^{\circ}\text{C}$, rectal temperature greater than $38\,^{\circ}\text{C}$, or the fluctuation of the body temperature within a day is than $1.0\,^{\circ}\text{C}$.

Causes and Mechanism of the Disease

1. Fever due to External Wind-cold or Wind-heat If parents do not give proper care, infants and small children can easily contract external wind-cold pathogens due to physical weakness, poor ability to fight against external pathogens, and the inability to change their own clothing accordingly. When the external pathogen invades the body surface, a suppressed *wei*-yang (i.e. defensive yang) causes fever.

2. Yin Deficiency with Internal Heat Yi deficient heat occurs when the child is physically weak, either due to congenital factors or malnutrition after birth, or experiences yin damage due to chronic disease. Any of these factors would cause lung and kidney deficiency, further leading to yin damage, so that fever occurs.

3. Excess Heat in the Lung and Stomach Lung and stomach heat patterns are result of congested heat due to excessive obstruction of the lung and the stomach caused by erroneous treatment or damage from improper food.

4. Fever due to Qi Deficiency Fevers that result from qi deficiency start with fatigue from overstrain, improper diet, or untreated chronic illness, poor conditioning, any of which can result in insufficient central qi, and an internal yin fire.

Clinical Manifestations

1. Fever due to External Wind-cold or Wind-heat Among patients with wind-cold pattern, the symptoms are fever, aversion to cold, headache, no sweating, stuffy nose, runny nose, tongue is light red with thin white coating, tight floating pulse, and red finger venules. In patients presenting with the wind-heat pattern, there can be fever, slight sweating, dry mouth, yellow nasal discharge, thin yellow tongue coating, rapid floating pulse, and purplish red finger venules.

2. Yin Deficiency with Internal Heat The fever occurs in the afternoon, feverish feeling in palms and soles, skinniness, mental fatigue, night sweats, reduced food intake, and red peeling tongue coating. The pulse is thready, rapid, and weak, while the finger venules are light purple.

3. Excess Heat in the Lung and Stomach High fever, red complexion, shortness of breath, no appetite, constipation, irritability, and thirst with desire for water. The tongue is red and dry, the pulse is rapid and strong, and the finger venules are dark purple.

4. Fever due to Qi Deficiency Low grade fever after exertion, low voice, no desire to speak, fatigue, spontaneous sweating occurring with slight movement, loss of appetite, emaciation, and postprandial diarrhea. The tongue is pale with thin white coating, while the pulse is deficient or deep, thready and weak, and the finger venules are light.

Treatment

1. Fever due to External Wind-cold or Wind-heat

(1) *Treatment Principles*: Clearing heat, releasing the exterior, and dispersing the exterior pathogens.

(2) *Prescription*: Pushing *cuán zhú* (gathering bamboo), *kǎn gōng* (kan trigram palace), and kneading *tài yáng* (EX-HN 5) 30 times each. Clearing *tiān hé shuǐ* (celestial river water) 200 times. For wind-cold pattern, add maneuvers of pushing *sān guān* (trigate) 200 times, pinch-kneading *èr shàn mén* (two-panel door) 30 times, pinching *fēng chí* (GB 20) five times. For wind-heat pattern, add pushing *jí* (spine) 100 times.

(3) *Modifications*: If additional symptoms include cough, sound of sputum, and rapid breathing, add push-kneading *dàn zhōng* (RN 17), kneading *fèi shù* (BL 13, 肺俞) and *fēng lóng* (ST 40, 丰隆), revolving *nèi bā guà* (inner eight trigram). When other symptoms include abdominal distention and fullness, no appetite, belching, acid reflux, and vomiting (not milk), add kneading *zhōng wǎn* (RN 12), push-kneading *bǎn mén* (board gate), simultaneous parting-pushing *fù yīn yáng* (abdominal yin yang), and pushing the *tiān zhù* (celestial pillar). While additional symptoms are irritability, restlessness, disturbed sleep, and startling, add methods such as clearing *gān jīng* (liver meridian), pinch-kneading *xiǎo tiān xīn* (minor celestial heart), and pinch-kneading *wǔ zhǐ jié* (five distal knuckles).

2. Yin Deficiency with Internal Heat

(1) *Treatment Principles*: Nourishing yin and clearing heat.

(2) *Prescription*: Supplementing *pí jīng* (spleen meridian) and *fèi jīng* (lung meridian), and kneading *shàng mǎ* (riding horse) 300 times each. Clearing *tiān hé shuǐ* (celestial river water) 200 times. Pushing *yǒng quán* (KI 1) 300 times. Press-kneading *zú sān lǐ* (ST 36), and revolving *láo gōng* (PC 8) 200 times each.

(3) *Modifications*: If irritability and sleeplessness exist, add the clearing *gān jīng* (liver meridian) and *xīn jīng* (heart meridian) methods, press-kneading *bǎi huì* (DU 20). If spontaneous or night sweating exist, add kneading *shèn dǐng* (kidney apex), and supplementing *shèn jīng* (kidney meridian) .

3. Excess Heat in the Lung and Stomach

(1) *Treatment Principles*: Clearing and draining internal heat, rectifying qi, and promoting digestion.

(2) *Prescription*: Apply the maneuvers of clearing *fèi jīng* (lung meridian), *wèi jīng* (stomach meridian) and *dà cháng* (large intestine) 300 times each. Perform the kneading *bǎn mén* (board gate) methods 50 times, the revolving *nèi bā guà* (inner eight trigram) method 100 times, the clearing *tiān hé shuǐ* (celestial river water) method 200 times, the retreating *liù fǔ* (six *fu*-organs) maneuver 300 times, and the kneading *tiān shū* (ST 25) method 100 times.

4. Fever due to Qi Deficiency

(1) *Treatment Principles*: Fortifying the spleen, boosting qi, and clearing the heat.

(2) *Prescription*: Supplementing *pí jīng* (spleen meridian) and *fèi jīng* (lung meridian), revolving *nèi bā guà* (inner eight trigram), rubbing *fù* (abdomen), simultaneous parting-pushing *shǒu yīn yáng* (hand yin yang), kneading *zú sān lǐ* (ST 36), kneading *pí shù* (BL 20) and *fèi shù* (BL 13) 200 times each. Perform the maneuvers of the clearing *tiān hé shuǐ* (celestial river water) and *dà cháng* (large intestine) for 100 times each.

(3) *Modifications*: If there are abdominal distension and poor appetite, add revolving *bǎn mén* (board gate), bilateral outward-pushing *fù yīn yáng* (abdominal yin yang), and rubbing *zhōng wǎn* (RN 12). If loose stool or diarrhea with undigested food residue exists, add rubbing *fù* (abdomen) counterclockwise, pushing *qī jié gǔ* (seven segmental bones) upwards, supplementing the large intestine meridian, and pushing from *bǎn mén* (board gate) to the wrist crease. If there are nausea and vomiting, add pushing *tiān zhù gǔ* (celestial pillar bone) and *zhōng wǎn* (RN 12), pushing from the wrist crease to *bǎn mén* (board gate), and kneading the right *duān zhèng* (straighten-up).

Prevention and Care

1. Wear proper clothing to child cool or warm according to the ambient temperature, maintain adequate air circulation in the room, and avoid promoting sweating by covering the child with a heavy quilt.

2. Encourage the child to drink water, pay attention to nutrition, eat more fruits to keep the mouth and tongue moist, and maintain regular urination and bowel movement.

3. The food should be soft, easy to digest, and light, such as rice soup, porridge, and dairy products. At the same time, the diet should be rich in protein, but without too much meat and greasy food. Eat often with small quantity, and overeating should be avoided.

Section 7   Cough

Among children, cough is a common symptom that indicates illness of the lung, as well as a protective reflex of the respiratory tract. It may be a symptom of acute or chronic bronchitis and other diseases.

Causes and Mechanism of the Disease

1. Cough from External Wind-cold or Wind-heat   Although a fragile organ, the lung controls respiration, governs purification and descent, connects the throat, uses the nose as its orifice, and is responsible for the skin and body hair. As the organ above other four *zang*-organs, it governs the whole surface of the body. Thus, if the body contracts an external pathogen, the lung is the first of the *zang*-organs to be attacked. The case is especially true in children, owing to their still-developing physique and qi, weak body constitution, and insufficient *wei* level defensive function. When wind-cold or wind-heat invades the body, the pathogen tightens the muscles, causing the lung qi to be unable to diffuse or be purified as well as the generation of phlegm. In other cases, children may contract a dryness pathogen that affects their airways, resulting in throat discomfort, and a scorching of lung fluids to create a sticky sputum, further leading to cough.

2. Cough due to Internal Damage   It is often due to physical weakness of the child, incompletely cured chronic external pathogenic invasion that depletes the healthy qi. In either way, the result is a lung yin deficiency, so that counterflow of lung qi goes upwards. Another cause is that the child's spleen and stomach are weak and easily damaged by food or milk, resulting in deficient cold of the spleen and stomach, so that they fail to transport water. Endogenous water-dampness, therefore, becomes stagnant and transforms to phlegm. It travels up and is stored in the lung, obstructing the airway, resulting in the failure of lung qi to diffuse, eventually leading to cough.

Modern medicine believes that cough is due to respiratory inflammation, or stimulation to the respiratory mucosa by foreign bodies, other physical factors, or chemical factors, cough caused by the cough center action. Cough is a protective reflex, so that foreign object or secretions can be dispelled from the body.

Clinical Manifestations

1. Wind-cold Cough   A productive cough that happens more often in winter and spring with heavy, dull and sluggish sound, nasal congestion, runny nose, aversion to cold, fever, and headache. The color of the tongue body is light red with thin white coating, while the pulse is floating and tight with floating red finger venules.

2. Wind-heat Cough   Sluggish cough with thick yellow phlegm not easily to be expectorated, sticky nasal discharge, sore and swollen throat, fever, sweating, constipation, and yellow urine. The tongue is red with thin yellow coating, while the pulse is floating and

rapid with floating purple finger venules.

3. Cough due to Internal Damage   Dry cough that lasts for a period of time with very little or no sputum, feverish feeling in palms and soles, hot flashes in the afternoon, thirst, dry throat, loss of appetite, emaciation, and fatigue. The tongue is red and dry with little coating, while the pulse is thready and rapid with stagnant purple finger venules.

Treatment

1. Wind-cold Cough

(1) *Treatment Principles*: Scattering wind, dissipating cold, diffusing lung qi, and relieving cough.

(2) *Prescription*: Pushing *cuán zhú* (gathering bamboo) and *kàn gōng* (kan trigram palace), kneading *tài yáng* (EX-HN 5), clearing *fèi jīng* (lung meridian), and opening *tiān mén* (celestial gate) 200 times each. Revolving *nèi bā guà* (inner eight trigram), push-kneading *dàn zhōng* (RN 17), pushing *sān guān* (trigate), kneading *wài láo gōng* (EX-UE 8), kneading *zhǎng xiǎo héng wén* (small crease of the palm), and knead-scrubbing *fèi shù* (BL 13) 100 times each.

2. Wind-heat Cough

(1) *Treatment Principles*: Scattering wind, clearing heat, dissolving phlegm and relieving cough.

(2) *Prescription*: Pushing *cuán zhú* (gathering bamboo) and *kàn gōng* (kan trigram palace), kneading *tài yáng* (EX-HN 5), and opening *tiān mén* (celestial gate) 200 times each. Retreating *liù fǔ* (six *fu*-organs) and clearing *fèi jīng* (lung meridian) and *tiān hé shuǐ* (celestial river water) 200 times each. Pushing *dàn zhōng* (RN 17), and kneading *zhǎng xiǎo héng wén* (small crease of the palm) and *fèi shù* (BL 13) 100 times each.

3. Cough due to Internal Damage

(1) *Treatment Principles*: Nourishing yin, clearing and moisten the lung, fortifying the spleen, and dissolving phlegm.

(2) *Prescription*: Supplementing *pí jīng* (spleen meridian) and *fèi jīng* (lung meridian) 200 times each. Revolving *nèi bā guà* (inner eight trigram), push-kneading *dàn zhōng* (RN 17), kneading *rǔ páng* (aside of the nipple, 乳旁), *rǔ gēn* (ST 18), *zhōng wǎn* (RN 12) and *fèi*

shù (BL 13), press-kneading *zú sān lǐ* (ST 36) 100 times each.

(3) *Modifications*: For chronic cough with weak constitution and shortness of breath, add supplementing *shèn jīng* (kidney meridian), and pushing *sān guān* (trigate) for 200 times each. For those of yin-deficiency pattern, add kneading *shàng mǎ* (riding horse) 200 times. For those having difficulty in coughing up the phlegm, add kneading *fēng lóng* (ST 40) and *tiān tū* (RN 22) to enrich yin, relieve cough and dissolve phlegm.

Prevention and Care

1. Pay attention to climate change, keep warm, and prevent the invasion of exterior pathogens.

2. Eat less spicy, greasy and fatty food, and food with heavy taste to prevent dryness damaging the lung.

3. Before the external pathogen is released, avoid greasy food and diet rich in animal content. If cough is not completely healed, avoid food that are too salty or too sour.

4. Avoid food and other factors, such as soot, dust, shouting, and crying, all of which can be irritating to the throat.

5. Rest well, drink plenty of water, and eat food that is not too rich after recovering from the illness.

Section 8   Pediatric Muscular Torticollis

Pediatric muscular torticollis is the deformity characterized by the head tilting to the ipsilateral shoulder or forward, resulting in the face rotating to the contralateral side. Generally it refers to the muscular torticollis caused by abnormal contracture of one side of the sternocleidomastoid muscle.

Cause and Mechanism of the Disease

The main pathology of muscular torticollis is fibrotic contracture of the sternocleidomastoid muscle, with apparent fibroblast proliferation and myofibrosis initially. Eventually it will be replaced by connective tissue if not treated. The etiology has not been fully confirmed, yet, there are many theories.

1. Most think it is related to injury. During labor, if one side of the baby's sternocleidomastoid muscle is suppressed and torn in the birth canal or by obstetric forceps that causes bleeding, the hematoma will become organized and lead to contracture within the muscle.

2. Some believe it is the result of ischemic changes of the sternocleidomastoid muscle. If, during the delivery, the head position of the baby is not ideal, obstruction of the blood supply on one side of the sternocleidomastoid muscle, results in ischemic damage.

3. Others think it is not related to the birth delivery. Rather, when the fetus is in the womb, the head has been tilted to one side all the time.

Clinical Manifestations

In the early stage, fusiform-shaped lump on one side of the neck may be found, and in some cases, may disappear after six months. Later, the ipsilateral sternocleidomastoid muscle gradually starts to contracting, becomes tense, and develops a cord-like change. As the result, the child's head tilts towards the ipsilateral side, and chin rotates to the contralateral side. A small number of the children may only have a lump that has a bone spur-shaped change around the attachment point of the ipsilateral sternocleidomastoid muscle on the clavicle. If the condition is not treated, it would affect the development of the face of the ipsilateral side. Moreover, even the healthy half of the face will also develop adaptive changes, causing the face to be asymmetric. In advanced cases, compensatory thoracic scoliosis generally would appear.

Treatment

1. *Treatment Principles*: Relaxing the sinews, invigorating blood, softening hard masses, and dissolving swelling. The treatment should be mostly localized on the neck.

2. *Prescription*: The child should lie in a supine position. The practitioner applies push-kneading the ipsilateral sternocleidomastoid muscle and grasping it 300 times. Next, hold the shoulder of the affected side with one hand, and hold the head with the other hand, push the child's head to the contralateral side of the shoulder slowly, and extend the affected sternocleidomastoid muscle gradually. Repeat the procedure multiple times. Lastly, use the push-kneading maneuver on the affected sternocleidomastoid muscle 300 times.

Appendix

Breathing Exercise for *Tuina* Physician and Preventative Methods

Chapter **Thirteen**

Do-It-Yourself *Tuina*

Section 1   Mind-Calming Method

In do-it-yourself health maintenance *tuina*, mind-calming method has actions such as calming the shen (mind, spirit), tranquilizing the heart, and awaken the brain. Therefore, it can be used to delay senescence and retain sufficient essence and spirit.

1. Combing Five Meridians   Slightly bend and separate five fingers with the middle finger placed on the anterior hairline, directly on the path of the *du mai*. The index and ring fingers should follow the bladder meridian on the lateral sides of the *du mai*, while the thumb and the little finger should lay on the Gallbladder meridian on the head. The pads of the fingers should stay on the surface of the scalp. Then, move the hand with fingers follow their assigned meridians from the front hairline all the way to the back of the neck unidirectionally for about 50 times.

2. Tapping with Ten Fingers   Slightly flex all ten fingers to tap the scalp from the front to the back of the head until there is a sense of warmth and relaxation.

3. Press-kneading the Forehead   Have the thenar muscle connect fully to the forehead, and induce the subcutaneous tissue to passively move with clockwise press-kneading about 100 times.

4. Press-kneading *Tài Yáng* and *Fēng Chí*   Use the pads of the index fingers to press-knead both *tài yáng* (EX-HN 5, 太阳) acupoints about 100 times. Then, place pads of thumbs on *fēng chí* (GB 20, 风池) of both sides, which is right at the lower edge of the occipital bone, and perform inward press-kneading about 100 times.

5. Grasping *Xīn Jīng* (Heart Meridian)   Place the thumb of one hand under the armpit of the other arm, and other four fingers on the medial side of the upper arm to perform   grasping methods about 100 times.

6. Press-kneading *Shén Mén* and *Nèi Guān*   Use the pad of one thumb to press-knead *shén mén* (HT 7, 神门) and *nèi guān* (PC 6, 内关) of the other arm, each point for about 30 seconds.

7. Tapping the Drum and Stirring the Sea   Place palms on each side of the ears with the root of the palm facing the front, and fingers pointing to the back. Then, tap the occipital area three times with the index, middle and ring fingers of both hands. Next, take palms away from the ears suddenly. Perform the procedure nine times. Afterwards, use the tongue to lick the upper and lower gum from left to right and right to left for nine times each direction, and swallow the saliva slowly three times.

Section 2   Stomach-Strengthening Method

The actions of the stomach-strengthening method include fortifying the spleen, harmonizing the stomach, warming the meridians and dissipating cold, so that it can be used to regulate gastrointestinal function.

1. Rubbing Upper Abdomen   Place either palm in the center of the upper abdomen. Then, rub it counterclockwise with small circles and transition to large circles 36 times. Next, rub it clockwise with large circles and transition to small circles 36 times.

2. Swing-pushing the Stomach *Fu*-organ Lie in a supine position, flex the lower limbs, and overlap hands on *zhōng wǎn* (RN 12). Use abdominal breathing, perform swing-pushing upwards with overlapped palms upon exhaling, and relax upon inhaling. Do this 36 times.

3. Simultaneous Yin and Yang Parting Pushing Either sit or lie in a supine position with hands opposite each other, place the entire of both palms under the xiphoid, push from the outward along the costal arch to the hypochondrium using moderate force, and gradually move to the lower abdomen nine times.

4. Rubbing the Margin of the Left Ribs Place the right palm on the margin of the ribs at the left upper abdomen, and rub them clockwise about 100 times.

5. Kneading *Tiān Shū* Either sit or lie in a supine position, place the index and middle fingers close together, place them on the left and right *tiān shū* (ST 25, 天枢), and perform kneading simultaneously, clockwise and counterclockwise 36 times each way.

6. Rubbing Lower Abdomen Rub the lower abdomen counterclockwise with a palm until the abdomen has a warm feeling, and the abdominal heat is better.

7. Pressing the Abdomen Place four fingers of one hand close together on *zhōng wǎn* (RN 12), and use regular abdominal breathing method. Press down with medium force during the inhalation, and perform circular kneading upon exhaling 36 times.

8. Press-kneading *Zú Sān Lǐ* Press-kneading both *zú sān lǐ* (ST 36) using the thumbs for about one minute.

Section 3   Qi-Rectifying Method

The self-care *tuina* method of loosening the chest and rectifying qi has varied effects including loosening the chest to rectifying qi, reversing counterflow of qi to benefit diaphragm, enhancing the function of the heart and lung, and improving the body's disease-resistant ability.

1. Press-kneading *Tiān Tū* Use the pad of the middle finger to press-knead *tiān tū* (RN 22, 天突) for about 100 times.

2. Press-rubbing *Dàn Zhōng* Place a palm on *dàn zhōng* (RN 17), use the point as the center, and perform clockwise press-rubbing about 100 times.

3. Press-kneading the Left *Wū Yì* Press-kneading of the left *wū yì* (ST 15, 屋翳) with the pad of the middle finger clockwise about 100 times.

4. Press-kneading the Left *Zhé Jīn* Press-kneading of the left *zhé jīn* (GB 23, 辄筋) with the pad of the middle finger clockwise about 100 times.

5. Palm-rubbing the Precordium The area accepting the treatment starts from *tiān tū* (RN 22), goes straight down along the sternum to the xiphoid. Use the root of a palm to rub one direction or back and forth about 100 times.

6. Rubbing the Chest Place the right palm between the two nipples with the fingertips obliquely pointing towards the navel. First, start push-rubbing from below the left breast, continue the maneuver, and circle back to the starting position, which brings the root of the palm to face the navel, start push-rubbing from below the right breast, continue the maneuver, and circle back to the starting point. Thus, the route of the operation shapes as a horizontal figure 8. Do this 36 times.

7. Finger-smearing the Intercostal Surface Area Spread the five fingers of each hand, place them the intercostal surface spaces, and smear top-down and bottom-up 5 times.

8. Squeezing *Nèi Guān* Be seated, and use the right thumb to press the left *nèi guān* (PC 6, 内关), while the remaining four fingers hold the dorsal side of the wrist. Use the pad of the thumb and apply moderate force to press in the direction of the wrist, then in the direction of the elbow nine times in each direction. Next, do it on the opposite side.

Section 4   Liver-Soothing Method

The actions of liver-soothing method in self-care *tuina* have actions such as regulating and smoothing qi movement, and harmonizing and benefiting meridians and collaterals, so that liver-soothing methods have the ability to rectify emotions, benefit the liver, and harmonize the gallbladder.

1. Soothing the Ribs   Be seated, place two palms on each side below the armpits, and fill in the intercostal spaces on the surface with fingers spreading out. First, use the left palm to perform simultaneous parting-pushing to the right until reaching the sternum at the level of the navel. Next, have the right palm to do the same maneuver to the left until reaching the sternum at the level of the navel. Do this on alternate sides nine times.

2. Kneading *Dàn Zhōng*   Remain seated, place either hand on *dàn zhōng* (RN 17) with four fingers close together, and perform kneading maneuver to the point with moderate force clockwise and counterclockwise, 36 times in each direction.

3. Scrubbing the Hypochondrium   Remain seated, and place both hands on the sternum with fingers close together with the left hand above the right. Then, scrub the hypochondrium horizontally along the ribs, and gradually move down to the floating ribs. Next, have the right hand above the left, and continue the maneuver until the area feels warm.

4. Flicking *Yáng Líng*   Remain seated, place two thumbs on *yáng líng quán* (GB 34) of each side respectively, and have other fingers to hold the legs to provide the support to the thumbs. First, knead on both sides for one minute, and flick the tendon of the area horizontally three to five times with appropriate force, causing the area to radiate soreness or numbness.

5. Pinch *Tài Chōng*   Be seated, use the tips of both thumbs on both *tài chōng* (LV 3) points respectively, and apply moderate power to press and pinch the points for about one minute, causing soreness and numbness. Then, use the pads of the thumbs to gently knead the points.

6. Scrubbing the Lower Abdomen   Either lie down or be seated, place the palms on the lateral sides of the ribs, and pushing-scrub obliquely to the direction of the lower abdomen until the palms reach the pubic bone. Perform the procedure back and forth 36 times.

7. Point-pressing *Zhāng Mén*   Place the tips of both middle fingers on both sides of the *zhāng mén* (LR 13, 章门) respectively, and press with moderate force for about one minute until there is soreness or numbness on both sides.

8. Kneading *Qī Mén*   Either lie down or be seated, place the root of the left palm on the right *qī mén* (LR 14, 期门) points, apply some force, and perform kneading clockwise and counterclockwise, 36 times in each direction. Then use the right hand to perform the same procedure on the opposite side.

Section 5   Essence-Boosting Method

In self-care *tuina*, essence-boosting method benefits the kidney qi, strengthens tendons, and promotes bone health. Thus, it helps to prevent and treat problems of the kidney system defined by Chinese medicine effectively to a certain extend.

1. Foulage *Yǒng Quán*   Sitting cross-legged, scrub palms until they are warm, place them on *sān yīn jiāo* (SP 6, 三阴交) of each side, and start scrubbing them, pass the ankle, and continue to the root of the big toes. Perform the maneuver back and forth until the warm sensation are obvious. Then, perform foulage on both *yǒng quán* (KI 1, 涌泉) until the areas of both feet are warm.

2. Rubbing the House of the Kidney   Place the palms on both sides of *shèn shù* (BL 23), perform circular press-rubbing from lateral to medial sides simultaneously for a total of 36 times.

3. Kneading the Life Gate   Place the index and middle fingers close together, on *mìng mén* (DU 4), and perform circular kneading maneuver, clockwise then counterclockwise, 36 times in each direction.

4. Scrubbing the Lumbosacral Area   Lean forward, flex the elbows and place both palms on both sides of the back. Use the whole palm or the hypothenar eminence of both sides to scrub back and forth, starting from the middle back to the sacral area until the area feels warm thoroughly.

5. Rubbing *Guān Yuán* Use either palm, and make *guān yuán* (RN 4, 关元) the center of a circle. Rub the lower abdomen counterclockwise and clockwise, each direction for 36 times, and then press the acupoint for three minutes.

6. Scrubbing the Lower Abdomen Place palms under both the lateral sides of the chest, and pushing-scrub obliquely towards to the pubic bone back and forth until the area feels thoroughly warm.

7. Vibration to the Ears First, push-scrub ears with palms from the front to the back 36 times. Next, use thumbs and index fingers to hold the earlobes and shake them 36 times. Then, insert index fingers into the external auditory meatus, perform rapid vibrations, suddenly pull out, and do this nine times.

8. Tighten-up the Perineum Stay calm, relax the whole body, and breathe using abdominal breathing technique which makes the abdominal wall out during inhaling and in during exhaling. Also, contract the muscles of the perineum during exhaling and relax those muscles during inhaling 36 times.

Chapter **Fourteen**

Exercises for *Tuina* Therapists

Section 1   Basic Stances

The most common basic stances include the attention stance, horse stance (middle stance), bow stance, cat stance, and flat stance in the exercises for *tuina* therapists. Through repetitive practice of these stances, the strength, explosive force and endurance of the muscles in the lower limbs will improve overtime.

1. Stand at Attention (*Bing Bu*)

(1)Keep the head straight, eyes looking forward, tongue against the upper palate, chin slightly lowered, and calm the mind.

(2)Breath naturally with serene facial expression, relax the shoulders, the chest slightly out, and back straight.

(3)The abdomen should be sucked in, arms should be naturally dropped, and the feet should be together.

(4)The whole foot needs to be planted on the ground, knees relaxed, and legs straight (Fig. 14-1).

2. Horse Stance (*Ma Bu*, Front Stance)

(1)Keep the upper body in upright pose, chest and back straight, stomach sucked in, buttock tightened, toes pointing slightly inward, and heels pointing outward.

(2)Next, have the left foot step shoulder-width or a bit greater to the left with toes pointing to the front, and soles firmly on the ground. Then, make toes slightly adduct inward, knees and hip flex for about 45°, or the thigh and calf form an angle close to 90° into half squat. The knees slightly point inward but do not to go beyond the tip of the toes.

(3)Keep the body's center of gravity midway between the feet, and have both hands at the sides, or make fists to place them on the lateral side of the waist.

If the distance between the feet is shoulder width, have the knee and hip flexed to squat, it is called the minor horse stance (Figure 14-2). Conversely, if the distance between the feet is double the shoulder width with the knees flexed, in squat position, thigh and calf forming a 90° angle, it is known as the major horse stance, also known as suspending crotch.

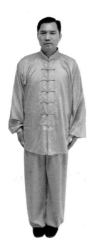

Figure 14-1   Stand at Attention

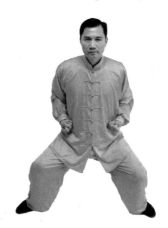

Figure 14-2   Horse Stance

3. Bow and Arrow Stance (*Gong Jian Bu*, Bow Stance) (Fig. 14-3)

(1)Have the upper body facing the front, chest out, waist straight, and buttock tucked up. Flex the knee of the leg in the front make it like a bow, with the thigh and calf forming a close to 90° angle. The leg on the back should be fully extended, so that it is as straight as an arrow.

(2)Have the eyes looking forward, make fists and hold them palms up at the lateral side of the waist. The basic requirements of this stance is to have the two legs shoulder width apart and the feet about shoulder and a half long. The soles of the feet should be firmly on the ground.

(3)The front knee, which is vertical to the sole of the feet, should be flexed, and form a half squat, while the thigh of the same leg should almost be in parallel with the ground, toes slightly pointing to the medial side.

(4)The knee of the leg on the back should remain extended, toes abducted to form a 45° to 60° angle, obliquely pointing to the front.

If the right leg is the front leg, then it is a right bow and arrow stance; otherwise, it is a left bow and arrow stance.

the left and right feet, with feet firmly on the ground. The center of gravity should stay in the middle, the knees need to be straight, and the tip of the toes point towards the medial side of the legs. The directions would make an inner square stance (Figure 14-4). If the two feet are close together, toes pointing out to form a 45° angle, legs straight, and the center of gravity of the body staying in the middle, then it is called a outer square stance (Figure 14-5).

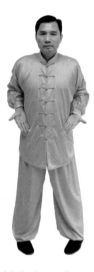

Figure 14-4   Inner Square Stance

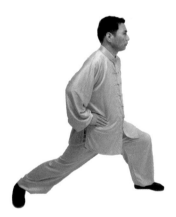

Figure 14-3   Bow and Arrow Stance

4. Square Stance (*Ba Zi Bu*)   Stand with the upper body upright, chest out, waist straight, abdomen sucked in, and buttocks tucked up. The stance requires a distance approximately twice of the foot length between

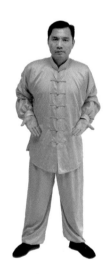

Figure 14-5   Outer Square Stance

5. Empty Stance (*Xu Bu*)   Stand with the upper body upright, chest out, waist straight, and abdomen sucked in and buttock tucked up. The stance requires one leg in the front and the other to the back, while the latter should have hip and knee flexed and be in squatting position with the whole foot on the ground, toes slightly pointing outwards. The front knee should be flexed slightly, with the tip of the toe gently touching the ground, and the body's center of the gravity falling on the leg on the back (Figure 14-6) . If the left foot is in front, it is called the left empty stance; otherwise, it is the right empty stance.

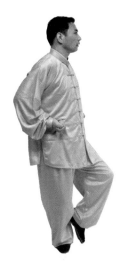

Figure 14-7   T- Stance

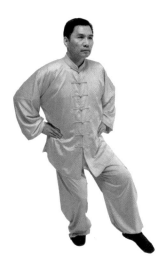

Figure 14-6   Empty Stance

6. T-Stance (*Ding Bu*)   Keep the upper body upright, chest out, waist straight, abdomen sucked in, and buttock tucked up. The stance requires that both legs be straight with the toes of the leg on the back slightly pivot outwards, while the other leg steps slightly to the front to make the heel one fist away from the arch of the rear foot. Both feet are firmly on the ground with the center of the gravity falling on the rear leg. The front foot and the rear one are perpendicular to each other, making a T-stance (Figure 14-7) .

7. Crouch Stance (*Pu Bu*)   Keep the upper body upright, chest out, waist straight, and hip relaxed. The basic requirement of this stance is to have the legs away from each other, so that one leg lays flat, close to the ground, the whole sole of the foot stick firmly on the ground, and the tip of the toes pivot inward. At the same time, the other leg is flexed making a full squat, thigh touching the posterior side of the calf, buttock close to the calf, knees and toes slightly abducted, and the whole foot firmly on the ground. Both hands should make fists and placed them on the lateral sides of the waist, while the body slightly turns to the straight leg, eyes looking at the anterior side of the same leg. This is the so-called crouch stance. If the left leg is straight, it is left crouch stance; otherwise, it is right crouch stance (Figure 14-8).

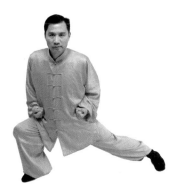

Figure 14-8   Crouch Stance

8. Rest Stance (*Xie Bu*) Chest out, and waist straight. The basics of this stance require the legs to be crossed, close together and make a full squat, the foot of one leg fully sticking on the ground with the toes pointing outwards, while the knee of the other leg is close to the lateral side of the opposite leg and the hip sitting near the heel. Make fists, hold them on each side of the waist with the center of the palm facing up, and eyes look straightly towards the anterior left. If the left foot is in the front, then it is a left rest stance; otherwise, it is a right rest stance (Figure 14-9).

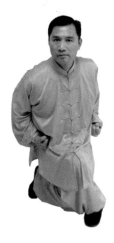

Figure 14-9 Rest Stance

Section 2 The Sinew Transforming Classic

The Sinew Transforming Classic (*Yì Jīn Jīng*, 易筋经) is an ancient Chinese practice, created by Bodhidharma who came to China from India in the 6th century. *Yì* (易) literally means change, *Jīn* (筋) refers to tendons, muscles, and sinew and bones, while *Jīng* (经) means a method; here, it means a way to change the tendons and bones. The goals of practicing *Yì Jīn Jīng* are regulating the *zang-fu* organs, and meridians and collaterals, and making a stronger physique.

I. Characteristics of the *Yì Jīn Jīng*

All twelve forms of *Yì Jīn Jīng* need to be executed with four extremities and the body thoroughly flexed, extended, adducted, and abducted, so that bones and joints can be exercised in all directions as much as possible. The form impacts the spine, tendons and bones through "stretching tendons and pulling bones". Such exercise requires physical relaxation, and natural breathing, while the moves should be even and smooth without gasping and disruption. The mind should remain calm and serene, and change following the changes of physical movements. In other words, the moves need to guide qi movements, so that the intention follows the physical body, and goes along with qi. The moves, whether symmetrical or asymmetrical, require coordination between the four limbs and torso, the upper limbs and lower limbs, and the left and right side of the body; thus, the body moves as an organic whole. The speed of the movement should be even and slow, and muscles relaxed with moderate, light and light. At the same time, the moves should be gentle yet firm. During practice, the stances introduced in section I can be applied.

II. Practice Method of *Yì Jīn Jīng*

(I) Skanda Presenting the Pestle

1. Starting Position Stand upright with the whole body relaxed. Keep the head straight as if trying to balancing an object on the head. Have the eyes to look forward implicitly, shoulders and elbows naturally hang, chest in, and back straight. At the same time, suck in abdomen, straighten up waist, and stand with feet together. The facial expression should be natural, the mind should be calm, and the breath should be moderate. The starting position of all forms begin with this position (Figure 14-10).

2. Palms Together at the Chest Level Left foot steps shoulder width to the left. Slowly abduct both arms until shoulder high with palms facing down. Rotate both wrists to have palms move forward and gradually move together. Then, flex the elbows, rotate the arms and wrists towards the chest with fingertips pointing upwards with both wrists and elbows at the shoulder level.

3. Rotating the Arms in Front of the Chest   Perform medial rotation of both arms, have the fingertips pointing to the chest, and make them level with *tiān tū* (RN 22, 天 突) located in the middle of the suprasternal fossa.

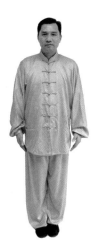

Figure 14-10   Starting Position

4. Arching the hands to Hold the Ball
Slowly rotate the forearm outwards with the elbow lowering down until both hands pointing upwards. Next, move both arms outwards slowly separating them, and making a ball-holding posture in front of the chest. Next, relax shoulders, allow the elbows to hang, slightly flex the fingers, and make palms facing each other, about 15 cm apart. The eyes should look straight forward, and the intention should stay between the two *láo gōng* (PC 8, 劳宫) acupoints (Figure 14-11).

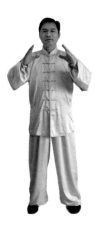

Figure 14-11   Arching the Hands to Hold the Ball

5. Closing Move   Take a deep breath first, and then exhale slowly, while both arms drop to the sides. Then, have the left foot move to the right, and finally stand in upright position.

(II) Monster Conquering Pestle

1. Pressing down with Both Hands   Step the left foot shoulder width to the left, press down with both hands, palms facing downwards and fingers pointing forward.

2. Flipping Palms and Lifting up the Hands   Flip both hands with palms facing up at the same time, raise them to the front of the chest, extend the arms forward slowly until they are at shoulder level (Figure 14-12).

3. Raising Arms Laterally   Open the arms to the sides of the body and keep them straight at shoulder level with palms facing up. Flip wrists, have the palms facing down and knees straight, lift heels up, stand on toes, and lean slightly forward and eyes widely open. Keep the lower limbs straight, with strength to the medial aspect the legs. Stand still, and keep the intention at *láo gōng* (PC 8, 劳宫) points of both hands (Figure 14-13).

4. Closing Move   Take a deep breath first, and exhale slowly while bringing the hands back to the sides. At the same time, put heels down, have the foot step back to be close to the left, and stand upright.

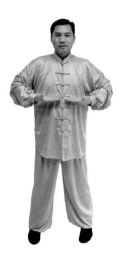

Figure 14-12   Flipping Palms and Lifting up the Hands

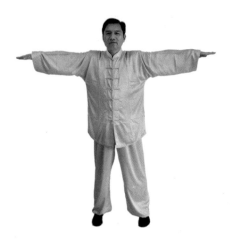

Figure 14-13   Raising Arms Laterally

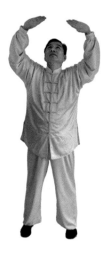

Figure 14-14   Supporting the Heavenly Gate with Palms

(III) Supporting the Heavenly Gate with Palms

1. Lifting the Palm to the Chest Level   Step the left feet shoulder-width to the left, and calm the mind and breath for a moment. Palms face up, raise the fingers slowly to the chest.

2. Flipping Palms and Lifting up   Rotate the wrists, turn the palms up, and raise arms over the head. Do not bend backwards.

3. Supporting the Heavenly Gate with Palms   Keep the four fingers of each hand close together, thumbs abducted, the webs between the thumbs and index fingers facing each other, and palms facing the heavenly gate while both arms raising up with implicit strength and eyes looking at the dorsal side of the palms. At the same time, raise the heels off the ground, and feel the power go through both lower limbs and waist (Figure 14-14).

4. Closing Move   Switch from palms to fists, dorsal side facing front, pull both fists slowly to the waist, and coordinate the action with a deep inhale. Then, lower both hands to the sides with slowly exhale, and at the same time put both heels on the ground slowly. Lastly, step the left foot back to be close to the right foot and stand upright.

(IV) Picking the Stars

1. Holding the Fists to Protect the Waist   Step the left foot shoulder width to the left, and make fists both sides with the thumbs tucked in the center of the palms. Then, raise fists to the waist level with the center of the palms facing up (Figure 14-15).

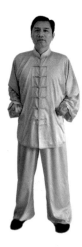

Figure 14-15   Stretching the Arms with Bow Stance

2. Stretching the Arms with Bow Stance   Step the left foot to the left anterior side to make a left bow stance, while the left fist changes to palm and extends the left arm to the left front corner at the level of head with the palm facing up, eyes looking at the left hand. At the same time, cover *mìng mén* (DU 4, 命门) with the dorsal side of the right hand. The acupoint *mìng mén* is located right below the second lumbar spinous process.

3. Hook with Empty Stance (*Xu Bu*)   Shift the center of gravity back to the right, turn the upper body to the right, and flex the right knee. At the same time, swing the left hand horizontally to the right with eyes following the left hand. Next, turn the upper body to the left, and slightly withdraw the left foot to make a empty stance. Then, swing left hand as the body turning to the left, make it hook-shaped, and raise it up to the anterior top of the head. The tip of the hook should point to the glabella, and eyes should be looking at the center of the hooked palm (Figure 14-16).

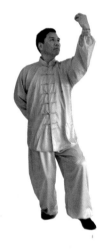

Figure 14-16   Hook with Empty Stance

4. Closing Move   Slowly inhale and exhale as the left foot returns to the starting position. The hook-shaped left hand changes to an open palm, and goes down anteriorly drawing an imaginary arc, while the right hand switches from fist to palm and falls down to the lateral side of the body. Repeat step 2 to 4 on the opposing side with mirrored movements.

(V) Drag Nine Cattle's Tails Backwards

1. Raising Hands with Horse Stance Move left foot further left until slightly more than shoulder-width apart. Raise both arms

laterally to above head, with palms facing each other. Flex knees to squat, and change palms to fists and push downward between the legs, with the dorsal side of the fists facing each other.

2. Left and Right Split Pushing   Lift both fists to the front of the chest and   change them to palms. Then perform left and right split pushing. Dorsiflex both wrists and fully extend both arms with palms facing out (Figure 14-17).

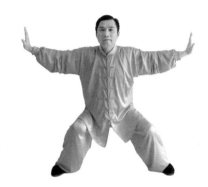

Figure 14-17   Left and Right Split Pushing

3. Drag Nine Cattles Backwards   Make a bow stance of the left side, switch the palms to fists, use left hand to draw a circumference to the anterior of the body. Next, flex left elbow to make it semicircular, make a forceful external rotation to pull backwards. Clench the fist to make a forceful external rotation with the fist right below the eyebrows, while both eyes focus on the fist. Hold the left elbow ahead of the left knee perpendicularly, while the knee is not ahead of the left tiptoes perpendicularly. Right hand draws a circumference and move to the posterior of the body. The right arm makes an internal rotation with a reverse force. The upper body bends to the chest, makes it closer to the thigh. Then straighten the back and bend backwards. All the other postures remain the same (Figure 14-18).

4. Closing Move   Take a deep breath, and slowly exhale. At the same time, withdraw the left foot. Place the open hands at the sides of the body, and stand upright (same movement in both directions, opposite direction).

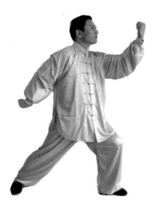

Figure 14-18   Drag Nine Cattles Backwards

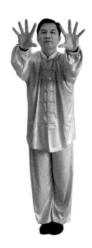

Figure 14-19   Lift the Heels and Showing off the Wings

(VI) Sticking out the Claws and Showing off the Wings

1. Making a Fist to Protect the Waist   Stand upright with both feet close together. Both hands should make a fist, with the center of the palms facing up, and hold them closely to both sides of the waist respectively.

2. Lifting the Palms and Pushing Forward   Raise both fists up to the front of the chest, change to palms and push forward with the center of the palm facing up, and fingers facing forward. The arms should be straight at the shoulder level.

3. Lifting the Heels and Showing off the Wings   Extend the elbows, dorsiflex the wrists to their maximum, have the fingers pointing up, and abduct the index fingers, so that the physical power can reach all the way through the palms to the fingers. Focus on the fingertips, image that the head is supporting an object, keep the chest out and stomach in. At the same time, raise the heels with legs straight. Next, along with inhaling, both hands make tight fists and adduct to the anterior of the chest, at the same time both heels slowly fall back to the ground. Perform this procedure seven times (Figure 14-19).

4. Closing Move   Take a deep breath, move the fists back to the   front of the chest, and exhale slowly. At the same time, lower both arms to the sides,.

(VII) Nine Ghosts Saber

1. Up and Crossing   Step the left foot shoulder-width to the left, hands crossed in front of the chest with the left hand stacked in front of the right hand.

2. Lifting up and Pressing down   Rotate both wrists with the left palm facing the front and lifting the left arm over the head, while the right palm facing down and pressing it towards the posterior of the body (Figure 14-20).

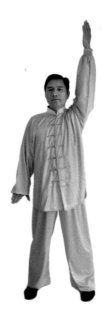

Figure 14-20   Lifting up and Pressing down

3. Opposite Pulling of the Arms and the Neck Flex the left elbow and hold the occipital area with the left hand. At the same time, move the right hand to the back, go upwards as much as possible to reach the lower part of the left shoulder blade and touch it firmly. Push the head forward with the left palm holding the occipital area with the left elbow flexed, simultaneously attempt to push backwards with the neck. With the left arm and the neck creating opposing forces, turn the body to the left, and look towards the left front corner (Figure 14-21).

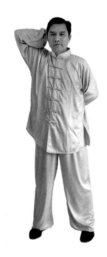

Figure 14-21 Opposite Pulling of the Arms and the Neck

4. Closing Move Withdraw both hands, turn the body to the starting position, move the arms to the side, hold them up to level with the shoulders with palms facing downwards. Take a deep breath, and exhale slowly while moving arms downwards. The arms continue to move until they return to their natural position. Move the left foot back to the right foot and stand straight. The right side of the movement should mirror the left side.

(VIII) Triple Accelerated Squats

1. Raising Arms with Palms-up Move the left foot to the left. The starting position between the two palms should be slightly wider than the shoulders. Lift arms forward with arms straight and shoulder width apart, palms facing up until the arms reach shoulder height (Figure 14-22).

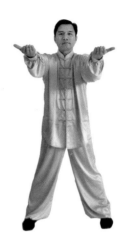

Figure 14-22 Raising Arms witth Palms-up

2. Horse Stance Squatting Rotate the palms internally until the palms face down. Next, abduct the elbows, flex the legs, squat down slightly and make a high horse stance with two palms pressing down simultaneously above the knees. At the same time, pronounce a low pitch "*hi*" while making a long exhale.

3. Triple Accelerated Squats Straighten the legs slowly while the flipping the palms and lifting up at the same time, as if lifting a thousand poundweight. Stop the palms at slightly higher than the shoulder. Next, flex knees to squat slowly at the second time, while both palms turning down, fingers naturally separated, the webs between the thumbs and index fingers facing each other, as if there is a ball floating on the water surface to be grabbed. Note that the second squat should be in a lower horse stance than the first one. At the same time, press down with the palms above the lateral side of the knees, upper body straight, adducting elbows tightly. Make eyes widely open, pronounce a low pitch "*hi*" while making a long exhale. Repeat this step and the squat this time should make an even lower horse stance (Figure 14-23).

4. Closing Move Take a deep breath first, and then slowly exhale, while the body and legs slowly straighten, palms up to shoulder level, then flip down, bring the arms to both sides. Bring the left foot back to the right and stand upright.

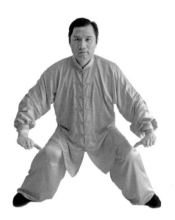

Figure 14-23   Triple Accelerated Squats

(IX) Blue Dragon Probing with the Claws

1. Starting Position   Step shoulder width to the left with the left foot. Lift both arms laterally to the shoulder level. Make fists, adduct and flex the arms, place the fists firmly on *zhāng mén* (LR 13, 章门) of both sides with the palmar sides facing up.

2. Turning and Probing with the Claws Loosen the right fist to make it claw-like, lift it up to the shoulder level. Turn the body to the left while extending the right arm to the left at the same time, as if a dragon is reaching out with the right claw. The intention and the focus of the eyes should follow the right hand, while the left fist remains unchanged (Figure 14-24).

3. Bending and Probing Downwards   Adduct the right arm towards the body. Bend the body, lowering it slowly through the right leg, and gradually get closer to the anterior of the left foot. At the same time, the claw-shaped right hand should follow the body to move downward, with the palmar side facing down.

4. Blue Dragon Probing with the Claw With the body bent and barely above the ground, move the body to the right foot

gradually, and the claw-shaped right hand follows to draw an imaginary semicircle. Both the heels shall firmly stay on the ground (Figure 14-25).

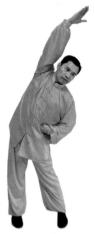

Figure 14-24   Turning and Probing with the Claws

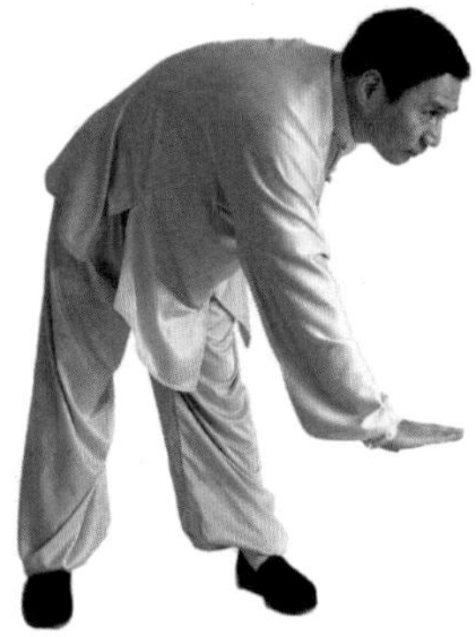

Figure 14-25   Blue Dragon Probing with the Claws

5. Closing Move   With horse stance, take a deep breath, then exhale slowly. Turn the body to face straight forwards.The right hand should be changed to an open palm from the claw-shape and draw an imaginary semicircle from the left to right. Next, slowly straight up the upper body as the right hand move up along the lateral side of the right leg. Then, make the palm back to a fist and place it to the right lateral lumbar area.

6. Repeat step 2 to 5 on the opposite side.

(X) Hungry Tiger Pouncing on the Prey

1. Probing with Bow Stance   Make a big step with the left foot forward with the right leg keeping firmly planted to form a left bow stance. Then, extend both arms from the side of the body, pounce forward with both hands. The hands should be level with the shoulders, palms forward, wrist dorsiflexed, as if they are a tiger's claws. The pouncing should be powerful, mimicking a hungry tiger.

2. Extending the Palms and Stacking the Feet   Put both hands on the ground with the left foot between them. Stack the left foot on top of the right heel. Shift the body weight backwards with feet firmly on the ground and chest leaning against the legs. At the same time, tighten chest and abdomen with arms extended and the head between arms (Figure 14-26).

3 Probing Forward and Returning   Curve the body above the ground, starting with the head, and following with the neck, chest, abdomen, and legs, and ending with the head facing up, eyes looking forward, chest out, waist relaxed and buttocks tightened. Reverse the order to return to the position in which the chest leans against the leg. Repeat it several times (Figure 14-27).

4. To Receive   In the hip high back low, the first deep breathing, and then slowly exhaled; right foot from the left heel up and down, step forward halfway, left foot with half a step, two feet into a parallel, slowly get up, his hands recovered on both sides

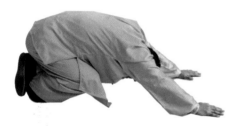

Figure 14-26   Extending the Palms and Stacking the Feet

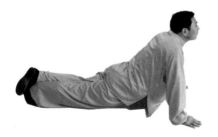

Figure 14-27   Probing Forward and Returning

(XI) Bow and Beat the Drum

1. Holding the Pillow with Horse Stance   Step to the left, slightly more than double shoulder width, both palms face up, and abduct both arms upwards to go beyond the head with the palms facing each other.

At the same time, flex both knees to make a horse stance. Next, have the fingers of both hands interlaced, flex the elbows, and slowly move the arms down, to support the occipital area of the head but with an opposing force with the back of the head with the eyes looking straight forwards (Figure 14-28).

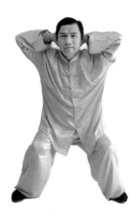

Figure 14-28   Holding the Pillow with Horse Stance

2. Bending the Waist with Knees Straight   Slowly bend forward and keep the lower limbs straight. Hold the head with both hands strongly, lower the head to go between the knees with the heels firmly staying on the ground and the eyes looking to the back.

3. Striking the Heavenly Drum   Cover the ears completely with the palms, and the four fingers on the occipital areas of both sides [i.e. *yù zhěn* (BL 9, 玉枕)]. Flick the *yù zhěn* area with both sides of the fingers for 24 times, and the sound of the pounding can be heard (Figure 14-29).

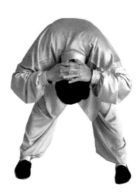

Figure 14-29   Striking the Heavenly Drum

4. Closing Move Take a deep breath and straighten the waist at the same time. Then slowly exhale with the hands move away from the occipital area and the palms facing down at the same time. Bring both arms back to the sides, move the left foot to the right, and return to an upright position.

(XII) Turning the Tail and Shaking the Head

1. Hold the Fingers and Lift-up Stand in upright position with feet close together and fingers of both hands crossed in front of the lower abdomen. Then, turn the palms upwards and lift them to chest level. Next, rotate the wrists outward until the crossed palms face the sky, continue to lift them up, extend both elbows above the head with power, and keep the arms raised, palms facing up, and eyes looking straight forward.

2. Bend Left and Right Turn the body turn 90° to the left, bend the body towards the left front corner, push the palms to the ground at the left front corner near the left foot, and keep knees straight and heels fixed on the ground. Concurrently, raise the head and look forward to the left. Then, return to standing position slowly, and lift hands up above the head. Mirror the same movements to the opposite side (Figure 14-30, Figure 14-31).

3. Bend Backwards and Forwards Bend the arms, head, and spine backwards to reach the anatomical limit. The knees should slightly bend with both feet on the ground, while the whole body is as taut as a tightened bow string with eyes looking up. Breathe naturally without holding it. Next, bend forward with palms facing down, force the palms to the anterior aspect of the feet with palms as close to the ground as possible. At the same time, the head bends backwards to look up, the lower limbs are straightened, and the heels are staying on the ground (Figure 14-32, Figure 14-33).

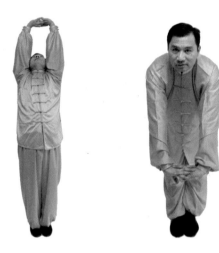

Figure 14-32 Bend Backwards and Forwards (1)   **Figure 14-33** Bend Backwards and Forwards (2)

4. Closing Move The movement should be synchronized with breathing, so that while inhaling deeply, straighten the upper body and lift the palms to the anterior aspect of the lower abdomen. Then, while exhaling deeply, bend the upper body until the palms reaches the ground and are able to push against it. Repeat for four times. Finally, straighten the waist, separate the hands, and slowly move the arms back to the sides of the body. Bring the left foot back to the right.

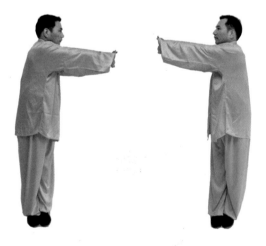

Figure 14-30 Bend Left and Right (1)   **Figure 14-31** Bend Left and Right (2)

Indexes

Index I.

Maneuvers

Index II.

Common Physical Examinations

Index III.

Diseases

Index IV.

Pediatric *Tuina* Acupoints

图书在版编目（CIP）数据

推拿学 = Theory and Practice of *Tuina*：英文 /
张伯礼，世界中医药学会联合会教育指导委员会总主编；
王之虹，王金贵主编；（美）段颖哲，（美）林楠，（美）
克里斯·杜威 (Chris Dewey) 主译 . —北京：中国中
医药出版社，2019.10
世界中医学专业核心课程教材
ISBN 978 – 7 – 5132 – 5730 – 5

Ⅰ . ①推…　Ⅱ . ①张…　②世…　③王…　④王…　⑤段…
⑥林…　⑦克…　Ⅲ . ①推拿—中医学院—教材—英文
Ⅳ . ① R244.1

中国版本图书馆 CIP 数据核字（2019）第 212142 号

中国中医药出版社出版

北京经济技术开发区科创十三街 31 号院二区 8 号楼
邮政编码　100176
传真　010-64405750
山东临沂新华印刷物流集团有限责任公司印刷
各地新华书店经销

开本 787×1092　1/16　印张 16.25　字数 835 千字
2019 年 10 月第 1 版　2019 年 10 月第 1 次印刷
书号　ISBN 978 – 7 – 5132 – 5730 – 5

定价　148.00 元
网址　www.cptcm.com

社 长 热 线　010-64405720
购 书 热 线　010-89535836
维 权 打 假　010-64405753

微信服务号　zgzyycbs
微商城网址　https://kdt.im/LIdUGr
官 方 微 博　http://e.weibo.com/cptcm
天猫旗舰店网址　https://zgzyycbs.tmall.com

如有印装质量问题请与本社出版部联系（010-64405510）